DIETARY MAGNESIUM: NEW RESEARCH

DIETARY MAGNESIUM: NEW RESEARCH

ANDREW W. YARDLEY
EDITOR

Nova Science Publishers, Inc.
New York

For permission to use material from this book please contact us:
Telephone 631-231-7269; Fax 631-231-8175
Web Site: http://www.novapublishers.com

Library of Congress Cataloging-in-Publication Data

Dietary magnesium : new research / Andrew W. Yardley, editor.
p. ; cm.
Includes bibliographical references and index.
ISBN 978-1-60692-109-8 (hardcover)
1. Magnesium in the body. 2. Magnesium--Metabolism. 3. Magnesium deficiency diseases. I. Yardley, Andrew W.
[DNLM: 1. Magnesium--metabolism. 2. Magnesium Deficiency. 3. Nutritional Requirements. QU 130 D565 2008]
QP535.M4D54 2008
669'.723--dc22

2008033234

Published by Nova Science Publishers, Inc. ✢ New York

Contents

Preface

Magnesium is the fourth most abundant mineral in the body and is essential to good health. Approximately 50% of total body magnesium is found in bone. The other half is found predominantly inside cells of body tissues and organs. Only 1% of magnesium is found in blood, but the body works very hard to keep blood levels of magnesium constant. Magnesium is needed for more than 300 biochemical reactions in the body. It helps maintain normal muscle and nerve function, keeps heart rhythm steady, supports a healthy immune system, and keeps bones strong. Magnesium also helps regulate blood sugar levels, promotes normal blood pressure, and is known to be involved in energy metabolism and protein synthesis. There is an increased interest in the role of magnesium in preventing and managing disorders such as hypertension, cardiovascular disease, and diabetes. Dietary magnesium is absorbed in the small intestines. Magnesium is excreted through the kidney. This new book presents the latest research in the field.

Short Communication - Magnesium (Mg) is the most abundant intracellular divalent cation and free cytoplasmic Mg can modulate the activity of a number of cellular enzymes, including key enzymes in phospholipase C signalling pathway which are initiated by antigen receptors on lymphocytes. The concentration of Mg may change after the cell activation. Lymphocytes have a role in the pathogenesis of COPD and recent studies indicate their abnormal function. As result of the above findings we determined the concentrations of total magnesium (tMg) and ionised magnesium (iMg) in isolated mononuclear cells (MNC) by using group of 46 COPD stable phase patients (past smokers, current smokers and non-smokers) and 61 control subjects (24 healthy smokers and 37 healthy non-smokers). Due to the antagonism of magnesium towards calcium we determined in the same sample the concentrations of the total (tCa) and ionised calcium (iCa). We found an increased of biologically active iMg in isolated MNC of the COPD patients compared to the group oh healthy non-smokers (median 22.09 μmol/10^9 cells, CI 5.67-50.00 vs. median 17.02 μmol/10^9 cells, CI 10.84-38.89, $p<0.05$) and increased concentration of tCa (36.01 μmol/10^9 cells, CI 4.81-82.14 vs. 18.18 μmol/10^9 cells, CI 3.84-74.66, 17.99 μmol/10^9 cells, CI 2.77-33.33, $p<0.05$) compared to the group of healthy non-smokers and healthy smokers respectively.

In isolated MNC of the patients the ratio of total calcium/total magnesium (tCa/tMg) was significantly increased (2.55, CI 0.57-6.33) compared to the group of healthy non-smokers (1.48, CI 0.20-6.22) and healthy smokers (1.51, CI 0.17-3.84). The MNC iMg value in COPD patients shows significant correlation with iCa (r=0.94, p=0.0000) and tMg with tCa (r=0.41, p=0.0237). Above study findings indicates that differential in the magnesium mobilization response has an impact on the resulting cellular response and will regulate cellular response to given stimulus.

Chapter 1 - Magnesium is an essential mineral with several dietary sources including whole-grains, green leafy vegetables, legumes, and nuts. Emerging evidence indicates that high magnesium intake from diet or supplements may favorably affect a cluster of metabolic abnormalities including insulin resistance, hypertension, and dyslipidemia, known as metabolic syndrome. The metabolic syndrome is prevalent worldwide and is associated with increased risks of major chronic diseases, such as type 2 diabetes mellitus (DM), cardiovascular diseases (CVD), nonalcoholic fatty liver diseases, polycystic ovary syndrome, and certain forms of cancer. In observational studies, magnesium intake has been inversely associated with chronic inflammation, dyslipidemia, insulin resistance, hypertension, type 2 DM, CVD, and colorectal cancer. Some small clinical trials with short durations appeared to support the potential efficacy of magnesium supplementation in the prevention and/or treatment of metabolic syndrome in human populations, although the long-term benefits and safety of magnesium treatment remain to be determined in future large-scale, well-designed randomized controlled trials with long follow-up periods. This article provides a systematic review of the current literature from human population studies on dietary magnesium intake and a host of metabolic disorders, focusing primarily on the role of magnesium intake in the development of metabolic syndrome, type 2 DM, hypertension, CVD, and colorectal cancer.

Chapter 2 - Asthma is a chronic, inflammatory disorder of the airways leading to airflow limitation. Its worldwide rise, mainly in developed countries, is a matter of worldwide concern. Inflammation of the bronchial mucosa and bronchial hyperresponsiveness are the hallmark features of asthma of all severities. Nocturnal asthma (NA) frequently occurs and would concern two thirds of asthmatics. But, it remains controversial whether NA is a distinct entity or is a manifestation of more severe asthma. Generally, it is considered as an exacerbation of the underlying pathology. The pathological mechanisms likely involve endogenous circadian rhythms with pathological consequences on both respiratory inflammation and hyperresponsiveness. A decrease in blood and tissue magnesium levels is frequently reported in asthma and often testifies to a true magnesium depletion.

The link with magnesium status and chronobiology are well established. The quality of magnesium status influences directly the Biological Clock (BC) function, represented by the suprachiasmatic nuclei. Reversely, BC dysrythmias influence the magnesium status. Two types of magnesium deficits must be clearly distinguished: deficiency corresponding to an insufficient intake which can be corrected through mere nutritional Mg supplementation and depletion due to a dysregulation of the magnesium status which cannot be corrected through nutritional supplementation only, but requests the more or less specific correction of the dysregulation mechanisms. Both in clinical and in animal experiments, the dysregulation mechanisms of magnesium depletion associate a reduced magnesium intake with various types of stress including biological clock dysrythmias. The differentiation between Mg depletion forms with hyperfunction of BC (HBC) and forms with hypofunction of BC (hBC) is seminal and the main biological marker is melatonin (MT) production. We hypothesize that, magnesium depletion with HBC or hBC may be involved in chronopathological forms of asthma. Nocturnal asthma would be linked to HBC, represented by an increase in MT levels. The corresponding clinical forms associate diverse expressions of nervous hypoexcitability: depression, nocturnal cephalalgia (*i.e.* cluster headaches), dyssomnia mainly advanced sleep phase syndrome, some clinical forms of chronic fatigue syndrome and fibromyalgia. The main comorbidities are depression and/or asthenia. They take place during the night or the "bad" seasons (autumn and winter) when the sunshine is minimum. The corresponding chronopathological therapy relies on phototherapies with sometimes additional psychoanaleptics. Conversely, asthma forms linked to hBC are less frequently studied and present a decrease in MT levels. They associate various signs of nervous hyperexcitability: anxiety, diurnal cephalalgia (mainly migraine), dyssomnia, mainly delayed sleep phase syndrome and some clinical forms of chronic fatigue syndrome and fibromyalgia. The treatment relies on diverse forms of "darkness therapy", possibly with the help of some psycholeptics. Finally, the treatment of asthma involves the maintenance of conventional dosing schedule of anti-asthma drugs, a balanced magnesium intake and the appropriate treatment of the chronopathological disorders.

Chapter 3 - Magnesium deficiency in pregnant women is frequently seen because of inadequate or low intake of magnesium. Magnesium deficiency during pregnancy can induce not only maternal and fetal nutritional problems, but also consequences that might last in offspring throughout life. Many epidemiological studies have disclosed that restricted fetal growth, i.e. intrauterine growth retardation (IUGR), is associated with an increased risk of insulin resistance in adult life.

We previously postulated that intracellular magnesium of cord blood platelets is lower in the small for gestational age group than in the appropriate for gestational age group, suggesting that intrauterine magnesium deficiency may result in IUGR.

Taken together, intrauterine magnesium deficiency in the fetus may lead to or program the insulin resistance after birth.

We hypothesize that intrauterine magnesium deficiency may induce metabolic syndrome in later life. Intracellular magnesium of the cord blood platelet may be a marker of early fetal growth, and can be used as a novel predictor of adult diseases. Low intracellular magnesium may represent the prenatal programming of insulin resistance and may have lifelong effects on metabolic regulation.

Chapter 4 - People with metabolic syndrome, a cluster of obesity, high blood pressure, dyslipidemia, and hyperglycemia, have at increased risk for cardiovascular disease and diabetes. Although components of the metabolic syndrome are related with inappropriate dietary patterns, the role of dietary constituents in the pathogenesis of the syndrome is poorly understood.

Evidence show that low dietary intakes of magnesium contributes to development of insulin resistance, a major component of the metabolic syndrome, supporting the hypothesis that suboptimal intake of magnesium might play a significant role in the development of the syndrome. On the other hand, recently has been reported that magnesium depletion is independently associated to low chronic inflammatory syndrome, suggesting that hypomagnesemia and low-grade inflammation are interactive risk factors for the metabolic syndrome and chronic disease.

Cross-sectional analyses of data from population based studies show that intake of magnesium is inversely related with the prevalence and incidence of metabolic syndrome. In addition, data from controlled randomized clinical trials provide evidence that oral magnesium supplementation restores serum magnesium levels decreasing inflammation and improving insulin sensitivity, high blood pressure, lipid profile, and serum glucose levels.

Nonetheless, to determine whether low dietary intake of magnesium is associated with an increased risk for the metabolic syndrome and, its potential usefulness in the prevention strategies of cardiovascular disease and diabetes requires confirmation, and further research.

We review the clinical evidence that show the association between dietary intake of magnesium and the metabolic syndrome; furthermore, we present results from a randomized double-bind clinical trial showing the efficacy of oral magnesium supplementation in the reduction of inflammation.

Chapter 5 - An increasing body of evidence suggests that low vitamin D status may impair both insulin secretion and action, ultimately increasing the risk of type 2 diabetes mellitus (DM). Experimentally, vitamin D repletion improves insulin sensitivity and insulin secretion in animal studies of rats. Cross-sectional studies in humans suggest an inverse association between circulating vitamin D levels and impaired glucose tolerance, insulin resistance, and risk of type 2 diabetes. Prospective data, albeit limited, also indicate an inverse association between intake of dietary and supplemental vitamin D and type 2 diabetes risk. Calcium and magnesium may exert both independent and interactive effects on the risk of type 2 diabetes through metabolically related pathways. Genetic variants of these pathways, including the vitamin D receptor (VDR) pathway and calcium and magnesium homeostasis related pathways, also appear to play a role in affecting the risk of type 2 diabetes in humans.

Chapter 6 - Plant and crop nutrition drives all terrestrial food-webs. Nutrient composition of crops can be manipulated through agronomy and genetics to optimize the delivery of essential minerals to humans and livestock. Our aim is to dissect and exploit the physiological and genetic bases for magnesium homeostasis in plants. Understanding how plants regulate Mg uptake from the rhizophere, as well as transport and cycling could have significant implications for plant nutrition and human health. With the knowledge of genes governing Mg homeostasis, it will be possible to reduce the need for fertilisers and to develop crops that grow efficiently on nutrient-poor soils. Furthermore, biofortification strategies through conventional breeding and transgenic approaches could lead to Mg-rich edible parts of crops, which would offer humans improved sources of this essential cation and overcome mineral malnutrition.

Chapter 7 - The ruminal epithelium is a stratified squamous epithelium that has evolved to display functions essential for the unique ability of cows and sheep to ferment dietary components like carbohydrates and protein, and to selectively absorb nutrients and minerals for the production of milk. A characteristic property of this tissue is its pronounced ability to transport magnesium against an electrochemical gradient. Absorption of magnesium is reduced by dietary elevation of ruminal potassium, leading to hypomagnesaemia that can reach clinical significance. Studies of the intact tissue and of isolated cells suggest that cellular magnesium uptake is decreased by apical depolarization of the ruminal membrane, resulting in both a lower cytosolic concentration and transepithelial transport of the element.

Another characteristic feature of this unusual epithelium is the expression of a sodium-conducting channel with functional properties that are clearly distinct from the epithelial sodium channel (ENaC) found in most mammalian epithelia. Thus, it has not been possible to demonstrate direct regulation of ruminal sodium transport by aldosterone, and the effects of amiloride are clearly limited to an inhibition of the sodium proton exchanger (NHE3) expressed by this tissue. Studies at the level of the animal and the tissue suggest that sodium conductance is enhanced by depolarization of the apical membrane. Recent *in vitro* studies have demonstrated that ruminal epithelial cells express non-selective cation channels in the apical membrane that are regulated by changes in cytosolic magnesium. We propose that the reduction in ruminal magnesium uptake observed after ingestion of high potassium fodder may be related to a role for magnesium in a signaling cascade that leads to an increase in the permeability of this non-selective cation channel for sodium, thus enhancing absorption of this ion from the rumen and restoring ruminal osmolarity, while contributing to the retention of potassium.

Chapter 8 - The role of trace elements in the pathogenesis of liver cirrhosis and its complications is still not clearly understood.

Zinc, copper, manganese and magnesium are essential trace elements whose role in liver cirrhosis and its complications is still a matter of research.

Zinc is associated with more than 300 enzymatic systems. Zinc is structured part of Cu-Zn superoxide dismutase, important antioxidative enzyme. Zinc acts as an antioxidant, a membrane and cytosceletal stabilizator, an anti-apoptotic agent, an important co-factor in DNA synthesis, an anti-inflammatory agent, etc. Copper is an essential trace element which participates in many enzymatic reactions. Its most important role is in redox processes. Reactive copper can participate in liver damage directly or indirectly, through Kupffer cell's stimulation. Scientists agree that copper's toxic effects are related to oxidative stress. Manganese is a structural part of arginase, which is an important enzyme in the urea metabolism. Manganese acts as an activator of numerous enzymes in Krebs cycle, particularly in the decarboxilation process.

Magnesium is important for the protein synthesis, enzyme activation, oxidative phosphorilation, renal potassium and hydrogen exchange etc.

Since zinc, copper, manganese and magnesium have a possible role in the pathogenesis of liver cirrhosis and cirrhotic complications, the aim of our study was to investigate the serum concentrations of mentioned trace elements in patients with liver cirrhosis and compare them with concentrations in controls.

Serum concentrations of zinc, copper, manganese and magnesium were determined in 105 patients with alcoholic liver cirrhosis and 50 healthy subjects by means of plasma sequential spectrophotometer. Serum concentrations of zinc were significantly lower (median 0.82 vs. 11.22 μmol/L, $p<0.001$) in patients with liver cirrhosis in comparison to controls. Serum concentrations of copper were significantly higher in patients with liver cirrhosis (median 21.56 vs. 13.09 μmol/L, $p<0.001$) as well as manganese (2.50 vs. 0.02 μmol/L, $p<0.001$). The concentration of magnesium was not significantly different between patients with liver cirrhosis and controls (0.94 vs. 0.88 mmol/L, $p=0.132$). There were no differences in the concentrations of zinc, copper, manganese and magnesium between male and female patients with liver cirrhosis. Only manganese concentration was significantly different between Child-Pugh groups ($p=0.036$). Zinc concentration was significantly lower in patients with hepatic encephalopathy in comparison to cirrhotic patients without encephalopathy (0.54 vs. 0.96 µmol/L, $p=0.002$). The correction of trace elements concentrations might have a beneficial effect on complications and maybe progression of liver cirrhosis. It would be recommendable to provide analysis of trace elements in patients with liver cirrhosis as a routine.

In: Dietary Magnezium: New Research
Editor: Andrew W. Yardley

ISBN 978-1-60692-109-8

Short Communications

Magnesium Concentration in Mononuclear Cells of COPD Patients in Stable Phase

N. Ruljančić*[1], S. Popović-Grle[2], V. Rumenjak[3], B. Sokolić[4], A. Malić[1], M. Mihanović[1] and I. Čepelak[5]

[1]Clinical Laboratory, "Sveti Ivan" Psychiatric Hospital,
Jankomirska 11, 10090 Susedgrad, Croatia

[2]Documentation and Reference Centre for Pulmonary Diseases,
University Hospital for Lung Diseases "Jordanovac",
Jordanovac 104, Zagreb, Croatia

[3]Department of Clinical Chemistry and Transfusion,
General Hospital "Sveti Duh", Sveti duh bb, Zagreb, Croatia

[4]Department for Clinical Biochemistry,
University Hospital for Treatment of Infectious Diseases"Dr. Fran Mihaljević",
Mirogojska 8, Zagreb, Croatia

[5]Department of Medical Biochemistry and Haematology,
Pharmaceutical-Biochemical Faculty,
University of Zagreb, A. Kovačića1, Croatia

Abstract

Magnesium (Mg) is the most abundant intracellular divalent cation and free cytoplasmic Mg can modulate the activity of a number of cellular enzymes, including key enzymes in phospholipase C signalling pathway which are initiated by antigen receptors on lymphocytes. The concentration of Mg may change after the cell activation. Lymphocytes have a role in the pathogenesis of COPD and recent studies indicate their abnormal function. As result of the above findings we determined the concentrations of

* Address for correspondence: Nedjeljka Ruljančić, Clinical Laboratory, "Sveti Ivan" Psychiatric Hospital, Jankomirska 11, 10000 Zagreb. Croatia. Fax: 00385 1 3794 116. Tel: 00385 1 3430059; E-mail: n_ruljancic@yahoo.com

total magnesium (tMg) and ionised magnesium (iMg) in isolated mononuclear cells (MNC) by using group of 46 COPD stable phase patients (past smokers, current smokers and non-smokers) and 61 control subjects (24 healthy smokers and 37 healthy non-smokers). Due to the antagonism of magnesium towards calcium we determined in the same sample the concentrations of the total (tCa) and ionised calcium (iCa). We found an increased of biologically active iMg in isolated MNC of the COPD patients compared to the group oh healthy non-smokers (median 22.09 μmol/10^9 cells, CI 5.67-50.00 vs. median 17.02 μmol/10^9 cells, CI 10.84-38.89, $p<0.05$) and increased concentration of tCa (36.01 μmol/10^9 cells, CI 4.81-82.14 vs. 18.18 μmol/10^9 cells, CI 3.84-74.66, 17.99 μmol/10^9 cells, CI 2.77-33.33, $p<0.05$) compared to the group of healthy non-smokers and healthy smokers respectively.

In isolated MNC of the patients the ratio of total calcium/total magnesium (tCa/tMg) was significantly increased (2.55, CI 0.57-6.33) compared to the group of healthy non-smokers (1.48, CI 0.20-6.22) and healthy smokers (1.51, CI 0.17-3.84). The MNC iMg value in COPD patients shows significant correlation with iCa ($r=0.94$, $p=0.0000$) and tMg with tCa ($r=0.41$, $p=0.0237$). Above study findings indicates that differential in the magnesium mobilization response has an impact on the resulting cellular response and will regulate cellular response to given stimulus.

Introduction

COPD is characterised by chronic local, and according to the latest data, systemic inflammation and oxidative stress. Various studies have shown that the lung inflammatory response is characterised by:

1. Increased numbers of neutrophils, macrophages and T-lymphocytes with CD8+ predominance.
2. Augmented concentrations of proinflammatory cytokines.
3. Evidence of oxidative stress [1].

It is currently accepted that an excessive/inadequate inflammatory response of the lungs to variety of noxious inhaled gases or particles (mostly cigarette smoke) is a key pathogenic mechanism in COPD [2]. Several studies have shown alteration in various circulating inflammatory cells including neutrophils and lymphocytes in COPD [3,4,5,6]. Circulating lymphocytes in patients with COPD have been less investigated than circulating neutrophils. Under normal conditions, the majority of lung T-cells is relatively hyporesponsive and become functional only after undergoing activation process. Recent studies indicate abnormal lymphocyte function in COPD [7]. Mg participates in immune response in numerous ways: as cofactor for immunoglobulin synthesis, C3 convertase, immune cell adherence, macrophage response to lymphokines, T helper-B cell adherence [8]. Recent data indicate that the concentration of free cytoplasmic magnesium may also change during the process of lymphocyte activation [9].

The majority of investigations determined the concentration of magnesium in serum or plasma, as only 1% of the magnesium is in blood plasma. This does not reflect the true state of the supply of the organism with magnesium. With regard to cells it is considered that different types of cells have different kinetic interchange of magnesium and other electrolytes.

It is still not completely clear which type of cells best reflect the status of magnesium in the organism [10,11,12].

Because of the ever increasing number of patients with COPD in the world and the aforementioned role of magnesium in inflammations, in this study the concentrations of total and ionised magnesium were determined (tMg and iMg) in the mononuclear cells (MNC) of patients with COPD. As magnesium is a known antagonist toward calcium [13] the concentration of total and ionised calcium (tCa and iCa) and the ratios of both forms of magnesium and calcium, were determined, in the same groups of patients and healthy subjects.

Materials and Methods

Subjects

The examination was performed on 46 patients with stable COPD (13 women and 33 men, mean age 66 years, range 44-80 years). Control subjects was 37 non-smokers, (3 women and 21 man age 49 years, range 33-63 years), and 24 healthy smokers, (6 women and 31 men, mean age 53 years, range 40-72 years).

Approval for the study was given by the local Ethics Committee and all of the subjects gave their informed consent.

The subjects completed a questionnaire which contained questions on smoking, blood pressure and possible other diseases. For all subjects spirometry and standard laboratory tests in blood and urine were performed on the same day. Healthy subjects were included in the study on the basis of the values of standard blood and urine tests in a referent interval and normal finding of spirometry.

Subjects with COPD, treated in the Clinical Hospital for Lung Diseases "Jordanovac", Zagreb, had been in the stable phase of the disease for at least three months, without hospitalisation and without change in therapy. The group of patients with COPD comprised 11 non-smokers and 34 smokers with forced expiratory volume (FEV_1) 30% - 70% of the predicted value. Table 1 shows the pulmonary function test of patients group with COPD.

Table 1. Pulmonary function test for patients with COPD, healthy control non-smokers and smokers

	COPD X (+/-SD)	Healthy non-smokers X (+/-SD)	Healthy smokers X (+/-SD)
FEV1 %	49.26 (14.58)	103.19 (18.41)	102.12 (19.54)
FEV1/FVC x100	51.29 (9.75)	80.83 (5.45)	81.53 (6.57)

FEV1% - forced expiratory volume in 1 sec.

FEV1/FCV - ratio of forced expiratory volume in 1 sec. and forced volume capacity.

According to the GOLD classification patients were classified in grade 2 and 3 COPD. Therapy consisted of a combination of β_2-agonist, anticholinergic and xanthic preparations, without corticosteroids. Subjects with diabetes, kidney disease, arterial hypertension, heart diseases, gastrointestinal diseases, endocrine diseases and asthma were excluded from the investigation. Subjects were taking drugs such as calcium antagonists, diuretics, digoxin, laxatives, antibiotics, or who consumed more than 50g alcohol daily, and those taking vitamin and mineral preparations, were also excluded from the investigation.

Samples

The blood of patients with COPD and healthy volunteers was taken in the morning between 7-10 hrs, and on the same day spirometry was performed. Sample was obtained by taking 10 ml of blood in a plastic test-tube with vacuum, coated with anticoagulant Li-heparin 15 000 IU/L (Venosafe, Terumo) and centrifuged for 10 minutes at 600g. The MNC obtained was stored at -20°C until analysis.

The MNC obtained were modified by the method of isolation according to Bojum [14]:

Blood is taken into a plastic test tube coated with anticoagulant Li-heparin 15000 IU/L (Venosafe, Terumo). 10 ml blood is mixed with 2.6 ml freshly prepared solution of dexstran (Dextran 500, 50g/L) in a glass test-tube and left to stand for 60 min. at room temperature. Plasma rich in leukocytes is carefully layered on solution Ficoll-Paque-plus (<0.12 EU/ml Amersham Pharmacia Biotech AB) ratio 2:1 and centrifuged at 400g 35 min. Because of the gradient of density during centrifugation MNC is situated between the layer of Ficoll-Paque solution and the plasma. The upper layer of plasma is removed and the layer of MNC is transferred to the test tube for centrifugation. The remaining part of the Ficoll-Paque solution and plasma in the MNC layer is removed by rinsing with approximately 6 ml cold solution of NaCl (9g/L) and centrifuging at 500 g for 10 min. Finally, removal of erythrocytes is carried out successively by adding 3 ml cold distilled water, mixing for 45 seconds and then adding 3 ml of cold NaCl (18 g/L) and mixing for a further 45 seconds. The suspension is centrifuged for 10 min. at 500 g. The procedure of removing the erythrocytes is performed at least three times. The MNC sediment is suspended in 1 ml of cold NaCl (9g/L) and the cells counted on a haematological counter (Nihon Kohden Mek 5100). The remaining suspended cells are sonicated with an ultrasound homogenisation (Cole-Parmer 4710), holding the eppendorf test tube in ice, 3x30 seconds, in intervals of 45 seconds. Such a lysate of cells is divided into 0.5 ml in two eppendorf test tubes and stored at -20°C until analysis.

Methods

The concentration of tMg and tCa was determined in MNC by the method of atomic absorption spectrophotometry (Atomic absorption spectrophotometer 2380, Perkin Elmer). The concentration of iMg and iCa in MNC was determined by the method of direct potenciometry on analyser Nova Ultra Stat Profile M (Nova Biomedical, USA Ltd.). Normalised values were taken at a temperature of 37°C and pH 7.4.

Procedure for Spirometry

Before starting the measurements the patient's height and weight was measured without shoes. The test was performed in a seated position. After applying noseclips, the subject was instructed to take a full inspiration, hold it briefly then exhale through a mouthpiece into the spirometer as forcefully and completely as possible. The test was repeated a minimum of three times, maximum eight times, until two reproducible efforts were obtained. The two largest FVCs and FEV_1s had to show <5% variability. After the spirometry measurement, according to standard procedure, the patient inhaled 400 μg of salbutamol from the MDI. After 30 minutes, spirometry was repeated three times and the highest FEV_1 value recorded. Before testing, regularly prescribed bronchodilators were withheld for 6 hours for inhaled short acting ß2-agonist, 12 hours for long acting ß2-agonist, 6 hours for inhaled anticholinergics, 12 hours for short acting theophylline preparations and 24 hours for long acting theophylline preparations. Bronchodilatory test was considered negative if the FEV_1 value after salbutamol was less than 200 ml and/or 12% before testing. Reference values were used according to ECCS, 1983 [15].

Statistical Methods

Mean values of parameters for each group of subjects are presented in medians and ranges. Differences between the examined and control groups were tested by non-parametric Mann-Whitney U test. A p-value of <0.05 was taken significant.

Results

Table 2. presents median and analogous ranges in concentration of magnesium, calcium, and their ratio in MNC of the subjects.

In MNC patients with the COPD concentration of iMg was significantly higher in relation to the control group of healthy non-smokers (median 22.09 μmol/10^9 cells, CI 5.67-50.00 vs. median 17.02 μmol/10^9 cells, CI 10.84-38.89, $p<0.05$). A statistically significant increase in the concentration of tCa was found in MNC of patients with COPD compared to the control group of healthy non-smokers and healthy smokers (36.01 μmol/10^9 cells, CI 4.81-82.14 vs. 18.18 μmol/10^9 cells, CI 3.84-74.66, 17.99 μmol/10^9 cells, CI 2.77-33.33, $p<0.05$). Concentration of the tCa in MNC within COPD patients was increased in relation to the control group of non-smokers and healthy smokers, with no change in its ionising form.

The tCa/tMg ratios in MNC of COPD patients were greater (2.55. CI 0.57-6.33) then control group of non-smokers (1.48, CI 0.20-6.22) and smokers (1.51, CI 0.17-3.84). This indicates relative tMg deficiency with regard to the concentration of tCa.

In addition to above, the concentration of tMg was not changed in MNC of COPD patients compared to both control groups. There was no change in the concentration of iMg in MNC of the patients with COPD compared to the control group of smokers.

Table 2. Median and ranges for concentration of magnesium and calcium and their ratios in COPD patients and control subjects of healthy non-smokers and healthy smokers

analyts	COPD (n=46)	Healthy non-smokers (n=37)	Healthy smokers (n=24)
	MNC (μmol/10^9 cells)	MNC (μmol/10^9 cells)	MNC (μmol/10^9 cells)
iMg	22.09* (5.67-50.00)	17,02 (10,84-38,89)	20.29 (9.35-30.00)
tMg	13.09 (4.96-36.36)	13,42 (7,50-26,09)	12.31 (6.5-20.00)
iCa	33.73 (10.63-107.14)	28,35 (16,90-77,78)	34.21 (18.12-61.9)
tCa	36.01•* (4.81-82.14)	18,18 (3,84-74,66)	17.99 (2.77-33.33)
iCa/iMg	1.63• (1.22-2.15)	1,70 (1,26-2,15)	1.81 (1.44-2.27)
tCa/tMg	2.55•* (0.57-6.33)	1,48 (0,20-6,22)	1.51 (0.17-3.84)

*Statistically significantly differences compared to the control group of healthy non-smokers; $p<0.05$.
•Statistically significantly differences compared to the control group of healthy smokers; $p<0.05$ Mann-Whitney U test; (tMg and tCa) concentration of total magnesium and calcium; (iMg and iCa) concentration of ionized magnesium and calcium.

There is also no statistically significant difference in any parameters between smokers (past smokers and current smokers) and non-smokers in the group of patients with COPD. Because of that but also because of the fact that the number of non-smokers was low a group of patients with COPD which included past smokers, current smokers and non-smokers was used in order to determine a statistically significant difference. In addition, The MNC iMg value in COPD patients shows significant correlation with iCa ($r=0.94$, $p=0.0000$) and good correlation of tMg with tCa ($r=0.41$, $p=0.0237$). This results show that there is a possibility that a differential Mg mobilization response will have an impact on resulting Ca increase and both cations will regulate cellular response to given stimulus.

Conclusion

The most recent definition of COPD has introduced the concept that inflammation is a key event in the pathogenesis of the disease, highlighting the need for a better knowledge of the mechanisms involved in the perpetuation of the inflammatory response [7]. COPD is characterised by local chronic inflammation involving the airways, parenchyma and blood vessels of the lungs. In this different parts of the lungs macrophages, T-lymphocytes (mainly CD8+) and neutrophils occur in an increasing number [2].The analysis of bronchial biopsies and lung parenchyma obtained from COPD patients compared with those from smokers with normal lung function and non smokers has provided new insight on the role of the different inflammatory and structural cells. Their signalling pathways and mediators, contribute to a better knowledge of the pathogenesis of COPD [16]. Cigarette smoke produces an innate immune response that, in those smokers who develop COPD, persists and is coupled with an adaptive immune response, involving T and B-cells [7]. According to GOLD standards [15, 17] parameters such as FEV_1 and pO_2 are generally used for diagnosis and determination of the degree and prognosis of COPD. More recently there was an increasing amount of data which indicates that COPD is not only a disease of the lungs but also a systemic inflammatory disease which includes activation of inflammatory cells, increased concentration of primary proinflammatory and anti-inflammatory cytokines [1].

Circulating lymphocytes in patients with COPD was less investigated than circulating neutrophils. Salueda et al [6] for example in the lymphocytes of patients with COPD compared to healthy non-smokers showed increased activity of cytochrom oxidase, terminal enzyme in the mitochondric electron transport chain. In study of Gupta et al [18] an alteration in alpha1- AT and T lymphocyte subsets in COPD patients suggested that interplay of these factors may be responsible for the progression of COPD.

Magnesium has an important role as cofactor in number of biochemical processes within cells, including the key enzymes in the phospholipase C (PLC) transmembrane signalling pathway. Activation of lymphocytes trough ligation of the antigen receptor complex initiates activation of PLC and Mg is cofactor for numerous enzymes in phosphatidilinositol metabolism. InsP3 mediates the release of Ca from intracellular stores into cytoplasm, while InsP4 and InsP3 mobilize extracellular Ca. Mg may thus regulate the cellular response to given stimulus [9]. The rise in Ca has important consequences for cell function and importance of Mg in activation of lymphocytes is well known [19,20,21]. As result of the above we have defined concentration of the tMg, tCa and their ionized form in MNC of patients with COPD and in control groups of smokers and non-smokers. Increased concentrations of tCa and tCa/tMg ratio in MNC of patients with COPD in this investigation suggest the conclusion of potentiated activity of calcium in these types of examined cells. Statistically significantly increased concentration of iMg was determined in MNC of patients with COPD compared to the group of healthy non-smokers. With our findings and an existing data found in literature on this subject [22] we can conclude that increase of tCa concentration in MNC results increase of the iMg concentration.

In our previous work on PMN (polymorphonuclear cells) of the COPD patients the concentration of tCa and the ratio of tCa/tMg increased compared to the control group of healthy non-smokers and healthy smokers. In the same work we found decreased biological active iMg in PMN compared to the group of healthy non-smokers (5.42, 1.98-17.31 $\mu mol/10^9$ cells vs. 7.50, 3.27-15.15 $\mu mol/10^9$ cells, $p<0.05$). There were no change in the concentration of tMg and iMg in the plasma of patients with COPD, while statistically significantly increased ratio tCa/tMg was determined compared to control group [23]. Above findings together with the MNC results indicates that there is relative tMg deficiency in both type of cells.

Depending on the cell type, iMg increase in MNC and decrease in PMN leads to conclusion that different types of cells have different distribution and regulation of iMg within these cells.

It is tempting to speculate that a differential Mg mobilization response will have consequences for the resulting cellular response. Current available techniques allow the experiments design to address these issues which will enable to clarify a differential iMg mobilization response in different type of cells.

The drugs used today in the treatment of stable COPD do not slow down the significant progression of the disease [24]. Based on the results of this study it can be hypothesised that the supplementation of magnesium salts to standard therapy, in patients with stable COPD, can improve the symptoms and possibly reduce the number of exacerbations of the disease. The hypothesis is justified by magnesium participation in oxidative stress defence reactions, regulation in leukocytes activation, and relaxing effect on smooth bronchial muscles.

In conclusion there is a need for the further longitudinal study and continued monitoring in order to determine effectiveness with magnesium salt therapy on the magnesium concentration in different cells and correlation with FEV1.

References

[1] Agusto AGN, Noguera A, Salueda J, Sala E, Pons J, Busquets X. Systemic effects of chronic obstructive pulmonary disease. *Eur. Respir. J.* 2003;21:347-360.

[2] Wouters E.F.M. Local and Systemic Inflamation in Chronic Obstructive Pulmonary Disease. *Preceedings of the American Thoracic Society* 2005;2:26-33.

[3] Burnett D, Hill SL, Chamba A Neutrophils from subjects with chronic lung disease show enhanced chemotaxis and extracellular proteolysis. *Lancet* 1987;2:1043-1046.

[4] Noguera A, Busquets X, Salueda I, Vilaverde JM, Mac Nee W, Agusto AGN. Expression of moleculs and G proteins in circulating neutrophils in chronic obstructive disease. *Am. J. Resp. Crit. Care Med.* 1998;158:1664-1668.

[5] Cross A, Erickson R, Ellis BA, Curnutte JT Spontaneuos activation of NADPH oxidase in cell free system:unexpected multiple effects of magnesium ion concentrations. *Biochem. J.* 1999;338:229-233.

[6] Salueda J, Garcia Palmer FJ, Gonzales G, Palou A, Agusto AG The activity of cytochrom oxidaze is increased in circulating lymphocytes of patients with Chronic obstructive disease, asthma and chronic artritis. *Am. J. Resp. Crit. Care Med.* 2000;161:32-35.

[7] Baraldo S, Oliani KM, Turato G, Zuin R, Saeta M The role of lymphocytes in the pathogenesis of asthma and COPD. *Curr. Med. Chemistry*. 2007;14:2250-2256.

[8] Galland L. Magnesium and immune function: an overview. *Magnesium* 1988;7(5-6):290-9.

[9] Rijkers GT, Henriquez N, Griffionen AW *Intracellular magnesium movements and lymphocyte activation*. 1993;6:205-213.

[10] Saris NEL, Mervaala E, Karppanen H, Khawaja J, Lewenstam A. Magnesium: An update on physiological, clinical and analytical aspects. *Clinica Chimica Acta* 2000;294:1-26.

[11] Elin RJ Magnesium: The fifth but forgotten electrolyte. *Am. J. Clin. Pathol.* 1994; 102:616-622.

[12] Ryschon TW, Rosenstein DL, Rubinov DR, Niemela JE, Elin RJ. Balaban RS. Relationship between skeletal muscles intracellular ionized magnesium and measurement of blood magnesium. *J. Lab. Clin. Med.* 1996;127:207-13.

[13] Iseri T, French JH Magnesium: Nature's physiologic calcium blocker. *Am. Heart J.* 1984;108:193-189.

[14] Boyum A. Isolation of mononucllear cells and granulocytes from human blood. *Scand. J. Clin. Lab. Invest.* 1986;21(97):77-89.

[15] American Thoracic Society. Lung function testing: selection of reference value and interpretative strategies. *Am. Rev. Respir. Dis.* 1991;144:1202-18.

[16] Di Stefano A, Caramori G, Ricciardolo FLM, Capelli A, Adcock IM, Donner CF. Cellular and molecular mechanisms in chronic obstructive pulmonary disease: an overview. *Clin. Exp. Allergy* 2004;34:1156-1167.

[17] Pauwels RA, Buist AS, Calverley PM, et al. Global strategy for the diagnosis, management, and prevention of chronic obstructive pulmonary disease: NHLBI/WHO Global Initiative for Chronic Obstructive Lung Disease (GOLD) Workshop summary. *Am. J. Respir. Crit. Care Med.* 2001;163:1256-1276.

[18] Gupta J, Chattopadhaya D, Bhadoria DP, Qadar Pasha, Gupta VK, Kumar M, Dabur R, Yadav V, Sharma GL. T lymphocytes subset profile and serum alpha 1 antitrypsin in pathogenesis of chronic obstructive disease. *Clinical and experimental imm*unology 2007:149;463-469.

[19] Hunziker N. Mg and its role in allergy, In: *Metal ions in biological systems*, eds. H. Sigeland A. Sigel, pp 531-547. New York:Mareel Dekker.

[20] McCoy H, Kenney LA. Mg and immune function: recent findings. *Magnes. Res.* 1992;5:281-293.

[21] McKee MD, Cecco SA, Niemela JE, Cormier J, Kim CJ, Steinberg SM, Rehak NN, Elin RJ, Rosenberg SA. Effects of interleukin 2 therapy on lymphocyte magnesium levels. *J. Lab Clin. Med.* 2002;139(1):5-12.

[22] Rijkers GT, Griffioen AW. Changes in free cytoplasmic magnesium following activation of human lymphocytes. *Biochem. J.* 1993;289:373-7.

[23] Ruljančić N, Popović-Grle S, Rumenjak V, Sokolić B, Malić A, Mihanović M, Čepelak I. COPD: Magnesium in the plasma and polymorphonuclear cells of patients during a stable phase. *COPD* 2007;4:41-47.

[24] Buhl R, Farmer SG. Future Direction in the pharmacologic Therapy of Chronic Obstructive Disease. *The proceedings of American Thoracic Society* 2005;2:83-93.

In: Dietary Magnezium: New Research
Editor: Andrew W. Yardley

ISBN 978-1-60692-109-8

Chapter I

Magnesium Intake, the Metabolic Syndrome, and Chronic Disease: A Critical Review of Epidemiologic Studies

*Yiqing Song**
Division of Preventive Medicine, Department of Medicine,
Brigham and Women's Hospital and Harvard Medical School,
Boston, MA

Abstract

Magnesium is an essential mineral with several dietary sources including whole-grains, green leafy vegetables, legumes, and nuts. Emerging evidence indicates that high magnesium intake from diet or supplements may favorably affect a cluster of metabolic abnormalities including insulin resistance, hypertension, and dyslipidemia, known as metabolic syndrome. The metabolic syndrome is prevalent worldwide and is associated with increased risks of major chronic diseases, such as type 2 diabetes mellitus (DM), cardiovascular diseases (CVD), nonalcoholic fatty liver diseases, polycystic ovary syndrome, and certain forms of cancer. In observational studies, magnesium intake has been inversely associated with chronic inflammation, dyslipidemia, insulin resistance, hypertension, type 2 DM, CVD, and colorectal cancer. Some small clinical trials with short durations appeared to support the potential efficacy of magnesium supplementation in the prevention and/or treatment of metabolic syndrome in human populations, although the long-term benefits and safety of magnesium treatment remain to be determined in future large-scale, well-designed randomized controlled trials with long follow-up periods. This article provides a systematic review of the current literature from

* Address correspondence to: Dr. Yiqing Song, Division of Preventive Medicine, Brigham and Women's Hospital, 900 Commonwealth Avenue East, Boston, MA 02215, USA. Phone: 617-278-0913, Fax: 617-731-3843; email: ysong3@rics.bwh.harvard.edu

human population studies on dietary magnesium intake and a host of metabolic disorders, focusing primarily on the role of magnesium intake in the development of metabolic syndrome, type 2 DM, hypertension, CVD, and colorectal cancer.

Introduction

Magnesium is an essential mineral critical for many metabolic functions in the body. Magnesium is primarily found in many unprocessed foods, such as whole grains, green leafy vegetables, legumes, and nuts [1-3]. The Dietary Reference Intake (DRI) for magnesium is 420 mg per day for adult men (over age 30) and 320 mg per day for women (over age 30) [1-3]. Surveys indicate that the average magnesium intake in the US general population is far below the DRI, particularly among adolescent girls, women, and the elderly [1, 3-5]. Because magnesium content tends to be lost substantially during the refining and processing of foods, the adoption of a "Western diet" characterized by low intake of vegetables and fruits and high intake of red and processed meat as well as other highly refined or prepared foods, is believed to contribute to suboptimal intake of dietary magnesium in the general population of industrialized countries [1-3].

Mg balance is regulated by the interaction among dietary magnesium intake, intestinal absorption, renal magnesium excretion, and magnesium exchange from bone [6, 7]. Magnesium deficiency refers to depletion of total body stores and is associated with several acute and chronic illnesses [7, 8]. Although serum magnesium may not reflect total body magnesium stores, serum magnesium levels are commonly used as the standard for defining magnesium deficiency (also known as hypomagnesemia) [8, 9]. Magnesium is a cofactor for hundreds of enzymes, particularly for those cellular reactions involved in the transfer, storage, and utilization of energy [3, 10, 11].Abnormalities in intracellular magnesium homeostasis have been hypothesized to be a link among insulin resistance, type 2 diabetes mellitus (DM), hypertension, and cardiovascular disease (CVD) [10]. However, a valid and feasible method for assessing intracellular magnesium (Mg) status is not available in clinical studies. The beneficial effects of magnesium intake may be explained by several mechanisms [see Figure (1)], including improvement of glucose and insulin homeostasis [12, 13], oxidative stress[10, 14, 15], lipid metabolism [16-19], vascular or myocardial contractility [10, 11, 20], endothelium-dependent vasodilation [10, 11, 14, 21], anti-arrhythmic effects [7, 22], anti-coagulant or anti-platelet effects [20, 21, 23, 24], and anti-inflammatory effects [25, 26]. Although numerous epidemiologic studies have extensively examined the association between magnesium intake and chronic disorders, most of them are ecologic or cross-sectional by design and are potentially confounded by other aspects of diet, lifestyle or socioeconomic factors. Their results need to be interpreted cautiously, although these data help to postulate hypotheses, implicating a role of magnesium in the etiology of metabolic abnormalities. In observational studies, prospective cohort design is considered optimal for the study of long-term dietary intake in the primary prevention of chronic diseases. However, prospective data for magnesium intake are relatively limited. In human intervention trials, a randomized double-blinded and placebo-controlled trial is considered the best approach to examine a cause-effect relation.

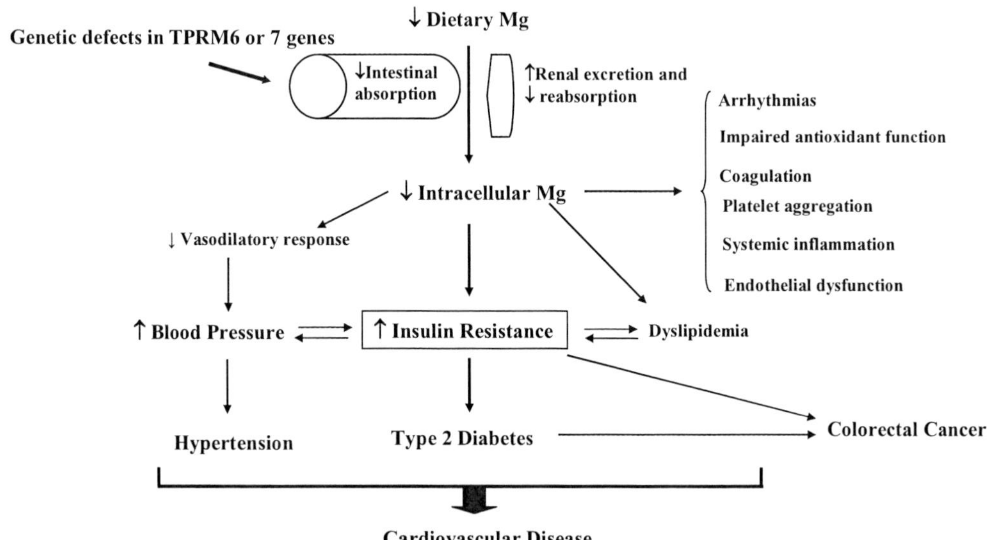

Figure 1. Scheme showing the possible mechanisms for a link between magnesium intake and chronic metabolic disorders.

However, short-term controlled trials are usually performed in the secondary prevention setting of chronic disease because of cost and logistical considerations. Oral magnesium supplementation with relatively infrequent side effects and no severe adverse effects may be effective in improving metabolic profiles in the general population. However, the long-term benefits and safety of magnesium treatment in metabolic abnormalities remain unclear with the lack of reliable data from large-scale, well-designed randomized controlled trials with long follow-up periods.

This review focuses on epidemiologic evidence on magnesium intake and the risk of developing metabolic syndrome-related chronic diseases, especially from prospective cohort studies and intervention trials, which help to elucidate the causal association between magnesium intake and these chronic diseases.

Magnesium Intake and Metabolic Syndrome Components

In recent years, emerging evidence has linked abdominal obesity, abnormal glucose metabolism, hypertension, and dyslipidemia (low high-density lipoprotein [HDL] cholesterol and elevated triglyceride) as a cluster of metabolic abnormalities defined as the metabolic syndrome [27, 28]. All components of the metabolic syndrome are risk factors for developing type 2 DM and CVD. As shown in Figure 1, adequate magnesium intake may protect against diabetes and CVD by improving these metabolic syndrome components.

Abdominal Obesity and Insulin Resistance

Obesity, particularly abdominal or visceral adiposity, has consistently been demonstrated as a fundamental cause of insulin resistance and type 2 DM [27, 29]. Some epidemiologic studies have examined directly the effects of whole grains on body weight and weight changes [30-32]. The observed associations between improved insulin sensitivity and components in whole grains including magnesium have been attributed, at least in part, to the beneficial effects of whole grains on body weight or weight changes. However, few studies have specifically examined the direct effect of magnesium intake on body weight.

Experimental data support a role of magnesium in glucose and insulin homeostasis [6, 10, 33]. Although the underlying mechanisms are not well understood, several pathways, affecting insulin secretion and action, have been proposed to explain the influence of magnesium status on insulin resistance. First, intracellular magnesium balance is critical for peripheral glucose utilization [34, 35] and insulin receptor-mediated signaling [36]. Magnesium also plays a role in glucose-stimulated insulin secretion in pancreatic β cells through its effects on cellular calcium homeostasis and/or oxidative stress [10, 37].

Epidemiologic evidence suggests an important role of magnesium in insulin sensitivity. Some cross-sectional studies have shown an inverse association between plasma or erythrocyte magnesium levels and fasting insulin levels in both diabetic patients and apparently healthy individuals [38, 39]. Several epidemiologic studies have also found an association between dietary magnesium intake and insulin homeostasis quantified by insulin clamp technique [40]. Similarly, a significant inverse association between dietary magnesium intake and fasting insulin concentrations was observed in several population-based cross-sectional studies [38, 41-43]. However, as in any cross-sectional studies, the observed associations cannot be established as causal.

Several short-term metabolic studies and small randomized trials have specifically examined the efficacy of magnesium supplementation in improving insulin sensitivity among nondiabetic individuals but the results have varied. Rosolova et al. have reported a relationship between plasma magnesium concentration and insulin-mediated glucose disposal [39, 44]. In a study of 18 nondiabetic participants, those with low levels of fasting plasma magnesium (< 0.80 mmol/L) had significantly higher plasma glucose and insulin concentrations after a 75-g oral glucose tolerance test (OGTT) and were more resistant to insulin-mediated glucose disposal reflected by higher steady state plasma glucose concentrations after a modification of insulin suppression test than those with high levels of plasma magnesium (> 0.83 mmol/L) [44]. Both groups were comparable in terms of sex, family history of diabetes, history of hypertension, cigarette smoking, alcohol consumption and steady-state insulin concentrations. Similar associations between plasma magnesium concentrations and insulin-mediated glucose disposal were also observed when the same investigators enrolled 98 healthy nondiabetic individuals [39]. One nonrandomized trial examined the effect of magnesium supplementation on insulin sensitivity in 12 nondiabetic participants with normal body weight [12]. Magnesium-deficient diet (<0.5 mmol/day) for 4 weeks led to approximately 25% reduction in an insulin sensitivity index determined by minimal model analysis using a modified intravenous glucose tolerance test [12]. Two randomized double-blind placebo-controlled trials have also assessed the effects of magnesium in both insulin secretion and action among nondiabetic participants [45, 46]. In one trial of 12 nonobese elderly participants, daily magnesium supplementation (4.5 g magnesium pidolate, equivalent to 15.8 mmol) for 4 weeks significantly improved glucose-induced insulin response and insulin-mediated glucose disposal [46]. In another randomized double-blind placebo-controlled trial, 60 apparently healthy participants who had low serum magnesium concentrations and insulin resistance assessed by the homeostasis model analysis for insulin resistance (HOMA-IR) were randomly allocated to receive either magnesium supplement (2.5 g/day magnesium chloride [12.5 mmol elemental magnesium]) or placebo [45]. Magnesium treatment for 3 months significantly improved insulin resistance as reflected by fasting glucose (5.8±0.9 to 5.0±0.6 mmol/L), insulin (103.2±56.4 to 70.2±29.6 mmol/L), and HOMA-IR (4.6±2.8 to 2.6±1.1, $P<0.0001$) [45]. Due to limited evidence, the beneficial effect of magnesium supplementation in improving insulin sensitivity in nondiabetic people has yet to be conclusively demonstrated and future long-term and well-designed controlled trials are warranted.

Dyslipidemia

Dietary magnesium may be related to lipid metabolism independent of its effects on insulin sensitivity. Malkiel-Shapiro (1956) et al. first reported that intramuscular injection of magnesium sulfate lowered serum β-lipoprotein in patients with coronary heart disease [47]. Animal studies have also suggested favorable effects of magnesium intake on lipid metabolism [16, 48-50]. For example, Altura and colleagues noted that magnesium supplements lowered serum cholesterol by 24% and triglycerides by 33% and attenuated the development of atherosclerotic lesions in cholesterol-fed rabbits [16]. Several hypothesized mechanisms have been proposed to explain the impact of magnesium on lipid profiles. As a cofactor for many rate-limiting enzymes critical for lipid metabolism, magnesium may decrease the activity of lecithin:cholesterol acyl-transferase (LCAT) [18] and HMG-CoA reductase, and increase lipoprotein lipase activity [51]. LCAT is an enzyme for the esterification of free cholesterol, which lowers LDL cholesterol (LDL-C) and triglyceride levels and raises HDL cholesterol (HDL-C) levels. HMG-CoA reductase is a rate-limiting enzyme in cholesterol biosynthesis. Lipoprotein lipase is responsible for the conversion of triglycerides to HDL-C and thus leads to a decrease in hepatic VLDL-triglyceride synthesis and secretion.

Because of limited data in humans, epidemiologic evidence for the role of magnesium in improving blood lipid profiles remains controversial. In a cross-sectional study of 192 Mexicans with metabolic syndrome and 384 age and sex-matched disorder-free controls, low serum magnesium levels were independently related to dyslipidemia (defined as fasting triglycerides ≥1.7 mmol/L and/or HDL-C <1.0 mmol/L) [52]. In the ARIC cohort of women and men free of CVD, serum magnesium intake was inversely related to serum triglycerides and positively related to LDL-C among whites while dietary magnesium intake was positively associated with plasma HDL-C among whites, independent of age and BMI [38].

Several trials have evaluated the effect of magnesium supplements on blood lipids among normal or hyperlipidemic patients. In the 1960s, a clinical trial reported that a combination of magnesium chloride and potassium chloride lowered α and β lipoproteins by 10% [53]. In a nonrandomized clinical trial, Davis et al. (1984) reported that an oral magnesium chloride (18 mmol/day) for 118 days significantly decreased total cholesterol, LDL-C, and VLDL cholesterol (VLDL-C) concentrations and increased HDL-C in 16 patients with hyperlipidemia [17]. Four randomized, double-blind, placebo-controlled trials have been conducted to evaluate the effects of oral magnesium supplementation on blood lipids among nondiabetic participants. Among 33 apparently healthy Japanese, oral supplementation of magnesium hydroxide (548 mg [9.82 mmol] for men and 411 mg [7.36 mmol] for women daily) for 4 weeks significantly increased HDL-C and apolipoprotein (apo) A1 and decreased serum LDL-C concentrations [18]. In the magnesium treatment group, HDL-C increased from 1.28±0.35 mmol/L to 1.37±0.34 mmol/L (7%); apoA1 from 1362±203 to 1386±195 mg/L (2%) while LDL-C decreased from 3.52±1.10 to 3.25±0.97 mmol/L (8%) after 4 weeks [18]. Magnesium supplementation also appeared to improve the lipid profile among hyperlipidemic patients with other overt chronic diseases. In a controlled trial by Rasmussen et al, 47 patients with ischemic heart disease and acute myocardial infarction (MI) were randomly allocated to either magnesium hydroxide (15mmol/day [360 mg]) or placebo for 3 months [19]. Magnesium supplementation led to a significant decrease in apo B (15%), minor increase of HDL-C (6%) and nonsignificant reduction in triglycerides and VLDL-C with no differences in apoA1 and LDL-C [19]. Magnesium supplementation was also observed to decrease total cholesterol and triglycerides in a trial of 30 patients with chronic renal insufficiency [54]. In contrast, one randomized, double-blind, placebo-controlled trial failed to demonstrate the efficacy of magnesium supplementation in improving lipid profile among healthy people [55]. In this trial of 50 normal volunteers, magnesium supplementation (magnesium oxide, 800 mg/day [20 mmol]) for 60 days did not result in any significant changes in lipid profile including total cholesterol, HDL-C, LDL-C, and VLDL-C concentrations, and triglycerides [55]. There is still insufficient evidence to draw definitive conclusions about the effect of magnesium supplementation on lipid metabolism in nondiabetic patients.

Indeed it is difficult to tease out the causal effect of magnesium on lipid metabolism independent of glucose and/or insulin homeostasis. One randomized double-blind placebo-controlled trial has examined the effect of magnesium supplementation on plasma lipid concentrations in people with insulin resistance [45]. Among 60 apparently healthy participants who had insulin resistance and low serum magnesium concentrations, magnesium supplementation (2.5 g/day magnesium chloride [12.5 mmol]) for 3 months significantly reduced total cholesterol (10.7%) and triglycerides (39.3%) and LDL-C (11.8%) and increased HDL-C (22.2%) [45]. Several studies (at least one nonrandomized trial and 6 randomized double-blind placebo-controlled trials) have focused on whether magnesium intake affects lipid profiles in diabetic patients [56-61]. A marked decrease in mean triglyceride levels after magnesium supplementation (300 mg/day elemental magnesium) was observed in one open trial of 9 patients with type 2 DM without insulin therapy [62]. In contrast, none of 6 randomized double-blind placebo-controlled trials found change in plasma lipids in type 2 DM patients after oral magnesium supplementation (15-30 mmol/day) from 6 weeks to 4 months [56-61]. Likewise, the effects of magnesium intake on plasma lipids in patients with type 1 DM were reported in an open study with 10 participants [63], but were not replicated in another double-blind, placebo-controlled study with 28 patients with type 1 DM [64]. Thus far, whether oral magnesium supplementation improves lipid profiles in diabetic participants remains unsettled.

Hypertension

A substantial body of research has accumulated for decades, implicating a pivotal role of magnesium intake in blood pressure (BP) regulation [11]. *In vitro* studies have shown that magnesium has multiple functions that may contribute to its antihypertensive effects [11]. Proposed underlying mechanisms include the inhibition of intracellular calcium mobilization as a calcium antagonist, attenuation of the adverse effect of sodium by stimulating activity of sodium-potassium (Na-K) ATPase or increasing urinary excretion of sodium, decreased release of catecholamine [11, 20], improvement of myocardial contractility and vascular smooth muscle tone [20], endothelium-dependent vasodilation [11, 21, 65], systemic inflammation [25, 26], and insulin secretion and action [10, 14].

The hypothetical relation between magnesium intake and BP was suggested by the results from ecologic studies that showed a negative correlation between water hardness and BP and hypertension [66, 67]. It should be noted that interpretation of such comparisons at population levels is always problematic because ecologic correlations based on grouped data at the population level may not reflect the corresponding association at the individual level due to confounding (known as ecological fallacy) [68]. In addition, the intake of magnesium from drinking water is negligible compared with total magnesium intake from diet [69] and thus may not be crucial in the prevention of magnesium deficiency.

The majority of epidemiologic data relating dietary magnesium to lower prevalence of hypertension is provided by numerous cross-sectional studies. Results from most, but not all cross-sectional studies suggest that magnesium intake reduces BP in diverse populations [65, 70]. Results from observational studies have been thoroughly reviewed elsewhere [70, 71]. A qualitative review of 29 observational studies concluded that there was an inverse association between dietary magnesium intake and BP, which was relatively consistent across studies using different study populations and sample sizes, various methodologies of diet assessment, and different statistical analyses [70]. However, the evidence from cross-sectional studies does not necessarily imply any causal relation due to the inherent limitation of this study design. Intriguingly, apparent gender and ethnic-differences were observed in some cross-sectional studies and deserve further investigation. For example, a Belgian study found a negative correlation between dietary magnesium and systolic BP in women only [72]. Simon et al. found a negative correlation between dietary magnesium intake and diastolic BP in white girls in 3 American cities, but not in African-American girls [73]. In a nationally representative sample of 6,046 white participants and 2,226 African-American participants in the National Health and Nutrition Examination Survey III (NHANES III), Ford et al. reported that a negative correlation between dietary magnesium intake and hypertension prevalence was more evident in African Americans than whites [74].

Prospective data on the relation of magnesium intake with the development of hypertension are very limited [75-77]. In the Women's Health Study, Song et al. reported that high intake of magnesium at baseline was modestly associated with a lower 10-year risk of incident hypertension among apparent healthy middle-aged and older US women [78]. Similar effects were observed among those nonsmokers with no history of diabetes or high cholesterol levels who were less likely to change diet. These data are similar to those from the Nurses' Health Study and the Health Professionals Follow-up Study, which have reported a significant inverse association between dietary magnesium intake and BP [75, 76]. In the Nurses' Health Study, Ascherio et al. observed an inverse relation of dietary magnesium with self-reported BP but not with the incidence of hypertension. After adjusting for age, BMI, and alcohol intake, the RR of incident hypertension was 1.10 (95% CI: 0.92-1.32; *P* for trend=0.56) and the average BP was 1.3/1.0 mm Hg lower in women with high intake (≥350 mg/d) than those with low magnesium intake (<200 mg/d) [79]. In contrast, the Atherosclerosis Risk in Communities (ARIC) study failed to detect a significant association between dietary magnesium and hypertension [77]. Although the ARIC study found a modest inverse association between serum magnesium levels and incident hypertension, the correlation between serum and dietary magnesium in this study was very low (correlation coefficient=0.053) [77]. In the Coronary Artery Risk Development in Young Adults Study (CARDIA) with follow-up of 15 years, dietary magnesium intake was inversely associated with incident hypertension (*P* for trend<0.01), but this association was substantially attenuated towards the null after adjustment for dietary factors including total energy, fiber, polyunsaturated fat, saturated fat and total carbohydrates [80]. Available evidence for the role of magnesium in primary prevention of hypertension is not compelling, but we cannot rule out a small effect of high magnesium intake in lowering blood pressure among normotensive people. To reconcile the discrepancies in the results from these previous prospective cohort studies, the data regarding the association between dietary magnesium intake and incidence of hypertension were pooled using a classic random-effect meta-analysis (Table 1) [81]. A χ^2 statistic was used to test between-study heterogeneity [82]. The summary estimate of RR is 0.88 comparing the highest category of dietary magnesium intake with the lowest category of intake (95% CI: 0.80-0.97; *P*=0.87 for between-study heterogeneity). Considering the partial influence shared by other highly correlated variables such as fiber, calcium, and potassium, dietary magnesium may have only a modest effect on the risk of hypertension.

Numerous small clinical trials have assessed the therapeutic effect of magnesium supplements in hypertension but yielded inconsistent results [70, 83]. Many sources of heterogeneity may have contributed to the inconsistency in these trials including small sample size, incomplete randomization, the lack of blinding in design, variable duration of follow-up, high rates of noncompliance, and differences in magnesium treatment protocols, magnesium formulation and dose, and study populations. In a recent meta-analysis of clinical trials between 1983 and 2001, Jee et al. identified 20 randomized trials with a sample size from 13 to 461 participants (median: 31 per trial) and a follow-up period from 3 to 24 weeks (median: 8.5 weeks) [83]. Their results showed that magnesium supplementation led to a small overall reduction in BP in a dose-dependent manner. For each 10 mmol/day (240 mg/day) increase in magnesium dose, systolic BP decreased by 4.3 mmHg (95% CI: -6.3 to –2.2; *P* for trend <0.001) and diastolic BP by 2.3 mmHg (95% CI: -4.9 to 0; *P* for trend=0.09)

[83]. Furthermore, the pooled results of 14 double-blind randomized trials among hypertensive patients showed that a 10 mmol/day (240 mg/day) increase in magnesium intake was associated with a decrease in both systolic BP (3.3 mmHg, 95% CI: -0.1 to 6.8) and diastolic BP (2.3 mmHg, 95% CI: -1.0 to 5.6) [83]. Overall, the evidence from these trials suggests a modest antihypertensive effect by magnesium supplementation, although additional research is needed to assess whether magnesium therapy is beneficial for the general population.

Table 1. Prospective Studies for the relationship between dietary magnesium intake and incident hypertension

Author (publication year), study cohort	Population	Incident cases	Follow-up, years	Multivariate RR and p for trend *
Witteman et al. (1989), NHS [75]	58218 (women)	3,275	4	0.78 (0.62-0.98), p=0.03
Ascherio et al. (1992), HPFS [76]	30681 (men)	1,248	4	0.89 (0.64-1.25), p=0.66
Peacock et al. (1999), ARIC [77]	7731 (4190 women and 3541 men)	822	6	0.99 (0.69-1.43) for women, p=0.73 0.98 (0.68-1.41) for men, p=0.68
He et al. (2006), CARDIA [80]	4637 (men and women)	932	15	0.87 (0.69-1.10), p=0.11
Song et al. (2006), WHS [78]	28349 (women)	8,544	10	0.93 (0.86-1.02) p=0.03

NHS, the Nurses' Health Study; HPFS, the Health Professionals Follow-up Study; ARIC, the Atherosclerosis Risk in Communities Study; CARDIA, the Coronary Artery Risk Development in Young Adults Study; and WHS, The Women's Health Study.

*Multivariate-adjusted relative risk (RR; 95% confidence interval, CI) represented those comparing the highest category with the lowest category of magnesium intake; p for trend indicated the linear trend across quartiles or quintiles of magnesium intake.

Systemic Inflammation and Endothelial Dysfunction

Although low-grade inflammation, as measured by C-reactive protein (CRP) with a high-sensitivity assay, has not been included in the definition of the metabolic syndrome, CRP levels have been associated with risk of CVD, insulin resistance, type 2 DM, hypertension, and features of the metabolic syndrome and with the metabolic syndrome itself [84]. Previous studies have also shown that CRP levels are positively correlated with many correlated metabolic components that are not incorporated into the metabolic syndrome definitions being used, such as endothelial adhesion molecules [85, 86], microalbuminuria [87], and impaired fibrinolysis [88]. Circulating concentrations of inflammatory cytokines have been highly correlated with insulin resistance and its related metabolic abnormalities. The underlying mechanisms by which magnesium intake influences systemic inflammation remains to be elucidated, although the most likely explanation is a causal link between magnesium homeostasis and insulin resistance [10, 14]. Alternatively, magnesium may influence insulin resistance through modulation of systemic inflammation.

Accumulating evidence from animal and human studies suggests that magnesium may also play a role in immune function [89]. A cross-sectional study of 371 non-diabetic, non-hypertensive obese Mexicans reported an inverse association between serum magnesium concentrations and high-sensitivity CRP concentrations [25]. It thus seems plausible to speculate that the beneficial effects of magnesium on chronic diseases may be partially mediated by its potential anti-inflammatory effect. Epidemiologic data, though very limited, have provided some cross-sectional evidence linking magnesium intake to systemic inflammation as reflected by elevated concentrations of CRP. The inverse association between magnesium intake and CRP was first reported in a large population of 11,686 apparently healthy women in the Women's Health Study [43]. In a large representative sample of US adults aged ≥20 years from the NHANES 1999-2000, individuals who consumed less than the recommended daily allowance (RDA) of magnesium were 1.48-1.75 times more likely to have elevated CRP (≥3.0 mg/L) than those who consumed ≥ RDA, with control for demographic and cardiovascular risk factors [90].

There is growing recognition that systemic inflammation and endothelial dysfunction may be two integral components of the metabolic syndrome, as common antecedents for the initiation of atherosclerosis and type 2 diabetes [91, 92]. Several lines of experimental evidence have also suggested that magnesium intake has beneficial effects on endothelial function [93-95]. Endothelial dysfunction has been closely related to insulin resistance [86, 92] and precedes the onset of early atherosclerotic CVD and type 2 DM [96]. Elevated plasma concentrations of soluble forms of endothelial adhesion molecules, released from shedding or proteolytic cleavage from the endothelial cell surface, are considered useful indicators of endothelial dysfunction/activation [92, 96]. Due to limited data, it is unclear whether magnesium intake is inversely related to circulating concentrations of endothelial biomarkers. In a recent cross-sectional study of 657 apparently healthy women from the Nurses' Health Study, Song et al found that magnesium intake was inversely associated with plasma concentrations of CRP and E-selectin, independent of age, BMI, smoking, physical activity, alcohol consumption, and postmenopausal hormone use. The multivariate adjusted geometric means for women in the highest quintile of dietary magnesium intake were 24% lower for CRP (1.70±0.18 vs. 1.30±0.10 mg/dL, P for trend =0.03) and 14% lower for E-selectin (48.5±1.84 vs. 41.9±1.58 ng/mL, P for trend=0.01) than those in the lowest quintile. Because of inherent limitations from observational study design and dietary measurement, their results are likely to reflect overall beneficial effects of magnesium intake from consuming magnesium-rich foods such as whole-grains, green leafy vegetables, legumes, and nuts on systemic inflammation and endothelial function.

Several lines of experimental evidence have also suggested that magnesium supplementation had beneficial effects on endothelial function [93]. In a randomized trial conducted in 35 patients with chronic heart failure, oral magnesium citrate 300 mg/day significantly reduced blood levels of CRP after 5 weeks (log CRP from 1.4±0.4 to 0.8±0.3; P<0.001), with a concomitant increase in intracellular magnesium levels (61±8 to 67±12 mmol/g cell protein; P=0.01) [97]. Future prospective studies or intervention trials are warranted to examine a causal effect of magnesium in systemic inflammation and endothelial function.

The Metabolic Syndrome

Metabolic syndrome comprises a constellation of metabolic abnormalities including visceral obesity, glucose intolerance, hypertension, and dyslipidemia [27, 28]. It is important to note that almost all epidemiologic studies of magnesium and the metabolic syndrome relied on the National Cholesterol Education Program (NCEP) Adult Treatment Program III (ATP III) diagnosis criteria [98], although there are other commonly used diagnosis criteria, such as those of the World Health Organization (WHO) [99], the European Group on Insulin Resistance (EGIR) [100], the American Association of Clinical Endocrinologists (AACE) [101], and the International Diabetes Federation (IDF) [102]. The evidence that magnesium favorably affects these metabolic abnormalities, though not entirely consistent, has led us to hypothesize that magnesium intake is related to a lower risk of metabolic syndrome. Regardless of diverse definitions used for the metabolic syndrome as an entity in different studies, this notion has been supported by epidemiologic evidence (summarized in Table 2).

Two cross-sectional studies have related serum magnesium level to metabolic syndrome and/or its components. In a cross-sectional population-based study of 192 individuals with metabolic syndrome and 384 matched healthy control subjects, low serum magnesium levels were associated with elevated risk of metabolic syndrome defined by the presence of at least two of the features (hyperglycemia, high BP, elevated fasting triglycerides, low HDL-C, and obesity) [52]. In another cross-sectional study, low levels of serum ionized magnesium were associated with the metabolic syndrome and serum magnesium level was inversely related to triglycerides and waist circumference. However, it remains controversial whether serum magnesium levels can reflect long-term magnesium intake or total magnesium status in the human body [103]. Serum magnesium did not appear to be correlated well with dietary magnesium intake and the intracellular magnesium pool; a biologically active portion of magnesium store [103, 104].

Magnesium intake has been observed to be associated with all features of the metabolic syndrome. Song *et al.* first reported an inverse relation between dietary intake of magnesium and the prevalence of metabolic syndrome among 11,686 apparently healthy American women in the Women's Health Study [43]. Compared with those who in the lowest quintile of magnesium intake, women in the highest quintile of intake had 27% lower risk of the metabolic syndrome according to the ATP-III criteria (OR: 0.73; 95% CI: 0.60-0.88; p for trend < 0.001). This inverse association also appeared to be more pronounced among women who were overweight and those who ever smoked. The authors suggested that a possible beneficial effect of magnesium intake on diabetes and cardiovascular disease might be related to its roles in ameliorating systemic inflammation and/or the development of the metabolic syndrome. Using data from the NHANES III, Ford *et al.* provided consistent evidence from a cross-sectional analysis that magnesium intake is inversely associated with the prevalence of the metabolic syndrome in both men and women [105].

Table 2. Epidemiologic evidence for the relationship between magnesium intake and the metabolic syndrome

Author, year Study Cohort	Participants	Age (range)	MetS definition	MetS proportion *	Magnesium categories and Multivariate RR (95%CI)	Adjusted variables
Song et al. (2005), WHS [84]	14719 US women (mostly Caucasian)	39-89	Modified NCEP ATP III criteria	Prevalence: 24.4%	Quintiles of dietary magnesium intake (mg/d) and ORs (95% CIs): Q1 (116-277): 1.00 (referent); Q2 (277-309): 0.89 (0.75-1.06); Q3 (309-341): 0.84 (0.70-1.02); Q4 (341-383): 0.78 (0.63-0.96); Q5 (383-837): 0.65 (0.52-0.83); (P for trend =0.0004) No significant associations with triglycerides	Age, smoking, exercise, total calorie, alcohol use, multivitamin use, parental history of myocardial infarction, dietary intakes of total fat, cholesterol, folate, glycemic load, and fiber.
Ford et al. (2007), NHANES III [105]	7669 Americans (3799 women and 3870 men)	26-82	NCEP ATP III criteria	Prevalence: 25.6%	Quintiles of dietary magnesium intake (men and women, mg/d) and Ors (95% CIs): Q1 (men≤221 and women≤164): 1.00 (referent); Q2 (222 to 292 and 165 to 213): 0.84 (0.58-1.23); Q3 (293 to 376 and 214 to 263): 0.76 (0.54-1.07); Q4 (377 to 465 and 264 to 336): 0.62 (0.40-0.98); Q5 (≥466 and ≥337): 0.56 (0.34-0.92); (P for trend <0.0001) No significant associations with individual metabolic syndrome components	Age, sex, race, education, smoking, CRP, alcohol use, physical activity, family history of early CHD, vitamin use, history of diabetes, fat, carbohydrate, fiber, total energy intake.

Author, year Study Cohort	Participants	Age (range)	MetS definition	MetS proportion *	Magnesium categories and Multivariate RR (95%CI)	Adjusted variables
He et al. (2006), CARDIA [80]	4637 (2363 Blacks and 2274 Whites)	18-30	NCEP ATP III criteria (Including diabetic cases)	13% incidence for 15 years of follow-up	Quartiles of total magnesium intake (median, mg/d) and ORs (95% CIs): Q1 (96.0): 1.00 (referent); Q2 (121): 0.98 (0.79-1.21); Q3 (147): 0.75 (0.59-0.96); Q4 (191): 0.69 (0.52-0.91); (P for trend<0.01) No significant associations with blood pressure and triglycerides.	Age, gender, race, education, smoking, physical activity, family history of diabetes, alcohol intake, dietary intakes of fiber, polyunsaturated fat, saturated fat, total carbohydrates, total energy with additional adjustment for each component of the metabolic syndrome at baseline.

WHS, The Women's Health Study; NHANES III, Third National Health and Nutrition Examination Survey; MetS, the metabolic syndrome; CARDIA, the Coronary Artery Risk Development in Young Adults Study; NCEP ATP III, the National Cholesterol Education Program (NCEP) Adult Treatment Panel III.

The multivariable OR of metabolic syndrome (according to the criteria of the ATP-III) for participants in the highest quintile of magnesium intake was 0.56 (95% CI: 0.34-0.92; p for trend=0.029) compared with those who in the lowest quintile of intake. The results remained after vitamin or mineral supplement users were excluded.

Recently, He *et al.* conducted a longitudinal study and prospectively examined the relations between magnesium intake and incident metabolic syndrome and its components (defined by the ATP-III definition) in American young adults [80]. During the 15 years of follow-up, the investigators documented 608 incident cases of the metabolic syndrome among 4,637 Americans, aged 18 to 30 years, who were free from metabolic syndrome and diabetes at baseline. After adjustment for potential confounders and baseline status of each component of the metabolic syndrome, magnesium intake was inversely associated with incidence of metabolic syndrome. The multivariable hazard ratio of metabolic syndrome for participants in the highest quartile was 0.69 (95% CI: 0.52-0.91; p for trend < 0.01) compared with those in the lowest quartile of magnesium intake. The inverse associations were not appreciably modified by gender and race (Caucasian and African American). Particularly, significant inverse relations were also observed between magnesium intake and fasting glucose level, waist circumference, and HDL cholesterol. All the data appeared to support the hypothesis that higher magnesium intake or a diet rich in magnesium is important to cardiometabolic health.

Magnesium Intake and Chronic Diseases

The available evidence from human populations suggests that dietary magnesium intake is associated with a host of metabolic syndrome-associated chronic diseases, including type 2 DM, CVD, and colorectal cancer.

Type 2 Diabetes Mellitus (DM)

A large body of data from clinical case studies and cross-sectional studies provided further evidence for the correlation between blood magnesium levels and type 2 DM [13, 38, 106-112]. Hypomagnesemia is common among patients with diabetes, especially those with poor metabolic control [108, 111, 113]. Polyuria caused by hyperglycemia, coupled with hyperinsulinemia, tended to increase renal excretion of magnesium or decrease renal re-absorption of magnesium, thereby resulting in hypomagnesemia in type 2 DM [114, 115]. Inadequate intake of dietary magnesium in diabetic patients may also cause hypomagnesemia [116]. However, these results are inconclusive in testing the hypothesis regarding the role of magnesium due to confounding by other aspects of diet, physical activity, smoking, obesity, socioeconomic status, and drug therapies such as hypoglycemic medication, diuretics, and insulin. Thus, whether low plasma magnesium is a cause or consequence of suboptimal glycemic control remains inconclusive.

Results from prospective studies of magnesium intake and risk of type 2 DM have been generally consistent (Figure 2). Previous reports from the Nurses' Health Study [117, 118], the Iowa Women's Health Study [119], the Health Professionals Follow-up Study [120], the European Prospective Investigation Into Cancer and Nutrition(EPIC)-Postdam Study [121], and the Black Women's Health Study [122] all indicated an inverse association between magnesium intake and risk of incident type 2 DM, although such an association was not found in the ARIC study with relatively small number of incident cases [123].

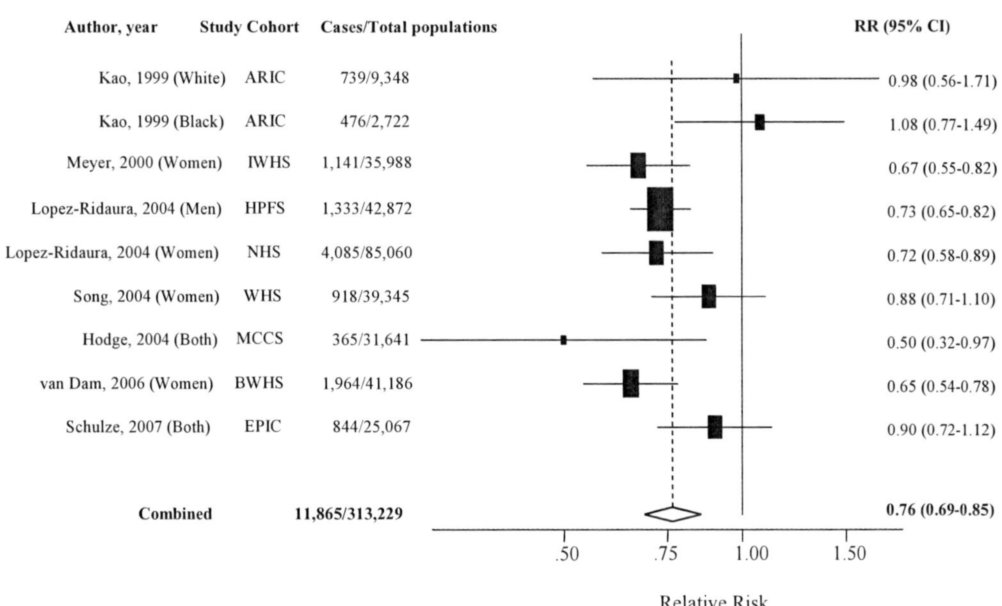

ARIC, the Atherosclerosis Risk in Communities Study; IWHS, Iowa Women's Health Study; HPFS, Health Professionals Follow-up Study; NHS, Nurses' Health Study; WHS, Women's Health Study; MCCS, Melbourne Collaborative Cohort Study; BWHS,Black Women's Health Study; EPIC, European Prospective Investigation Into Cancer and Nutrition-Postdam Study

Figure 2. A meta-analysis of prospective studies regarding the association between dietary magnesium intake and incidence of type 2 diabetes.

However, the prospective ARIC study showed an inverse association between serum concentrations of magnesium at baseline and subsequent risk of type 2 DM [123]. Since there is a lack of correlation between serum levels and dietary magnesium intake (r=0.06) [123-125], such an association may not reflect the impact of long-term magnesium intake.

When the data from these prospective cohorts were pooled (Figure 2), the summary estimate of RR was 0.76 comparing the highest category of dietary magnesium intake with the lowest category of intake (95% CI: 0.69-0.85; P= 0.04 for between-study heterogeneity). Our results were consistent with two recent meta-analyses that were independently conducted but did not include all the prospective studies available. In one meta-analysis of eight independent cohorts with 286,668 participants and 10912 diabetes cases, the overall RR for a 100 mg/day increase in magnesium intake was 0.85 (95% CI, 0.79-0.92; P= 0.002 for between-study heterogeneity). Results were similar for dietary magnesium (RR, 0.86; 95% CI, 0.77-0.95) and total magnesium (RR, 0.83; 95% CI, 0.77-0.89) [126]. In another separate meta-analysis of eight cohorts involving 271,869 participants and 9,792 cases, the RR for the highest category compared with the lowest category was 0.77 (95%CI, 0.72-0.84; *P*= 0.04 for between-study heterogeneity) for total magnesium intake [121]. Although cereal fiber that is always highly correlated with magnesium intake may explain in part the observed beneficial effect of magnesium intake, cereal fiber has been associated with a lower diabetes risk independent of magnesium in several previous cohort studies and meta-analyses [80, 121, 122]. Thus, the evidence from prospective cohort studies is strongly supportive of the role of magnesium intake in the development of type 2 DM.

In an earlier report from the Nurses' Health Study, women in the highest quintile compared with the lowest quintile of magnesium intake had a relative risk (RR) of 0.68 (95% confidence interval [CI], 0.45-1.01; *P* for trend=0.02) for women with a BMI less than 29 and 0.73 (95% CI, 0.53-1.02; *P* for trend=0.008) for women with a BMI of 29 or higher [117]. In another large cohort of 39,345 middle-aged and older US women participating in the Women's Health Study with an average of 6-year follow-up, this inverse association remained significant albeit only among women with a BMI of 25 or more (RR, 0.78; 95% CI, 0.62-0.99; *P* for trend=0.02) [43]. Because the extent to which magnesium intake influences insulin sensitivity may differ among women with different body weights, we speculated that the potential beneficial effects of high intake of magnesium may be greater among overweight persons who are prone to insulin resistance. It remains to be confirmed in future studies whether magnesium intake has differential beneficial effects in individuals with different levels of metabolic status.

There are as yet no clinical trials examining the efficacy of magnesium supplementation or consumption of major magnesium-rich foods on the primary prevention of type 2 DM. In the 1980s, several nonrandomized and uncontrolled trials for secondary prevention in diabetic patients showed that oral magnesium supplementation may improve glucose tolerance and reduce insulin requirement among patients with type 2 DM [62, 127-129]. Nine randomized controlled trials of oral magnesium supplementation have assessed diabetes-related phenotypes (e.g., glycemic control, or insulin sensitivity) among patients with type 2 DM [56, 57, 59-61, 127, 130-132]. A total of 370 patients with type 2 DM were enrolled in these 9 trials evaluating oral magnesium supplementation (median dose: 15 mmol/day [360 mg/day]) from 4 to 16 weeks (median:12 weeks) to improve diabetes control. Of them, four randomized double-blind trials showed beneficial effects by oral magnesium supplementation on glycemic control among patients with type 2 diabetes [59, 130-132]. By contrast, five randomized double-blind placebo-controlled trials showed no beneficial effects of oral magnesium supplementation on glycemic control among patients with type 2 DM [56, 57, 60, 61, 127]. Because almost all trials included small numbers of participants and were of relatively short duration, these randomized controlled trials have been underpowered to reliably assess the efficacy of oral magnesium supplementation. In addition, differences in study population, duration of diabetes, glycemic treatment, and intervention periods, coupled with different magnesium doses and formulations used, have led to difficulties in interpreting the potential benefits of oral magnesium supplementation for patients with type 2 DM. Oral magnesium supplementation as adjunct therapy may be effective in improving glycemic control among type 2 DM patients. Side effects were relatively infrequent among diabetic patients in the magnesium treatment group. No severe adverse effects, including cardiovascular events or deaths, were reported. The most common side effects were gastrointestinal symptoms including diarrhea and abdominal pain [56, 57, 59-61, 127, 130-132]. However, the long-term benefits and safety of magnesium treatment on glycemic control remain to be determined in future large-scale, well-designed randomized controlled trials with long follow-up periods.

Cardiovascular Disease

The relationship between magnesium and CVD has been studied extensively for nearly seventy years. The first evidence in the English literature can be traced to the 1935, when Zwillinger reported that intravenous magnesium sulfate suppressed digitalis-induced cardiac arrhythmia in humans [20]. Subsequently, many nonrandomized and uncontrolled clinical trials demonstrated that the use of different magnesium supplements, either oral or intravenous treatment, appeared to be protective against arrhythmias and death due to acute myocardial infarction (MI) or chronic heart failure [7, 20, 22]. Animal studies showed that magnesium deficiency accelerated the atherosclerotic process and magnesium supplementation suppressed the development of atherosclerosis [16, 133]. Several lines of evidence from earlier autopsy studies showed lower magnesium content in the myocardium of patients with sudden coronary deaths than in those who died of other causes such as accidents [134-137]. Proposed mechanisms include inhibition of intracellular calcium overload due to ischemia [10, 11, 20], preservation of energy-dependent cellular activity by conserving cellular ATP [6, 11, 14, 20], anti-arrhythmic effect [7, 22], improvement of myocardial contractility [10, 11, 20], decreased release of catecholamine [11], delayed progression of myocardial ischemia [20, 21], reduced reperfusion injury [10, 20, 21], improved lipid metabolism [16-19], and anti-coagulant or anti-platelet effects [20, 21].

In the late 1950s, the hypothesis that magnesium lowers the risk of CVD gained further support from ecologic studies. Since Kobayashi (1957) reported an inverse correlation between water hardness and the death rate from cerebrovascular disease in Japan [138], many ecologic studies in different geographic area and diverse populations showed similar correlations relating the hardness of drinking water to reduced cardiovascular mortality [20, 67, 139-141]. As discussed above, the difficulties in the use of ecologic data at the population level for making causal inferences at the individual level is widely recognized because of the potential confounding bias due to inherent limitations of the study design [68]. It has been pointed out that magnesium intake from drinking water is often negligible compared with magnesium intake from diet [69], and thus may not be crucial in the prevention of magnesium deficiency.

Some large population-based cross-sectional studies have also suggested a negative correlation between magnesium status and CVD phenotypes [38], [142]. Two large cohort studies have prospectively examined the relationship between serum magnesium levels and risk of developing coronary heart disease (CHD) [104, 143]. Higher serum magnesium concentrations have been associated with a lower risk of coronary heart disease in both the National Health and Nutrition Examination Survey I Epidemiologic Follow-up Study (NHEFS) [143] and the ARIC Study [104]. However, it is unclear whether such an association with serum magnesium reflects the impact of long-term dietary intake in the development of CVD.

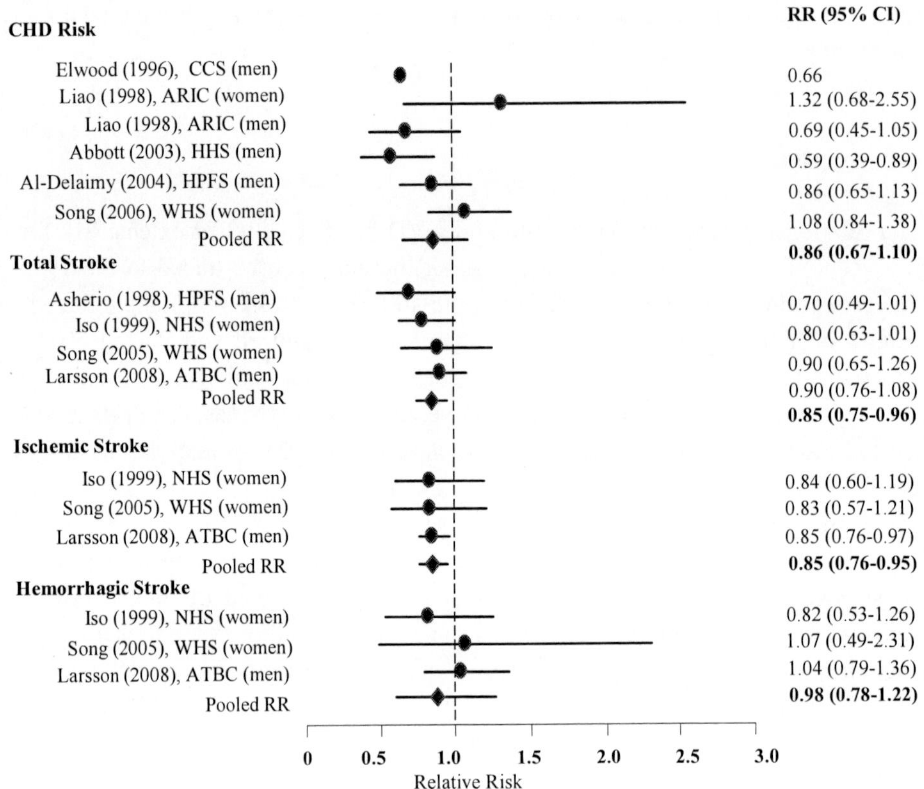

CCS, Caerphilly Cohort Study; ARIC, the Atherosclerosis Risk in Communities Study; HHS, Honolulu Heart Study; HPFS, Health Professionals Follow-up Study; NHS, Nurses' Health Study; WHS, Women's Health Study; ATBC, Alpha-Tocopherol, Beta-Carotene Cancer Prevention Study.

Figure 3. A meta-analysis of prospective studies regarding the association between dietary magnesium intake and incidence of cardiovascular disease.

Despite the data from ecologic and cross-sectional studies linking low magnesium intake and CVD, few epidemiologic studies have evaluated the role of magnesium intake in the primary prevention of CVD. Of note, an inverse association between dietary magnesium and the risk of CHD, though generally weak, has been observed in the Honolulu Heart Study [144] and the HPFS [145]. In the ARIC study with 13,922 middle-aged US adults with 4 to 7 years of follow-up, dietary magnesium assessed by 61-item food frequency questionnaire (FFQ) had a modest inverse association with risk of CHD in men but not in women. In contrast, neither the Caerphilly cohort of 2,172 men aged 45-59 with 10-year follow-up [146] nor the WHS of 39,876 women aged 39-89 with 10-year follow-up [147] found that dietary magnesium intake assessed by FFQ was associated with CHD risk after control for traditional CHD risk factors. When the data from these prospective cohorts were pooled (Figure 3), the random-effect pooled estimate of RR was 0.86 comparing the highest category of dietary magnesium intake with the lowest category of intake (95% CI: 0.67-1.10; P= 0.06 for between-study heterogeneity). Overall, the findings of cohort studies suggest that magnesium is unlikely to decrease substantially the risk of CHD, although a modest association cannot be ruled out. The efficacy of magnesium treatment on the secondary prevention of CVD, especially arrhythmias and mortality after acute MI, has received much attention in many small clinical trials [22].

The apparently conflicting trial results have led to extensive discussions on this issue in many systematic reviews [20, 22, 148], meta-analyses [149-152], and clinical commentaries [153-155]. In particular, three large secondary prevention trials in patients with MI have yielded inconsistent results. The first large randomized, double-blind, placebo-controlled study (The Second Leicester Intravenous Magnesium Intervention Trial, LIMIT2) showed that intravenous magnesium therapy before thrombolytic therapy caused a 24% relative reduction in mortality after 28 days following acute MI and a 25% lower incidence of left ventricular failure [156]. Subsequently, two large-scale randomized trials failed to support the efficacy of intravenous magnesium therapy for patients with acute MI [157, 158]. A critical examination of trial data with updated meta-analysis also raised serious doubts on the benefits of intravenous magnesium following MI [149]. Inconsistencies in the trial data may be due, in part, to differences in the time course of therapy and optimal dosage of magnesium for the prevention of CHD complications [153-155]. Thus, there is still considerable controversy about the true effect of magnesium therapy in the secondary prevention of CHD mortality or other complications.

Another area of controversy is the relationship between magnesium intake and the development and progression of stroke. Some animal studies [159-161], though not all [162], have suggested potential neuroprotective effects by magnesium supplementation in rodent stroke models. In addition to its cardiovascular effects, magnesium may also play a role in reducing cerebral ischemia, including inhibition of ischemia-induced glutamate release, N-methyl-D-aspartate receptor blockade, calcium entry via voltage gated channels antagonism, enhancement of mitochondrial calcium buffering, prevention of ATP depletion, and vasodilatation of cerebral blood vessels [163-165]. However, the relation between magnesium intake and stroke is less well studied in epidemiologic studies, especially large prospective studies. During 8 years of follow-up of the HPFS study with 328 strokes documented, dietary magnesium intake was inversely associated with risk of total stroke; the multivariate-adjusted RR was 0.70 (95% CI, 0.49-1.01) comparing the highest quintile of magnesium intake (median: 452 mg/day) with the lowest quintile (median: 243 mg/day). This inverse association was apparent among hypertensive men. Among 85,764 US women followed for 14 years, the Nurses' Health Study showed no significant associations between magnesium intake and total stroke and stroke subtype, although a modest effect of magnesium on ischemic stroke could not be excluded [166]. Both the WHS [147] and the Alpha-Tocopherol Beta-Carotene Lung Cancer Prevention Study (ATBC) [126] found that a high magnesium intake was associated with lower risk of ischemic stroke but not with hemorrhagic stroke. Because the number of incident cases of hemorrhagic stroke was small, each study individually was underpowered to address differential effects of magnesium intake on stroke subtypes. As shown in Figure 3, the pooled results appeared to be different for ischemic stroke (RR, 0.85; 95% CI, 0.76-0.95; P= 0.99 for between-study heterogeneity) and hemorrhagic stroke (RR, 0.98; 95% CI, 0.78-1.22; P= 0.65 for between-study heterogeneity) [126]. Different stroke subtypes have disparate pathophysiologies and may explain differential effects of magnesium intake on them. Overall, the evidence is still not convincing due to relatively limited data and further investigation in prospective studies with sufficient cases of incident stroke is warranted.

In addition, the efficacy of intravenous magnesium treatment in the secondary prevention of stroke has been suggested in some small pilot trials [165, 167] but was not confirmed in the IMAGES study (Intravenous Magnesium Efficacy in Stroke), an international, multicenter, double-blind, placebo-controlled trial [168]. Magnesium treatment given within 12 hours of stroke onset in 2589 patients failed to reduce mortality or disability at 90 days, although subgroup analyses suggested possible benefit in ischemic lacunar strokes [168]. Taken together, the evidence is not convincing and this area requires further investigation.

Colorectal Cancer

The possible beneficial effect of magnesium on patients with insulin resistance and type 2 diabetes have led to the hypothesis that magnesium deficiency contributes to the pathogenesis of colorectal cancer, which has been linked to insulin homeostasis. Magnesium may play an important role in regulating cell proliferation, differentiation, apoptosis, and angiogenesis [169]. Magnesium is also involved in maintaining genomic stability [170], inhibiting c-*myc* oncogene expression in the colon cancer cells [171], and potentially reducing toxic effects of bile acids on colonic epithelial cells [172]. Experimental data in animals have linked magnesium intake to colon cancer development. Magnesium supplementation in animals with experimentally induced colon cancer resulted in fewer colon tumors and smaller cryptal cells of the colon [65]. A recent population genetic study reported that magnesium intake was associated with a lower risk of colorectal adenoma in both men and women, suggesting that magnesium protects against colorectal carcinogenesis at an early stage [97].

Observational studies of the association between magnesium intake and colorectal cancer incidence are very sparse. Recently, the Swedish Mammary Screening Cohort Study (SMSC) and the Iowa Women's Health Study (IWHS) reported an inverse association between total magnesium intake and colon cancer risk [126, 173]. While the Swedish cohort study reported an inverse association with rectal cancer risk [126], the results from the IWHS suggested an inverse association with colon cancer. However, two recent large cohort studies did not replicate the observations. In the Women's Health Study, there was no significant association between magnesium intake and colorectal cancer incidence [174]. The Netherlands Cohort Study found no association, although the study observed statistically significant inverse trends in colorectal cancer across increasing quintiles of magnesium intake in overweight individuals [175].

When the data from these four prospective cohorts were pooled (Figure 4), the random-effect pooled estimate of RRs comparing the highest category of dietary magnesium intake with the lowest category of intake were 0.81 for total colorectal cancer (95% CI: 0.69-0.95; $P = 0.45$ for between-study heterogeneity), 0.81 (95% CI: 0.68-0.97; $P = 0.02$ for between-study heterogeneity) for colon cancer, and 0.84 (95% CI: 0.63-1.12; $P = 0.40$ for between-study heterogeneity) for rectal cancer. Overall, there is suggestive evidence for an inverse association between total magnesium intake and colon cancer incidence, although there was significant heterogeneity in the study results. Due to limited data, further investigation in large prospective cohort studies is warranted to elucidate the true role of magnesium in colorectal cancer development.

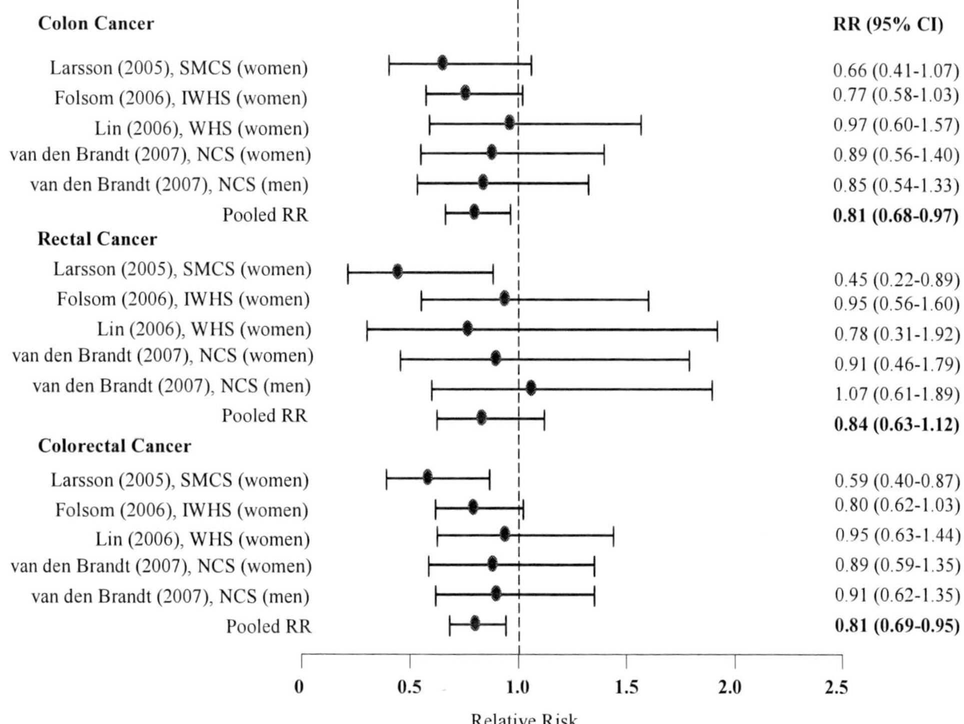

SMCS, Swedish Mammary Screening Cohort Study; IWHS, Iowa Women's Health Study; WHS, Women's Health Study; NCS, Netherlands Cohort Study.

Figure 4. A meta-analysis of prospective studies regarding the association between dietary magnesium intake and incidence of colorectal cancer.

Conclusion

In summary, biological and epidemiologic evidence suggest that magnesium may be an important nutrient required for human health. A large body of evidence has shown that high magnesium intake from diet or supplements may favorably affect a cluster of metabolic abnormalities including insulin resistance, hypertension, and dyslipidemia, known as metabolic syndrome. However, there are still many important questions in previous studies that require answers before we are able to obtain conclusive evidence.

First, errors in the dietary assessment, including potential dietary change over the course of follow-up and residual confounding by poorly measured or unmeasured variables and highly correlated nutrients, may have substantially limited the ability of large cohort studies to elucidate the causal effect of any single nutrient on disease risk.

While much uncertainty exists regarding the validity of epidemiologic studies, obviously, the best approach to confirm a cause-effect relation is to perform a double-blinded and placebo-controlled randomized trial. Nevertheless, conducting such a trial would be difficult for primary prevention of chronic diseases such as type 2 DM and CVD because of cost, logistical, and compliance issues. The evidence for the benefits of magnesium supplementation in the secondary prevention of chronic disease remains a matter of debate. It is obvious that future large well-conducted secondary prevention trials are warranted to unravel the efficacy and safety of magnesium supplements.

Few studies, especially intervention trials, have examined the relation between magnesium intake and these metabolic disorders that are not included in the metabolic syndrome definition such as oxidative stress, microalbuminuria [87], and impaired fibrinolysis [88]. It remains to be addressed whether or to what extent these abnormalities could be ameliorated by magnesium intake and contribute to the overall benefit of magnesium intake.

From a mechanistic perspective, there is compelling need for the development of a reliable method to measure total body magnesium store and levels of intracellular magnesium, or biologically active ionized or free magnesium. Extracellular magnesium levels are under tight homeostatic regulation in the human body. Thus, normal levels of serum magnesium are within a narrow range and do not correlate well with total magnesium status or with intracellular magnesium pool [103, 104]. However, serum magnesium concentrations are still the most commonly used metric to define magnesium deficiency in humans. More accurate, reliable, and affordable means to assess individual magnesium status in large population studies would provide more informative answers regarding magnesium intake and the risk of metabolic-related disorders.

The precise mechanisms underlying magnesium metabolism are far from clear. Recent genetic studies about links between a mitochondrial mutation, TRPM6 (an ion channel kinase of the "transient receptor potential" gene family) mutations, and hypomagnesemia have shed light on the underlying molecular basis for magnesium metabolism and helped identify genetic variants in modifying the metabolic effects of magnesium intake [176-178]. However, there are few population data available on common genetic susceptibility to magnesium deficiency in the general population. Recent studies have implicated the interaction of genetic variants in TRPM7 or TRPM6 with magnesium intake to affect disease risk. Future replication in large, well-defined, and population-based studies are warranted. In addition, the application of microarray technology in randomized-controlled setting will not only enable us to analyze the expression levels of thousands of genes simultaneously, but also afford us the opportunity to gain important insight into the molecular mechanism for complex biological systems of inflammation, insulin resistance, and metabolic abnormalities in response to magnesium supplementation.

In summary, available evidence suggests that higher intake of magnesium may contribute to a reduction in the risk of type 2 DM, hypertension, and CVD. In particular, the evidence for the beneficial effect of magnesium intake on risk of type 2 DM is relatively consistent and parallels the findings from metabolic studies showing the role of adequate magnesium status in improving insulin sensitivity. Until more definitive data are available, the collective evidence regarding the potential benefits of magnesium intake is consistent with prevailing dietary recommendations for primary prevention of type 2 DM, hypertension, and CVD by consuming foods rich in magnesium such as vegetables, whole grains, legumes, and nuts.

Refereces

[1] Cleveland LE, Goldman JD, Borrud LG. Data tables: Results from USDA's 1994 continuing survey of food intakes by individuals and 1994 diet and health knowledge survey. Beltsville, MD.: Agricultural Research Service, U.S. Department of Agriculture.; 1994.

[2] Groff JL, Gropper SS. Macrominerals. In: *Advanced Nutrition and Human metabolism*. California:Wadsworth, 2000, 371-400.

[3] Vaquero MP. Magnesium and trace elements in the elderly: intake, status and recommendations. *J. Nutr. Health Aging* 2002; 6:147-53.

[4] Pennington JAT, Young BE. Total Diet Study: nutritional elements. *J. Am. Diet. Assoc.* 1991; 91:179.

[5] Ford ES, Mokdad AH. Dietary magnesium intake in a national sample of US adults. *J Nutr.* 2003; 133:2879-82.

[6] Saris NE, Mervaala E, Karppanen H *et al.* Magnesium. An update on physiological, clinical and analytical aspects. *Clin. Chim. Acta* 2000; 294:1-26.

[7] Touyz RM. Magnesium in clinical medicine. *Front Biosci*. 2004; 9:1278-93.

[8] Innerarity S. Hypomagnesemia in acute and chronic illness. *Crit. Care Nurs.* Q 2000; 23:1-19; quiz 87.

[9] Gums JG. Magnesium in cardiovascular and other disorders. *Am. J. Health Syst. Pharm.* 2004; 61:1569-76.

[10] Barbagallo M, Dominguez LJ, Galioto A *et al.* Role of magnesium in insulin action, diabetes and cardio-metabolic syndrome X. *Mol. Aspects Med.* 2003; 24:39-52.

[11] Touyz RM. Role of magnesium in the pathogenesis of hypertension. *Mol. Aspects Med.* 2003; 24:107-136.

[12] Nadler JL, Buchanan T, Natarajan R *et al.* Magnesium deficiency produces insulin resistance and increased thromboxan synthesis. *Hypertension* 1993; 21:1024-1029.

[13] Paolisso G, Ravusin E. Intracellular magnesium and insulin resistance: results in Pima Indians and Caucasians. *J. Clin. Endocrinol. Metab.* 1995; 80:1382-1385.

[14] Paolisso G, Barbagallo M. Hypertension, diabetes mellitus, and insulin resistance: the role of intracellular magnesium. *Am. J. Hypertens* 1997; 10:346-355.

[15] Vitale JJ, Nakamura M, Hegsted DM. The effect of magnesium deficiency on oxidative phosphorylation. *J. Biol. Chem.* 1957; 228:573-6.

[16] Altura BT, Brust M, Bloom S *et al.* Magnesium dietary intake modulates blood lipid levels and atherogenesis. *Proc. Natl. Acad. Sci. USA* 1990; 87:1840-4.

[17] Davis WH, Leary WP, Reyes AJ, Olhaberry JV. mono-therapy with magnesium increases abnormally low high-density lipoprotein cholesterol: a clinical assay. *Curr. Ther. Res.* 1984; 36:341-346.

[18] Itoh K, Kawasaka T, Nakamura M. The effects of high oral magnesium supplementation on blood pressure, serum lipids and related variables in apparently healthy Japanese subjects. *Br. J. Nutr.* 1997; 78:737-50.

[19] Rasmussen HS, Aurup P, Goldstein K *et al.* Influence of magnesium substitution therapy on blood lipid composition in patients with ischemic heart disease. A double-blind, placebo controlled study. *Arch. Intern. Med.* 1989; 149:1050-3.

[20] Seelig MS, Heggtveit HA. Magnesium interrelationships in ischemic heart disease: a review. *Am. J. Clin. Nutr.* 1974; 27:59-79.

[21] Chakraborti S, Chakraborti T, Mandal M *et al.* Protective role of magnesium in cardiovascular diseases: a review. *Mol. Cell Biochem.* 2002; 238:163-179.

[22] Shechter M. Does magnesium have a role in the treatment of patients with coronary artery disease? *Am. J. Cardiovasc. Drugs* 2003; 3:231-9.

[23] Nadler JL, Malayan S, Luong H *et al.* Intracellular free magnesium deficiency plays a key role in increased platelet reactivity in type II diabetes mellitus. *Diabetes Care* 1992; 15:835-41.

[24] Paolisso G, Tirelli A, Coppola L *et al.* Magnesium administration reduces platelet hyperaggregability in NIDDM. *Diabetes Care* 1989; 12:167-8.

[25] Guerrero-Romero F, Rodriguez-Moran M. Relationship between serum magnesium levels and C-reactive protein concentration, in non-diabetic, non-hypertensive obese subjects. *Int. J. Obes. Relat. Metab. Disord.* 2002; 26:469-74.

[26] Song Y, Ford ES, Manson JE, Liu S. Relations of magnesium intake with metabolic risk factors and risks of type 2 diabetes, hypertension, and cardiovascular disease: A critical appraisal. *Current Nutrition and Food Science* 2005; 1:231-243.

[27] Wilson PW, Grundy SM. The metabolic syndrome: practical guide to origins and treatment: Part I. *Circulation* 2003; 108:1422-4.

[28] Wilson PW, Grundy SM. The metabolic syndrome: a practical guide to origins and treatment: Part II. *Circulation* 2003; 108:1537-40.

[29] Wilson PW, Kannel WB. Obesity, diabetes, and risk of cardiovascular disease in the elderly. *Am. J. Geriatr. Cardiol.* 2002; 11:119-23,125.

[30] Koh-Banerjee P, Franz M, Sampson L *et al.* Changes in whole-grain, bran, and cereal fiber consumption in relation to 8-y weight gain among men. *Am. J. Clin. Nutr.* 2004; 80:1237-45.

[31] Liu S, Willett WC, Manson JE *et al.* Relation between changes in intakes of dietary fiber and grain products and changes in weight and development of obesity among middle-aged women. *Am. J. Clin. Nutr.* 2003; 78:920-7.

[32] McKeown NM, Meigs JB, Liu S *et al.* Carbohydrate nutrition, insulin resistance, and the prevalence of the metabolic syndrome in the Framingham Offspring Cohort. *Diabetes Care* 2004; 27:538-46.

[33] Balon TW, Jasman AP, Scott S *et al.* Dietary magnesium prevents fructose-induced insulin insensitivity in rats. *Hypertension* 1994; 23:1036-1039.

[34] Kandeel FR, Balon E, Scott S, Nadler JL. Magnesium deficiency and glucose metabolism in rat adipocytes. *Metabolism* 1996; 45:838-843.

[35] Hall S, Keo L, Yu KT, Gould MK. Effect of ionophore A23187 on basal and insulin-stimulated sugar transport by rat soleus muscle. *Diabetes* 1982; 31:846-50.

[36] Suarez A, Pulido N, Casla A *et al.* Impaired tyrosine-kinase activity of muscle insulin receptors from hypomagnesaemic rats. *Diabetologia* 1995; 38:1262-1270.

[37] Giugliano D, Paolisso G, Ceriello A. Oxidative stress and diabetic vascular complications. *Diabetes Care* 1996; 19:257-267.

[38] Ma J, Folsom AR, Melnick SL *et al.* Associations of serum and dietary magnesium with cardiovascular disease, hypertension, diabetes, insulin, and carotid arterial wall thickness: the ARIC study. Atherosclerosis Risk in Communities Study. *J. Clin. Epidemiol* 1995; 48:927-940.

[39] Rosolova H, Mayer O, Reaven GM. Insulin-mediated glucose disposal is decreased in normal subjects with relatively low plasma magnesium concentrations. *Metabolism* 2000; 49:418-420.

[40] Humphries S, Kushner H, Falkner B. Low dietary magnesium is associated with insulin resistance in a sample of young, nondiabetic black Americans. American Journal of *Hypertension* 1999; 12:747-756.

[41] Fung TT, Manson JE, Solomon CG *et al.* The association between magnesium intake and fasting insulin concentration in healthy middle-aged women. *J. Am. Coll Nutr.* 2003; 22:533-8.

[42] Manolio TA, Savage PJ, Burke GL *et al.* Correlates of fasting insulin levels in young adults: the CARDIA study. *J. Clin. Epidemiol.* 1991; 44:571-8.

[43] Song Y, Manson JE, Buring JE, Liu S. Dietary magnesium intake in relation to plasma insulin levels and risk of type 2 diabetes in women. *Diabetes Care* 2004; 27:59-65.

[44] Rosolova H, Mayer O, Reaven G. Effect of variations in plasma magnesium concentration on resistance to insulin-mediated glucose disposal in nondiabetic subjects. *J. Clin. Endocrinol. Metab.* 1997; 82:3783-3785.

[45] Guerrero-Romero F, Tamez-Perez HE, Gonzalez-Gonzalez G *et al.* Oral magnesium supplementation improves insulin sensitivity in non-diabetic subjects with insulin resistance. A double-blind placebo-controlled randomized trial. *Diabetes Metab* 2004; 30:253-8.

[46] Paolisso G, Sgambato S, Gambardella A *et al.* Daily magnesium supplements improve glucose handling in elderly subjects. *Am. J. Clin. Nutr.* 1992; 55:1161-7.

[47] Malkiel-Shapiro B, Bersohn I, Terner PE. Parenteral magnesium sulphate therapy in coronary heart disease. A preliminary report on its clinical and laboratory aspects. *Med. Proc.* 1956; 2:455-462.

[48] Rayssiguier Y. Role of magnesium and potassium in the pathogenesis of arteriosclerosis. *Magnesium* 1984; 3:226-38.

[49] Rayssiguier Y, Gueux E, Weiser D. Effect of magnesium deficiency on lipid metabolism in rats fed a high carbohydrate diet. *J. Nutr.* 1981; 111:1876-83.

[50] Vitale JJ, White PL, Nakamura M *et al.* Interrelationships between experimental hypercholesteremia, magnesium requirement, and experimental atherosclerosis. *J. Exp. Med.* 1957; 106:757-66.

[51] Rayssiguier Y, Noe L, Etienne J *et al.* Effect of magnesium deficiency on post-heparin lipase activity and tissue lipoprotein lipase in the rat. *Lipids* 1991; 26:182-6.

[52] Guerrero-Romero F, Rodriguez-Moran M. Low serum magnesium levels and metabolic syndrome. *Acta Diabetol.* 2002; 39:209-13.

[53] Haywood J, Sylvester R. Effect of oral magnesium and potassium on serum lipids. *Clin Med.* 1962; 10:67.

[54] Kirsten R, Heintz B, Nelson K *et al.* Magnesium pyridoxal 5-phosphate glutamate reduces hyperlipidaemia in patients with chronic renal insufficiency. *Eur. J. Clin. Pharmacol*. 1988; 34:133-7.

[55] Marken PA, Weart CW, Carson DS *et al.* Effects of magnesium oxide on the lipid profile of healthy volunteers. *Atherosclerosis* 1989; 77:37-42.

[56] Eriksson J, Kohvakka A. Magnesium and ascorbic acid supplementation in diabetes mellitus. *Ann. Nutr. Metab*. 1995; 39:217-23.

[57] Eibl NL, Kopp HP, Nowak HR *et al.* Hypomagnesemia in type II diabetes: effect of a 3-month replacement therapy. *Diabetes Care* 1995; 18:188-192.

[58] Gilleran G, O'Leary M, Bartlett WA *et al.* Effects of dietary sodium substitution with potassium and magnesium in hypertensive type II diabetics: a randomised blind controlled parallel study. *J. Hum. Hypertens* 1996; 10:517-21.

[59] Rodriguez-Moran M, Guerrero-Romero F. Oral magnesium supplementation improves insulin sensitivity and metabolic control in type 2 diabetic subjects: a randomized double-blind controlled trial. *Diabetes Care* 2003; 26:1147-52.

[60] de Valk HW, Verkaaik R, van Rijn HJ *et al.* Oral magnesium supplementation in insulin-requiring type 2 diabetic patients. *Diabetes Med.* 1998; 15:503-507.

[61] Purvis JR, Cummings DM, Landsman P *et al.* Effect of oral magnesium supplementation on selected cardiovascular risk factors in non-insulin-dependent diabetics. *Arch. Fam. Med*. 1994; 3:503-8.

[62] Yokota K, Kato M, Lister F *et al.* Clinical efficacy of magnesium supplementation in patients with type 2 diabetes. *J. Am. Coll. Nutr*. 2004; 23:506S-509S.

[63] Djurhuus MS, Klitgaard NA, Pedersen KK *et al.* Magnesium reduces insulin-stimulated glucose uptake and serum lipid concentrations in type 1 diabetes. *Metabolism* 2001; 50:1409-17.

[64] Hagg E, Carlberg BC, Hillorn VS, Villumsen J. Magnesium therapy in type 1 diabetes. A double blind study concerning the effects on kidney function and serum lipid levels. *Magnes. Res.* 1999; 12:123-30.

[65] Yamori Y, Mizushima S. A reiview of the link between dietary magnesium and cardiovascular risk. *J. Cardiovascular Risk* 2000; 7:31-35.

[66] Dawson EB, Frey MJ, Moore TD, McGanity WJ. Relationship of metal metabolism to vascular disease mortality rates in Texas. *Am. J. Clin. Nutr*. 1978; 31:1188-1197.

[67] Stitt FW, Clayton DG, Crawford MD, Morris JN. Clinical and biochemical indicators of cardiovascular disease among men living in hard and soft water areas. *Lancet* 1973; 1:122-126.

[68] Schwartz S. The fallacy of the ecological fallacy: the potential misuse of a concept and the consequences. *Am. J. Public Health* 1994; 84:819-824.

[69] Rubenowitz E, Axelsson G, Rylander R. Magnesium in drinking water and death from acute myocardial infarction. *Am. J. Epidemiol*. 1996; 143:456-462.

[70] Mizushima S, Cappuccio FP, Nichols R, Elliott P. Dietary magnesium intake and blood pressure: a qualitative overview of the observational studies. *J. Hum. Hypertens* 1998; 12:447-453.

[71] Whelton P, Klag M. Magnesium and blood pressure: review of the epidemiological and clinical trial experience. *Am. J. Cardiol.* 1989; 63:26-30.

[72] Kesteloot H, Joossens JV. Relationship of dietary sodium, potassium, calcium, and magnesium with blood pressure. Belgian Interuniversity Research on Nutrition and Health. *Hypertension* 1988; 12:594-9.

[73] Simon JA, Obarzanek E, Daniels SR, Frederick MM. Dietary cation intake and blood pressure in black girls and white girls. *Am. J. Epidemiol.* 1994; 139:130-40.

[74] Ford ES. Race, education, and dietary cations: findings from the Third National Health And Nutrition Examination Survey. *Ethn. Dis.* 1998; 8:10-20.

[75] Witteman JC, Willett WC, Stampfer MJ *et al.* A prospective study of nutritional factors and hypertension among US women. *Circulation* 1989; 80:1320-1327.

[76] Ascherio A, Rimm EB, Giovannucci EL *et al.* A prospective study of nutritional factors and hypertension among US men. *Circulation* 1992; 86:1475-1484.

[77] Peacock JM, Folsom AR, Arnett DK *et al.* Relationship of serum and dietary magnesium to incident hypertension: the Atherosclerosis Risk in Communities (ARIC) Study. *Ann. Epidemiol.* 1999; 9:159-165.

[78] Song Y, Sesso HD, Manson JE *et al.* Dietary magnesium intake and risk of incident hypertension among middle-aged and older US women in a 10-year follow-up study. *Am. J. Cardiol.* 2006; 98:1616-1621.

[79] Ascherio A, Hennekens C, Willett WC *et al.* Prospective study of nutritional factors, blood pressure, and hypertension among US women. *Hypertension* 1996; 27:1065-1072.

[80] He K, Liu K, Daviglus ML *et al.* Magnesium intake and incidence of metabolic syndrome among young adults. *Circulation* 2006; 113:1675-82.

[81] DerSimonian R, Laird NM. Meta-analysis in clinical trials. *Control. Clin. Trials* 1986; 7:177-188.

[82] Petitti DB. *Meta-analysis, decision analysis, and cost-effectiveness analysis.* NewYork: Oxford University Press, Inc; 2000.

[83] Jee SH, Miller ER, 3rd, Guallar E *et al.* The effect of magnesium supplementation on blood pressure: a meta-analysis of randomized clinical trials. *Am. J. Hypertens* 2002; 15:691-696.

[84] Song Y, Liu S, Manson JE. High-sensitivity C-reactive protein and the metabolic syndrome. In: *The Metabolic Syndrome: Epidemiology, Clinical Treatment, and Underlying Mechanisms*. Hansen BC, Bray GA (Editors). Totowa, New Jersey: Humana Press; 2008. pp. 167-188.

[85] Bautista LE. Inflammation, endothelial dysfunction, and the risk of high blood pressure: epidemiologic and biological evidence. *J. Hum. Hypertens* 2003; 17:223-30.

[86] Pinkney JH, Stehouwer CD, Coppack SW, Yudkin JS. Endothelial dysfunction: cause of the insulin resistance syndrome. *Diabetes* 1997; 46 Suppl 2:S9-13.

[87] De Bakker PI, Graham RR, Altshuler D *et al.* Transferability of tag SNPs to capture common genetic variation in DNA repair genes across multiple populations. *Pac. Symp. Bio.comput*. 2006:478-86.

[88] Lipid, lipoproteins, C-reactive protein, and hemostatic factors at baseline in the diabetes prevention program. *Diabetes Care* 2005; 28:2472-9.

[89] Tam M, Gomez S, Gonzalez-Gross M, Marcos A. Possible roles of magnesium on the immune system. *Eur. J. Clin. Nutr*. 2003; 57:1193-7.

[90] King DE, Mainous AG, 3rd, Geesey ME, Woolson RF. Dietary magnesium and C-reactive protein levels. *J. Am. Coll. Nutr*. 2005; 24:166-71.

[91] Dandona P, Aljada A, Chaudhuri A *et al.* Metabolic syndrome: a comprehensive perspective based on interactions between obesity, diabetes, and inflammation. *Circulation* 2005; 111:1448-54.

[92] Schram MT, Stehouwer CD. Endothelial dysfunction, cellular adhesion molecules and the metabolic syndrome. *Horm. Metab Res*. 2005; 37 Suppl 1:49-55.

[93] Shechter M, Sharir M, Labrador MJ *et al.* Oral magnesium therapy improves endothelial function in patients with coronary artery disease. *Circulation* 2000; 102:2353-8.

[94] Pearson PJ, Evora PR, Seccombe JF, Schaff HV. Hypomagnesemia inhibits nitric oxide release from coronary endothelium: protective role of magnesium infusion after cardiac operations. *Ann. Thorac. Surg*. 1998; 65:967-72.

[95] Dickens BF, Weglicki WB, Li YS, Mak IT. Magnesium deficiency in vitro enhances free radical-induced intracellular oxidation and cytotoxicity in endothelial cells. *FEBS Lett.* 1992; 311:187-91.

[96] Price DT, Loscalzo J. Cellular adhesion molecules and atherogenesis. *Am. J. Med.* 1999; 107:85-97.

[97] Almoznino-Sarafian D, Berman S, Mor A *et al.* Magnesium and C-reactive protein in heart failure: an anti-inflammatory effect of magnesium administration? *Eur. J. Nutr.* 2007; 46:230-7.

[98] Executive Summary of The Third Report of The National Cholesterol Education Program (NCEP) Expert Panel on Detection, Evaluation, And Treatment of High Blood Cholesterol In Adults (Adult Treatment Panel III). *Jama* 2001; 285:2486-97.

[99] Alberti KG, Zimmet PZ. Definition, diagnosis and classification of diabetes mellitus and its complications. Part 1: diagnosis and classification of diabetes mellitus provisional report of a WHO consultation. *Diabet Med*. 1998; 15:539-53.

[100] Balkau B, Charles MA. Comment on the provisional report from the WHO consultation. European Group for the Study of Insulin Resistance (EGIR). *Diabet Med*. 1999; 16:442-3.

[101] Einhorn D, Reaven GM, Cobin RH *et al.* American College of Endocrinology position statement on the insulin resistance syndrome. *Endocr. Pract*. 2003; 9:237-52.

[102] Alberti KG, Zimmet P, Shaw J. The metabolic syndrome--a new worldwide definition. *Lancet* 2005; 366:1059-62.

[103] Reinhart RA. Magnesium metabolism. A review with special reference to the relationship between intracellular content and serum levels. *Arch. Intern. Med.* 1988; 148:2415-20.

[104] Liao F, Folsom AR, Brancati FL. Is low magnesium concentration a risk factor for coronary heart disease? The Atherosclerosis Risk in Communities (ARIC) Study. *Am. Heart J.* 1998; 136:480-90.

[105] Ford ES, Li C, McGuire LC *et al.* Intake of dietary magnesium and the prevalence of the metabolic syndrome among U.S. adults. *Obesity* (Silver Spring) 2007; 15:1139-46.

[106] Alzaid AA, Dinneen SF, Moyer TP, Rizza RA. Effects of insulin on plasma magnesium in noninsulin-dependent diabetes mellitus: evidence for insulin resistance. *J. Clin. Endocrinol. Metab.* 1995; 80:1376-1381.

[107] Levin G, Mather H, Pilkington TRE. Tissue magnesium status in diabetes mellitus. *Diabetologia* 1981; 21:131-134.

[108] Mather H, Nisbet JA, Burton GH *et al.* Hypomagnesemia in diabetes. *Clin. Chim. Acta* 1979; 95:235-242.

[109] McNair P, Christensen M, Christiansen C *et al.* Renal hypomagnesemia in human diabetes mellitus: its relation to glucose homeostasis. *Eur. J. Clin. Invest* 1982; 12:81-85.

[110] Paolisso G, Scheen A, D'Onofrio F, Lefebvre P. Magnesium and glucose homeostasis. *Diabetologia* 1990; 33:511-4.

[111] Resnick L, Altura BT, Gupta R *et al.* Intracellular and extracellular magnesium depletion in type 2 diabetes mellitus. *Diabetologia* 1993; 36:767-770.

[112] Yajnik CS, Smith RF, Hockaday TD, Ward NI. Fasting plasma magnesium concentrations and glucose disposal in diabetes. *Br. Med. J. (Clin. Res. Ed)* 1984; 288:1032-4.

[113] Sjogren A, Floren CH, Nilsson A. Magnesium, potassium and zinc deficiency in subjects with type II diabetes mellitus. *Acta Med. Scand.* 1988; 224:461-6.

[114] Djurhuus MS, Skott P, Hother-Nielson O *et al.* Insulin increases renal magnesium excretion: a possible cause of magnesium depletion in hyperinsulinaemic states. *Diabet Med.* 1995; 12:664-9.

[115] McNair P, Christensen MS, Christiansen C *et al.* Renal hypomagnesaemia in human diabetes mellitus: its relation to glucose homeostasis. *Eur. J. Clin. Invest* 1982; 12:81-5.

[116] Schmidt LE, Arfken CL, Heins JM. Evaluation of nutrient intake in subjects with non-insulin-dependent diabetes mellitus. *J. Am. Diet Assoc.* 1994; 94:773-4.

[117] Colditz GA, Manson JE, Stampfer MJ *et al.* Diet and risk of clinical diabetes in women. *Am. J. Clin. Nutr.* 1992; 55:1018-1023.

[118] Salmeron J, Manson JE, Stampfer MJ *et al.* Dietary fiber, glycemic load, and risk of non-insulin-dependent diabetes mellitus in women. *JAMA* 1997; 277:472-7.

[119] Meyer KA, Kushi LH, Jacobs DR, Jr. *et al.* Carbohydrates, dietary fiber, and incident type 2 diabetes in older women. *Am. J. Clin. Nutr.* 2000; 71:921-30.

[120] Salmeron J, Ascherio A, Rimm EB *et al.* Dietary fiber, glycemic load, and risk of NIDDM in men. *Diabetes Care* 1997; 20:545-50.

[121] Schulze MB, Schulz M, Heidemann C *et al.* Fiber and magnesium intake and incidence of type 2 diabetes: a prospective study and meta-analysis. *Arch. Intern. Med.* 2007; 167:956-65.

[122] van Dam RM, Hu FB, Rosenberg L *et al.* Dietary calcium and magnesium, major food sources, and risk of type 2 diabetes in U.S. black women. *Diabetes Care* 2006; 29:2238-43.

[123] Kao WH, Folsom AR, Nieto FJ *et al.* Serum and dietary magnesium and the risk for type 2 diabetes mellitus: the Atherosclerosis Risk in Communities Study. *Arch. Intern. Med.* 1999; 159:2151-2159.

[124] Djurhuus MS, Gram J, Petersen PH *et al.* Biological variation of serum and urinary magnesium in apparently healthy males. *Scand. J. Clin. Lab. Invest.* 1995; 55:549-58.

[125] Elin RJ. Assessment of magnesium status. *Clin. Chem.* 1987; 33:1965-70.

[126] Larsson SC, Bergkvist L, Wolk A. Magnesium intake in relation to risk of colorectal cancer in women. *JAMA* 2005; 293:86-9.

[127] Gullestad L, Jacobsen T, Dolva LO. Effect of magnesium treatment on glycemic control and metabolic parameters in NIDDM patients. *Diabetes Care* 1994; 17:460-1.

[128] Karppanen H, Tanskanen A, Tuomilehto J *et al.* Safety and effects of potassium- and magnesium-containing low sodium salt mixtures. *J. Cardiovasc. Pharmacol.* 1984; 6 Suppl 1:S236-43.

[129] Sjogren A, Floren CH, Nilsson A. Oral administration of magnesium hydroxide to subjects with insulin-dependent diabetes mellitus: effects on magnesium and potassium levels and on insulin requirements. *Magnesium* 1988; 7:117-22.

[130] de Lourdes Lima M, Cruz T, Carreiro Pousada J *et al.* The effect of magnesium supplementation in increasing doses on the control of type 2 diabetes. *Diabetes Care* 1998; 21:682-686.

[131] Paolisso G, Sgambato S, Pizza G *et al.* Improved insulin response and action by chronic magnesium administration in aged NIDDM subjects. *Diabetes Care* 1989; 12:265-9.

[132] Paolisso G, Scheen A, Cozzolino D *et al.* Changes in glucose turnover parameters and improvement of glucose oxidation after 4-week magnesium administration in elderly noninsulin-dependent (type II) diabetic patients. *J. Clin. Endocrinol. Metab.* 1994; 78:1510-4.

[133] Orimo H, Ouchi Y. The role of calcium and magnesium in the development of atherosclerosis. Experimental and clinical evidence. *Ann. NY Acad. Sci.* 1990; 598:444-57.

[134] Iseri LT, Alexander LC, Mc CR *et al.* Water and electrolyte content of cardiac and skeletal muscle in heart failure and myocardial infarction. *Am. Heart J.* 1952; 43:215-27.

[135] Chipperfield B, Chipperfield JR. Heart-muscle magnesium, potassium, and zinc concentrations after sudden death from heart-disease. *Lancet* 1973; 2:293-6.

[136] Johnson CJ, Peterson DR, Smith EK. Myocardial tissue concentrations of magnesium and potassium in men dying suddenly from ischemic heart disease. *Am. J. Clin. Nutr.* 1979; 32:967-70.

[137] Elwood PC, Sweetnam PM, Beasley WH *et al.* Magnesium and calcium in the myocardium: cause of death and area differences. *Lancet* 1980; 2:720-2.

[138] Kobayashi J. On geographical relationship between chemical nature of drinking water and death rate from apoplexy. *Berichte Ohara Inst Landwirtschaftliche Biol.* 1957; 11:12-21.

[139] Schroeder HA. Relations between hardness of water and death rates from certain chronic and degenerative diseases in the United States. *J. Chronic. Dis*. 1960; 12:586-91.

[140] Folsom AR, Prineas RJ. Drinking water composition and blood pressure: a review of the epidemiology. *Am. J. Epidemiol.* 1982; 115:818-32.

[141] Sauvant MP, Pepin D. Drinking water and cardiovascular disease. *Food Chem. Toxicol.* 2002; 40:1311-25.

[142] Tsuji H, Venditti FJ, Jr., Evans JC *et al.* The associations of levels of serum potassium and magnesium with ventricular premature complexes (the Framingham Heart Study). *Am. J. Cardiol.* 1994; 74:232-5.

[143] Ford ES. Serum magnesium and ischaemic heart disease: findings from a national sample of US adults. *Int. J. Epidemiol.* 1999; 28:645-51.

[144] Abbott RD, Ando F, Masaki KH *et al.* Dietary magnesium intake and the future risk of coronary heart disease (the Honolulu Heart Program). *Am. J. Cardiol.* 2003; 92:665-9.

[145] Al-Delaimy WK, Rimm EB, Willett WC *et al.* Magnesium intake and risk of coronary heart disease among men. *J. Am. Coll Nutr.* 2004; 23:63-70.

[146] Elwood PC, Fehily AM, Ising H *et al.* Dietary magnesium does not predict ischaemic heart disease in the Caerphilly cohort. *Eur. J. Clin. Nutr.* 1996; 50:694-7.

[147] Song Y, Manson JE, Cook NR *et al.* Dietary magnesium intake and risk of cardiovascular disease among women. *Am. J. Cardiol.* 2005; 96:1135-1141.

[148] Antman EM. Magnesium in acute myocardial infarction: overview of available evidence. *Am. Heart J.* 1996; 132:487-95; discussion 496-502.

[149] Higgins JP, Spiegelhalter DJ. Being sceptical about meta-analyses: a Bayesian perspective on magnesium trials in myocardial infarction. *Int. J. Epidemiol.* 2002; 31:96-104.

[150] Pogue J, Yusuf S. Overcoming the limitations of current meta-analysis of randomised controlled trials. *Lancet* 1998; 351:47-52.

[151] Teo KK, Yusuf S, Collins R *et al.* Effects of intravenous magnesium in suspected acute myocardial infarction: overview of randomised trials. *BMJ* 1991; 303:1499-503.

[152] Yusuf S. Meta-analysis of randomized trials: looking back and looking ahead. *Control Clin. Trials* 1997; 18:594-601; discussion 661 6.

[153] Antman EM. Magnesium in acute MI. Timing is critical. *Circulation* 1995; 92:2367-72.

[154] Borzak S, Ridker PM. Discordance between meta-analyses and large-scale randomized, controlled trials. Examples from the management of acute myocardial infarction. *Ann. Intern. Med.* 1995; 123:873-7.

[155] Seelig MS, Elin RJ, Antman EM. Magnesium in acute myocardial infarction: still an open question. *Can. J. Cardiol.* 1998; 14:745-9.

[156] Woods KL, Fletcher S, Roffe C, Haider Y. Intravenous magnesium sulphate in suspected acute myocardial infarction: results of the second Leicester Intravenous Magnesium Intervention Trial (LIMIT-2). *Lancet* 1992; 339:1553-8.

[157] Early administration of intravenous magnesium to high-risk patients with acute myocardial infarction in the Magnesium in Coronaries (MAGIC) Trial: a randomised controlled trial. *Lancet* 2002; 360:1189-96.

[158] ISIS-4: a randomised factorial trial assessing early oral captopril, oral mononitrate, and intravenous magnesium sulphate in 58,050 patients with suspected acute myocardial infarction. ISIS-4 (Fourth International Study of Infarct Survival) Collaborative Group. *Lancet* 1995; 345:669-85.

[159] Izumi Y, Roussel S, Pinard E, Seylaz J. Reduction of infarct volume by magnesium after middle cerebral artery occlusion in rats. *J. Cereb. Blood Flow Metab.* 1991; 11:1025-30.

[160] Marinov MB, Harbaugh KS, Hoopes PJ *et al.* Neuroprotective effects of preischemia intraarterial magnesium sulfate in reversible focal cerebral ischemia. *J. Neurosurg.* 1996; 85:117-24.

[161] Yang Y, Li Q, Ahmad F, Shuaib A. Survival and histological evaluation of therapeutic window of post-ischemia treatment with magnesium sulfate in embolic stroke model of rat. *Neurosci. Lett.* 2000; 285:119-22.

[162] Zhu HD, Martin R, Meloni B *et al.* Magnesium sulfate fails to reduce infarct volume following transient focal cerebral ischemia in rats. *Neurosci. Res.* 2004; 49:347-53.

[163] Lin JY, Chung SY, Lin MC, Cheng FC. Effects of magnesium sulfate on energy metabolites and glutamate in the cortex during focal cerebral ischemia and reperfusion in the gerbil monitored by a dual-probe microdialysis technique. *Life Sci.* 2002; 71:803-11.

[164] Nowak L, Bregestovski P, Ascher P *et al.* Magnesium gates glutamate-activated channels in mouse central neurones. *Nature* 1984; 307:462-5.

[165] Muir KW. Magnesium in stroke treatment. *Postgrad. Med. J.* 2002; 78:641-5.

[166] Iso H, Stampfer MJ, Manson JE *et al.* Prospective study of calcium, potassium, and magnesium intake and risk of stroke in women. *Stroke* 1999; 30:1772-9.

[167] Saver JL, Kidwell C, Eckstein M, Starkman S. Prehospital neuroprotective therapy for acute stroke: results of the Field Administration of Stroke Therapy-Magnesium (FAST-MAG) pilot trial. *Stroke* 2004; 35:e106-8.

[168] Muir KW, Lees KR, Ford I, Davis S. Magnesium for acute stroke (Intravenous Magnesium Efficacy in Stroke trial): randomised controlled trial. *Lancet* 2004; 363:439-45.

[169] Maier JA, Nasulewicz-Goldeman A, Simonacci M *et al.* Insights into the mechanisms involved in magnesium-dependent inhibition of primary tumor growth. *Nutr. Cancer* 2007; 59:192-8.

[170] Hartwig A. Role of magnesium in genomic stability. *Mutat. Res.* 2001; 475:113-21.

[171] Hwang DL, Yen CF, Nadler JL. Insulin increases intracellular magnesium transport in human platelets. *J. Clin. Endocrinol. Metab.* 1993; 76:549-553.

[172] Wang A, Yoshimi N, Tanaka T, Mori H. The inhibitory effect of magnesium hydroxide on the bile acid-induced cell proliferation of colon epithelium in rats with comparison to the action of calcium lactate. *Carcinogenesis* 1994; 15:2661-3.

[173] Folsom AR, Hong CP. Magnesium intake and reduced risk of colon cancer in a prospective study of women. *Am. J. Epidemiol.* 2006; 163:232-5.

[174] Lin J, Cook NR, Lee IM *et al.* Total magnesium intake and colorectal cancer incidence in women. *Cancer Epidemiol. Biomarkers Prev.* 2006; 15:2006-9.

[175] van den Brandt PA, Smits KM, Goldbohm RA, Weijenberg MP. Magnesium intake and colorectal cancer risk in the Netherlands Cohort Study. *Br. J. Cancer* 2007; 96:510-3.

[176] Schlingmann KP, Weber S, Peters M *et al.* Hypomagnesemia with secondary hypocalcemia is caused by mutations in TRPM6, a new member of the TRPM gene family. *Nat. Genet* 2002; 31:166-70.

[177] Walder RY, Landau D, Meyer P *et al.* Mutation of TRPM6 causes familial hypomagnesemia with secondary hypocalcemia. *Nat. Genet* 2002; 31:171-4.

[178] Wilson FH, Hariri A, Farhi A *et al.* A cluster of metabolic defects caused by mutation in a mitochondrial tRNA. *Science* 2004; 306:1190-4.

In: Dietary Magnezium: New Research
Editor: Andrew W. Yardley
ISBN 978-1-60692-109-8

Chapter II

Chronopathological Forms of Asthma due to Magnesium Depletion with Hypo- or Hyper-Function of the Biological Clock: Therapeutic Implications

***Jean Durlach*[*1], *Nicole Pagès*[2], *Pierre Bac*[3], *Michel Bara*[4] *and Andrée Guiet-Bara*[4]**

[1]SDRM, Université Pierre et Marie Curie, 75252 Paris Cédex 05, France
[2]Laboratoire de Toxicologie, Faculté de Pharmacie, Strasbourg, 67400 Illkirch-Graffenstaden, France
[3]Laboratoire de Pharmacologie, Faculté de Pharmacie, Paris XI, 92290 Chatenay-Malabry, France
[4]Laboratoire de Physiologie et de Pathologie, UPMC, 75252 Paris Cédex 05, France

Abstract

Asthma is a chronic, inflammatory disorder of the airways leading to airflow limitation. Its worldwide rise, mainly in developed countries, is a matter of worldwide concern. Inflammation of the bronchial mucosa and bronchial hyperresponsiveness are the hallmark features of asthma of all severities. Nocturnal asthma (NA) frequently occurs and would concern two thirds of asthmatics. But, it remains controversial whether NA is a distinct entity or is a manifestation of more severe asthma. Generally, it is considered as an exacerbation of the underlying pathology. The pathological mechanisms likely involve endogenous circadian rhythms with pathological consequences on both

* Address for correspondence: Dr. Jean Durlach, Président de la SDRM, Rédacteur en Chef de *Magnesium Research*, 64 Rue de Longchamp, 92200 Neuilly-sur-Seine, France. Tel. +33 1 40 88 38 69; Fax: +33 1 40 88 36 13; e-mail: jean.durlach@wanadoo.fr or Dr. N.PAGES, 12 Rue R. Thomas. 91400 Saclay, France. e-mail: nicole.pages4@wanadoo.fr

respiratory inflammation and hyperresponsiveness. A decrease in blood and tissue magnesium levels is frequently reported in asthma and often testifies to a true magnesium depletion.

The link with magnesium status and chronobiology are well established. The quality of magnesium status influences directly the Biological Clock (BC) function, represented by the suprachiasmatic nuclei. Reversely, BC dysrythmias influence the magnesium status. Two types of magnesium deficits must be clearly distinguished: deficiency corresponding to an insufficient intake which can be corrected through mere nutritional Mg supplementation and depletion due to a dysregulation of the magnesium status which cannot be corrected through nutritional supplementation only, but requests the more or less specific correction of the dysregulation mechanisms. Both in clinical and in animal experiments, the dysregulation mechanisms of magnesium depletion associate a reduced magnesium intake with various types of stress including biological clock dysrythmias. The differentiation between Mg depletion forms with hyperfunction of BC (HBC) and forms with hypofunction of BC (hBC) is seminal and the main biological marker is melatonin (MT) production. We hypothesize that, magnesium depletion with HBC or hBC may be involved in chronopathological forms of asthma. Nocturnal asthma would be linked to HBC, represented by an increase in MT levels. The corresponding clinical forms associate diverse expressions of nervous hypoexcitability: depression, nocturnal cephalalgia (*i.e.* cluster headaches), dyssomnia mainly advanced sleep phase syndrome, some clinical forms of chronic fatigue syndrome and fibromyalgia. The main comorbidities are depression and/or asthenia. They take place during the night or the "bad" seasons (autumn and winter) when the sunshine is minimum. The corresponding chronopathological therapy relies on phototherapies with sometimes additional psychoanaleptics. Conversely, asthma forms linked to hBC are less frequently studied and present a decrease in MT levels. They associate various signs of nervous hyperexcitability: anxiety, diurnal cephalalgia (mainly migraine), dyssomnia, mainly delayed sleep phase syndrome and some clinical forms of chronic fatigue syndrome and fibromyalgia. The treatment relies on diverse forms of "darkness therapy", possibly with the help of some psycholeptics. Finally, the treatment of asthma involves the maintenance of conventional dosing schedule of anti-asthma drugs, a balanced magnesium intake and the appropriate treatment of the chronopathological disorders.

Key words: asthma, magnesium deficiency, magnesium depletion, hyperfunction of the biological clock (HBC), hypofunction of the biological clock (hBC), melatonin, phototherapy, darkness therapy

Main Abbreviations

NA = nocturnal asthma
NNA = non nocturnal asthma
COPD = Chronic obstructive pulmonary disease
FEV_1 = forced expiratory volume in one second
PEF = Peak expiratory flow
BC = biological clock
SCN = suprachiasmatic nuclei
MT = melatonin

HBC = hyperfunction of the biological clock
NhE = neural hypo excitability
hBC = hypofunction of the biological clock
NHE = nervous hyperexcitability

Introduction

Asthma is an important health priority worldwide because of its high and increasing prevalence, its high morbidity and mortality despite effective treatment and innovative research developments and its direct or indirect costs [166, 336]. It affects approximately 5-12% of the population and is a frequent cause of emergency hospital admission [34, 135]. It is the most common inflammatory chronic disease in childhood [48, 155, 166, 258, 268, 302]. A number of distinct mechanisms underlie the development of this disorder [54]. The National Heart, Lung and Blood Institute has stratified asthma severity and distinguished between mild intermittent asthma and three categories of persistent asthma, mild, moderate and severe, including in this characterization the frequency of nocturnal awakenings [318]. While many asthma attacks are relatively mild and can be treated and controlled at home, some are more severe and may even require hospitalization.

The striking increase in prevalence and severity of asthma over recent decades in affluent societies and the rarity of this disease in less affluent populations confirms the importance of environmental factors in the cause of asthma, although which environmental factors are responsible is still not clear [86, 226]. Accumulating evidence points towards an important role of diet, obesity and gastrooesophageal reflux in determining the expression of the disease [17, 18, 155, 360]. Family studies show that genetic factors are also important in determining individual susceptibility to asthma [86, 340]. Finally, the role of psychological factors in the development and exacerbation of asthma, as well as in the precipitation and provocation of asthma attacks, is known [206, 366].

Asthma is a clinical syndrome consisting of chronic airway inflammation, airway hyperresponsiveness, and expiratory airflow limitation with recurring episodes of wheezing, dyspnea, tightness in the chest, and cough that reverses after bronchodilator treatment [318, 332]. The prognosis for asthma depends on the levels of obstruction and bronchial hyperresponsiveness [41, 302].

It has long been recognized that asthma presents a diurnal rhythm in the occurrence and severity of symptoms with nocturnal worsening between 4 AM and 8 AM [67, 224]. Up to 74% of asthmatics awaken at night at least once a week due to wheezing, chest tightness or cough [350]. This nocturnal aggravation appears to be related to an exaggerated response to a circadian rhythm in lung function observed in healthy individuals [67]. It is generally admitted that it would result from both several circadian rhythms and fading effect of medication administered at bedtime [30]. Nocturnal asthma (NA) indicate severe asthma and asthma deaths generally occurs between midnight and 8 AM [39]. However, it remains controversial whether NA is a distinct entity or is a manifestation of more severe asthma [53].

We showed recently that different manifestations linked to chronopathological forms of magnesium depletion were regularly observed in various, rather common pathologies including migraine, sudden infant death, multiple sclerosis or affective disorders [95, 96, 98, 99, 100, 102] that greatly improved from treatments based upon these chronobiological data [94]. For instance, photic cephalalgia (mainly migraine) often related to magnesium depletion with hypofunction of the BC may greatly improved after treatment correcting both magnesium imbalance and the chronobiological disorder by darkness therapies in addition to conventional treatments. At the opposite, seasonal affective disorder (SAD) or winter depression may be related to magnesium depletion with hyperfunction of the BC. Its treatment relies on correcting both magnesium imbalance and chronobiological disorder by light therapies [100, 102].

Two types of magnesium deficits exist: Magnesium *deficiency* corresponds to an insufficient intake which can be corrected through mere nutritional Mg supplementation whereas Mg *depletion* due to a dysregulation of the magnesium status cannot be corrected through nutritional supplementation only, and requests the more or less specific correction of the dysregulation mechanisms. *Depletion* is frequently due to the association of a reduced magnesium intake with various types of stress including biological clock dysrhythmias. The differentiation between Mg depletion forms with hyperfunction and forms with hypofunction of the Biological Clock (BC) is seminal and the main biological marker is melatonin (MT).

We hypothesize hereafter that some forms of nocturnal asthma (NA) would be linked to a Hyperfunction of the Biological Clock (HBC) where magnesium status could be implicated. We would show that some other forms of asthma among non-nocturnal asthma patients (NNA) could be, on the contrary, linked to a magnesium depletion with hypofunction of the Biological Clock (hBC). It may be assumed that all these asthma patients must be treated with the same conventional asthma treatment, the same balanced magnesium intake but will benefit from either light or darkness therapies according to their asthma chronobiological phenotype.

The aim of the present study is to consider (i) the frequency of magnesium depletion in asthma (ii) the two opposite forms of associated chronopathological disorders *i.e* hyper-function (HBC) or hypo-function (hBC) of the biological clock (BC) (iii) the interaction between magnesium and the various treatments with light (phototherapies) or dark ("darkness therapies") therapies on the chronopathological forms of magnesium depletion.

I. Magnesium Deficit in Asthma

Magnesium has been implicated in respiratory diseases although conclusions were too often drawn from effects of parenteral high pharmacological $MgSO_4$ doses [202, 325]. Its well-known muscle relaxing effect induce a reduction of bronchospasm and an increase in airways diameter [34, 36, 59, 72, 88, 142, 144, 150, 151, 170, 218, 245, 254, 256, 282, 283, 303, 311, 319, 325]. It relaxes bronchial smooth muscle *in vitro* [325] and bronchodilate asthmatic airways *in vivo* thus improving lung function in human patients [254, 319]. Potential mechanisms of the smooth muscle relaxation induced by magnesium **pharmacological doses** may be linked to (i) direct relaxation of bronchial smooth muscle,

[325] (ii) calcium channels blocking properties together with an activation of adenylate cyclase, both leading to inhibition of myosine kinase resulting in myorelaxation [47, 74, 303], (iii) inhibition of cholinergic neuromuscular transmission with decreased sensibility to depolarizing action of acetylcholine [79], (iv) increased beta receptor affinity favoring the effects of beta-2 mimetics [106, 285], (v) stabilization of mast cells and T-lymphocytes (vi) stimulation of nitric oxide and prostacyclin generation. Some of these effects may be responsible for the anti-inflammatory properties of magnesium [26, 47, 85, 151, 161, 243, 319]. In addition, magnesium favors many pulmonary immunological defense mechanisms [26] and intervenes in melatonin regulation [98, 102] (cf I.4).

I.1. Hypomagnesemia in Asthma

Relevant epidemiologic studies showed that plasma magnesium concentrations in asthmatics from various countries are generally lower compared to healthy controls [11, 17, 18, 257]. Serum total magnesium level under 0.74 mmol/L is almost always associated with more severe asthma and more hospitalizations while patients with mild or moderate asthma may have normal magnesium levels (0.82 ± 0.08 mmol/L) [11, 373]. Multiple regression analysis showed that severe asthma is the only factor associated significantly with hypomagnaesemia [11]. No effect is observed in chronic asthma for inhaled beta-agonist, inhaled steroid or theophylline therapy on serum Mg level [11]. No alteration in serum Mg level was observed during asthmatic attacks [110, 175] or histamine and methacholine challenge [85, 373].

I.2. Other Magnesium Disturbances in Asthma

A urinary magnesium significant loss (6.81 ± 3.9 vs. 2.79 ± 1.39 mmol/day, $p = 0.01$) was observed in placebo-treated persistent moderate asthmatic children [25] or babies suffering from bronchial obstructive bronchitis [26].

Tissue magnesium may also decrease, as shown by reduced erythrocyte levels during asthmatic attacks or histamine and methacholine challenge [85, 104, 373] which normalized in the symptom-free period [111].

Stable asthmatics have a low skeletal magnesium content which reveals the Mg deficiency in asthmatics [146]. This deficit in body stores is revealed by the parenteral loading test in some patients with stable bronchial asthma: the ratio of magnesium retention to urinary excretion and bronchial reactivity to inhaled methacholine is significantly inversely correlated with the erythrocyte magnesium level [149].

I.3. The Two Forms of Magnesium Deficits in Asthma

Hypomagnesemia has been implicated in chronic asthma through mechanisms involving modulation of inflammatory processes [52, 104] and regulation of bronchomotor tone [254, 319]. The magnesium deficit can be characteristic of an insufficient magnesium intake and of alterations in magnesium retention mechanisms as well. In addition, beta-2 agonists which are the first line of asthma therapy and theophylline can stimulate magnesium efflux in peripheral tissues [165, 177] leading to an aggravated magnesium deficit of the cells [25].

The various biological markers of magnesium deficit may not be due to magnesium deficiency, but testify to a clinical form of magnesium **depletion**. We have highlighted the possible importance of several types of magnesium depletion in the aetiopathogenesis of diverse diseases, particularly of magnesium depletion caused by the association between an insufficient intake of magnesium and a chronopathological stress [95, 96, 98, 99, 102].

1.3.1. Magnesium Deficiency

Magnesium d*eficiency* is linked to an insufficient intake and may be corrected through a physiological nutritional oral magnesium supplementation, over a long period of time. It is noteworthy that chronic magnesium deficiency in human beings is frequent. On all the continents a large part of the population has a dietary intake lower than the recommended dietary allowances (RDAs) for magnesium. The RDA for magnesium intake is 350 mg/day for an adult male, 280 mg/day for a female and 10-13 mg/kg/day for growing children [250]. The magnesium requirement of almost all healthy adults is 6 mg/kg/day [97]. In France 23% of women and 18% of men have dietary magnesium intakes lower than the 2/3 of the RDAs for Mg [42, 94, 97, 158, 294, 374].

A pharmacological magnesium therapy involving in clinical practice mainly oral or intravenous high doses of magnesium sulfate are completely inappropriate in that indication. It is reserved to some indications generally in emergency situations. These two magnesium treatments are basically different in nature and action. The first one is devoid of any toxicity. The second, causes a iatrogenic magnesium load, whatever the magnesium status, and may induce magnesium toxicity. It is a real scientific fraud and an ethical misconduct to fail to differentiate between the safety of a nutritional physiological oral magnesium supplementation and the potentially dangerous effects of high pharmacological doses. But this basic distinction between the two types of magnesium treatments is too often overlooked in papers on magnesium therapy.

Magnesium deficiency in asthma: Poor magnesium intake is associated with impairment of pulmonary function, objectived by a decrease in forced expiratory volume in one second (FEV_1) and a higher risk of both wheezing and airway hyperreactivity. Consequently, individuals with a low Mg intake may be at increasing risk of developing asthma or a chronic airflow obstruction [322]. A suboptimal intake of dietary nutrients such as Mg was recently recognized to be a potential risk factor for asthma, especially in childhood [18, 155]. The decrease in dietary Mg intake could be, at least in part, the reason of the increasing allergic diseases.

Atoxic nutritional magnesium therapy may palliate the coexistent magnesium deficiency. A beneficial effect of magnesium on lung function, airway reactivity or wheeze was observed in two observational studies [42, 158, 322] but not confirmed in others [50, 320]. These conflicting results could be attributable to the fact that supplementation is only effective in magnesium deficiency whereas it would be without effect in magnesium depletion [98]. Pharmacological magnesium treatment for chronic obstructive pulmonary diseases or asthma is not very efficient and may be potentially hazardous in that indication [98].

To sum up: Magnesium deficiency may be considered as an adjuvant nutritional disorder in asthma but asthma *per se* does not only depends on the deficiency

1.3.2. Magnesium depletion

Magnesium d*epletion* is due to a dysregulation of the magnesium status which cannot be corrected through nutritional supplementation only, but requires the most specific correction of the dysregulation mechanism. There exists as many clinical forms of magnesium depletion as many possibilities of the dysregulation of the magnesium status. But both in clinical therapeutics and in animal experiment, the dysregulation mechanisms of magnesium depletion frequently associates reduced magnesium intake with various types of stress [94, 95, 98, 102]. Among these, dysrhythmias by dysregulation of the Biological Clock must be considered.

Magnesium depletion in asthma: Many disturbances of magnesium levels clearly indicate magnesium deficit in asthmatic patients. Serum (or plasma) and erythrocyte magnesium are usually normal, but in both **severe** or **acute asthma,** lower erythrocyte magnesium is often reported while magnesium plasma remains unchanged. Decreases in Mg levels in both polymorphonuclear cells and muscles can be observed. Magnesium depletion in asthma may result from the coexistence of major magnesium deficits together with a chronobiological dysrythmia of the biological clock [11, 78, 84, 88, 90, 91, 94, 95, 104, 110, 111, 271, 284, 374).

I.4. Links between Magnesium Status and Chronobiology

Circadian rhythms are endogenously generated by the biological clock (BC) represented by the suprachiasmatic nuclei (SCN) of the anterior hypothalamus. The links with magnesium status and chronobiology are well established [98]. The quality of magnesium status influences directly the Biological Clock function.. Reversely, BC dysrythmias influence the magnesium status. A close relationship exists between BC and the magnesium status.

1. Magnesium from physiological to pharmacological concentrations can directly enhance melatonin secretion by stimulating serotonin N-acetyltransferase, the magnesium key enzyme for synthesis of melatonin (MT) and to enhance indirectly the production of MT through an increased activity of the SCN [91, 240, 241].
2. Magnesium deficiency may decrease MT production and SCN function [91, 92].
3. MT can decrease magnesemia through its effects on Mg distribution [73, 91].

Consequently it obviously appears that chronobiology and nutritional magnesium intake interact with a possible central magnesium regulation. MT production is controlled both by photoperiod and magnesium status. Light, through SCN, decreases MT production, darkness having the opposite effect [244, 276-278, 346-348]. Mg deficiency decreases MT production whereas Mg overload stimulates it [91, 96]. It could be assumed that a balanced magnesium status might be necessary for an optimal MT function and a darkness therapy effectiveness. Reversely MT might potentiate the effects of Mg therapy [3, 61, 96, 108, 112]. We will develop the clinical forms of magnesium depletion associating Mg deficiency with dysfunction of the Biological Clock (BC), either hyper- (HBC) or hypo-function (hBC) in

asthma. Finally, the interaction between magnesium and the various treatments with light or darkness therapies on the chronopathological forms of magnesium depletion will be discussed.

II. Chronopathological Forms of Asthma

II.1. Hyperfunction of the Biological Clock (HBC) in Asthma

HBC may be due to either **primary** disorders of BC (SCN and pineal gland) or **secondary** with an increased homeostatic response in the case of hyposensitivity to inducing light. This means that the biological clock behaves in homeostatic hyperfunction resulting in **Nervous hypoExcitability** (NhE). The corresponding clinical forms associate diverse expressions of NhE: depression, nocturnal cephalalgia without photophobia (*i.e.* cluster headaches), dyssomnia mainly advanced sleep phase syndrome (ASPS), some clinical forms of chronic fatigue syndrome and fibromyalgia. The main comorbidities are depression and/or asthenia. They take place during the night or the "bad" seasons (autumn and winter) when the sunshine is minimum. The therapy relies on classical asthma treatment, a balanced magnesium intake and sometimes additional psychoanaleptics and adequate chronopathological therapy [98-100, 102].

II.1.1. Clinical Form of Asthma with HBC: Nocturnal Asthma

Lung function in a healthy individual varies in a circadian rhythm, with peak lung function occurring near 4:00 PM (1600 hours) and minimal lung function occurring near 4:00 AM (0400 hours). An episode of NA is characterized by an exaggeration in this normal variation in lung function from daytime to nighttime, with diurnal changes in pulmonary function generally higher than 15%. There is also a circadian variation in bronchial hyperresponsiveness with an eightfold increase in bronchial reactivity overnight as opposed to a twofold increase in non nocturnal asthma (NNA) [227, 318]. Approximately, 75% of asthmatics suffering from nocturnal symptoms awakened one night per week, 64% three nights per week and 39% every night [350]. The occurrence of NA is associated with increased morbidity and inadequate asthma control, and has an important negative impact on quality of life [55, 225]. But, it remains controversial whether NA is a distinct entity or is a manifestation of more severe asthma [55]. According to the National Heart, Lung and Blood

Institute, NA is a variable exacerbation of the underlying asthma condition associated with increases in symptoms, need for medication, airway responsiveness, and/or worsening of lung function [224]. The distal lung units, specifically the collateral channels, may be selectively altered at night in NA, possibly because of smooth muscle contraction, inflammation and/or oedema [192].

The mechanisms by which nocturnal asthma develop remain unclear and may vary from patient to patient [55]. Several factors may contribute to NA (allergen exposure in bed, supine position, interruption of the bronchodilator therapy, gastro-oesophageal reflux, tenseness of the airways and secretion accumulation) but they do not constitute a general concept for the explanation of nightly exacerbation [221].

In patients with NA, circadian variations in airflow limitation are seen, with decreases in peak expiratory flow rate (PEF) and forced expiratory volume in one second (FEV_1). According to Sutherland et al. [332, 333], in this asthma phenotype, the circadian worsening in NA is associated with increased airway inflammation [226] increased airways responsiveness [227], and worsened airflow limitation [355]. Aggravation of dyspnoea at night, reduction of PEF when awaking [197, 354], bronchostriction mainly during rapid eye movement [310] have been reported. Many hormonal, neural, cellular and humoral factors show diurnal fluctuations which favour a constrictive bronchial response in the night [221]. The better marker that varies in a circadian rhythm is melatonin which increases during the nighttime (cf. II.1.2.1.). *In vitro* studies have shown exogenous melatonin to be pro-inflammatory in asthma but it is unknown whether endogenous melatonin levels are a controller of airway inflammation in nocturnal asthma [332]. Under physiological conditions, the melatonin level increases when the anti-inflammatory cortisol level is decreased. This suggests that melatonin levels may influence the secretion of hypothalamic-pituitary-adrenal axis thus inducing inflammation [184]. Other markers also show circadian fluctuations and correlate with the overnight decrement in lung function. For instance, nadirs in epinephrine and cortisol levels that occur in the body around 10 PM to 4 PM and elevated histamine and other mediator levels that occur between midnight and 4 AM play a major role in the worsening of asthma during the night [188]. The other circadian variations include alveolar tissue inflammation [189, 190], intrinsic adrenergic hormonal milieu changes [22], hypothalamic-pituitary-adrenal axis dysfunction [334], alterations of both the affinity and activity of glucocorticoid receptors [191] and ß-adrenergic receptors [349], increase in alveolar tissue CD4+ lymphocytes which play a pivotal role in eosinophil recruitment, increase in peripheral blood and alveolar eosinophil and macrophage number and function [22, 53, 118, 189, 190, 352.] (i) T-lymphocytes are though to play a major role in the pathogenesis of asthma by producing inflammatory cytokines and possibly chemokines allowing eosinophils to migrate from the blood through the vascular endothelium [122, 123, 190, 214, 332] (ii) Mast cells release after antigen activation TNF-α, arachidonic acid metabolites, proteases, histamine, serotonin and nitric oxide that contribute to cellular influx into the lung [229]. Interestingly, in agreement with our hypothesis, recent findings indicate that melatonin is also important in the control of cell recruitment from the bone marrow and the migration of the inflammatory cells to the lungs since pinealectomy in an experimental model of allergic airway inflammation in rats reduced the total cell number count in the lung and at the same time bone marrow proliferation that both returned to control levels after treatment with melatonin [229]. This could be related to the facts that T lymphocytes have cell surface G protein–linked and nuclear melatonin receptors [190]and macrophages and CD4+ lymphocytes have been proposed as major sites of melatonin's actions [129]. As a whole, melatonin is pro-inflammatory [332]. But, it is also reported that melatonin may also exert protective effects in inflammation as well as in other pathologies by stimulating several anti-oxidative enzymes and by inhibiting the inducible nitric oxide synthase (iNOS) activity in neutrophils and macrophages responsible for the overproduction of nitric oxide (NO) in μM range in inflammation [248]. However, a recent study on 5 nocturnal asthma subjects showed an increase in exhaled NO, with a circadian variation. The peak of NO was reached at 4 PM, the time of best pulmonary function [127] whereas exhaled NO decreased during the night. The authors suggest that the significant decrease in exhaled NO may reflect an important chronobiological defect in NO production which in view of its bronchodilator action could play a role in nocturnal exacerbations of asthma [127]. If this hypothesis is true, then melatonin would also act in a negative fashion by inhibiting iNOS. (iii) Cell influx includes eosinophils, neutrophils and lymphocytes capable of secreting various inflammatory mediators that lead to subsequent tissue damage, bronchoconstriction and airway hyperreactivity. Airway neutrophilia has been reported in severe persistent asthma which is often associated with increased nocturnal symptoms [172]. These human peripheral blood mononuclear cells may also synthesize melatonin [115]. Finally, matrix metalloproteinase-9 (MMP-9) expression increased in nocturnal sputum of severe asthma patients compared with patients with mild asthma or normal subjects. MMP-9 are responsible for remodelling of the extracellular matrix (ECM) and may facilitate leukocytes migration through the ECM and between endothelial cells [230]. Interestingly, we reported also an increase in MMP-9 in magnesium-deficient mice [262].

All these chronobiological events promote nocturnal worsening of asthma and increased nocturnal deaths [336].

II.1.2. Characteristics of HBC in Asthma

II.1.2.1. Biological Characteristic (increase in the Melatonin)

The major biological characteristic is represented by **an increase in the melatonin levels** in various fluids, corresponding to the elective marker of the biological clock [98, 333]. Plasma melatonin measurement has long been the reference, but salivary melatonin measurement was shown as a reliable, sensitive and easy method to monitor changes in the circadian rhythms of melatonin [358, 375].

A 1 hour delay of peak serum melatonin levels was reported in NA [333]. In this NA phenotype alone, melatonin levels are negatively correlated with overnight change in FEV_1 suggesting a chronopathological mechanism of asthma, melatonin being, in our opinion, only a biological marker. However, many recent data must be taken into account (i) melatonin is also synthetized by several other tissues of the body including the immune system [115], (ii) it may have a role in modulating airway function, since melatonin receptors have been shown to be present in the lungs of experimental animals [264], (iii) it exhibits immunoenhancing properties by regulating cytokine production of immunocompetent cells [56] (iv) it affects asthma severity because it enhances allergic airway inflammation [229] and airway smooth muscle tone in animal models [272, 359]. When melatonin was added *in vitro* to peripheral blood mononuclear call samples collected from patients with NA and healthy subjects at 4 P.M. and 4 A.M., an inflammatory response was observed with increased production of interleukin-1, intereukin-6 and tumor necrosis factor alpha at both times. In NA patients, the cytokine response could not be further stimulated at 4 A.M., as observed in non nocturnal asthma, suggesting chronic overstimulation *in vivo* [332].

Consistent with the concept of HBC is the common observation that pediatric active asthma abates when puberty occurs [251, 372], while melatonin levels decrease physiologically. This physiological decrease in melatonin corresponds to a real improvement of both NA prevalence and severity. Similarly, specific immunotherapy in children sensitized to pollens led to a significant improvement of their symptoms at the end of treatment and to a decrease in both melatonin and beta endorphin levels. These results suggest the disappearance of the opioid-melatonin system stimulating influence on the immune system [130]. Asthma is one of the most common medical conditions that can complicate pregnancy [147]. Various stresses in pregnant women may convert a simple Mg deficiency into *Mg depletion* including environmental factors such as smoking, viruses, pollens but the role of chronopathological stress appears to be too often neglected [100]. The measurement of melatonin levels in pregnant women was never reported to our knowledge but aggravations were reported in 16-22% of mild asthmatics and in 83% of severe asthmatics, the majority of them improving after delivery [132, 327]. This suggest an increase in melatonin levels during pregnancy which would return to the previous situation after delivery.

A beneficial effect of light (or at least cessation of darkness) on lung function was observed in two observational studies. In an intractable nocturnal asthma woman, resistant to various bronchodilators and steroids, significant improvement of asthma was observed by awakening the patient quietly at 3 AM (thus interrupting darkness) before the melatonin peak with inhalation of 2.5 mg salbutamol [298]. Similarly, phototherapy and partial sleep deprivation lead to an improvement in 4 asthmatics [215, 216].

An immediate and long term efficacy of the high mountains climate (1560 m) was reported in various allergic diseases including asthma, involving insolation as an important factor of asthma improvement [105]. Conversely, clear and consistent seasonal patterns are observed for asthma hospitalizations with an autumn peak, when light decreases (and viral infections increase) and a summer trough when light is maximum in the northern hemisphere [70, 126, 238].

II.1.2.2. The Clinical Forms of Neurohypoexcitability (NhE) Resulting from HBC are Both Central and Peripheral

All the clinical forms **of NhE resulting from HBC** may coexist with the same chronobiological characteristics: nocturnal and hibernal pathologies, increase in melatonin levels, and clear improvement by light. The major comorbidity is represented by depressive states and asthenia. We called that type of persons "photophile" patients, in that they are clearly improved during the daylight and the "nice seasons" [98].

II.1.2.2.1. The Central Forms Associate Psychic, Algic and Hypnic Manifestations:

a) Depression whose main type corresponds to the seasonal affective disorder (SAD) or winter depression. Psychic asthenia (psychasthenia) would somewhat represent a minor form of SAD. An important comorbidity of depression with asthma (31-34 % of asthma patients) was shown in random and representative population samples, rather than in a clinical sample [4, 135, 247]. Three specific symptoms, dyspnoea, wakening at night with asthma symptoms, and morning symptoms, are particularly strongly associated with depression. There was also a significant and clinically important impact on the quality of life of those who reported wakening at night, morning symptoms and dyspnoea. A link between asthma and respiratory disease and suicidal ideation and suicide attempts has been reported [139].

- **Sleep disturbances**. The changes which characterize NA have been reported not only to circadian events but also to sleep itself [224, 318]. The most **common sleep disturbances** among asthmatic patients were (i) obstructive sleep apnea representing a source of severe sleep fragmentation [28, 370] and (ii) advanced sleep phase syndrome with early morning awakening (51%), difficulty in maintaining sleep (44%) and daytime sleepiness (44%) [27, 35, 172].

In asthmatic shift workers, exacerbations took place during the daytime, when they slept. Circadian variation was intimately related to sleep (when melatonin increases) and virtually independent of solar time [66], but these results were repudiated later by the same group [154].

In a rat model of asthma, sleep (particularly rapid eye movement, REM) deprivation, reliably suppressed eosinophils in either the bronchoalveolar lavage fluid or the bronchial lamina propria, underlying the role of REM sleep in NA [167].

- **Cephalalgia** *without photophobia* (and even with photophilia) represents a nocturnal and hibernal disorder. It is the case of cephalalgia with obstructive sleep apnea periods and of cluster headaches [62]. The patient is healthier during the "nice" seasons [98, 202, 230].

II.1.2.2.2. The Peripheral Manifestations are Neuromuscular, Mainly Represented by Myalgia and Muscular Asthenia

Some clinical forms of the fibromyalgic syndrome with HBC associating to muscular troubles, depression, chronic fatigue syndrome, cephalalgia and dyssomnia may be a type of nervous hypoexcitability linked to HBC [152, 180, 183, 236, 274, 342].

In women with endometriosis, hypothyroidism, **fibromyalgia, chronic fatigue syndrome**, autoimmune diseases, allergies and **asthma** are significantly more common than in women in the general population [315]

II.2. Hypofunction of the Biological Clock in Asthma

II.2.1. Clinical Form of Asthma With hBC

Whereas nocturnal asthma gave rise to a great number of clinical and epidemiological studies, non nocturnal asthma (NNA) is rarely studied as a whole. We do not suggest that all the NNA are asthma with hBC but we hypothesize that among them, some forms may be related to hBC when they associate decreased melatonin levels and clinical symptoms of nervous hyperexcitability (NHE) *i.e.* anxiety ranging from generalized anxiety to panic attacks, diurnal cephalalgia (mainly migraine), dyssomnia, such as delayed sleep phase syndrome, some clinical forms of chronic fatigue syndrome and of fibromyalgia [98, 102]. They may be due to either primary disorders of the BC or to a secondary homeostatic response to light hypersensitivity. The organism responds to the pathogenic effect of this light hypersensitivity by protective reactive *photophobia*, whose mechanism is still unclear [217]. The treatment relies on diverse forms of darkness therapies, possibly with the help of some psycholeptics [98, 102].

II.2.2. Characteristics of hBC in Asthma

II.2.2.1. Biological Characteristic

The main biological marker of hBC is *a decrease in melatonin* (or its metabolite) *levels* in various fluids [98, 102]. An important decrease in the 24-h mean level and amplitude of both plasma melatonin [184] and salivary melatonin [114] was observed in mild intermittent or persistent and moderate to severe asthma patients. Chronic glucocorticotherapy reduced activity of the pituitary adrenal axis and suppressed melatonin rhythm [184, 203].

The decrease in amplitude (difference between the low daytime melatonin and the higher level at night) observed in asthma patients might be related to the pathological state of asthma [114]. The underlying mechanism of the decrease in melatonin parameters is unknown. However, in stressed rats, increased corticosterone may have a direct effect on pinealocytes or melatonin is more rapidly metabolized during the stress [21, 224].

II.2.2. 2. Clinical Characteristics

The clinical characteristics of the secondary forms of chronobiological NHE are of circadian as well as of seasonal type: the symptomatology is mainly *diurnal* and observed *in spring and summer*, when *light hyperstimulation is obviously maximum* during daylight or during the fair seasons. The clinical forms of NHE are both central and peripheral [95, 98, 99, 102].

II.2.2.2.1. The Central Forms Associate Psychic, Algic and Hypnic Manifestations

a) Nervous hyperexcitability: Migraine and chronic respiratory inflammation like rhinitis, sinusitis, and asthma have been reported to be the most commonly seen disorders in chemical sensitivity patients [376]. A chemical odor intolerance was also reported that would indicate a phenomenon of dishabituation leading to generalization with both hypersensitivity to light and odors) [51]. Dishabituation is the contrary of habituation, a physiological phenomenon characterized by a more or less gradual decrease of the responses to repetitive stimuli of constant parameters [237]. Dishabituation, corresponds first to a decrease in habituation leading to a rapid recovery of the initial sensory reactivity and secondly may even lead to potentiation (or sensibilization) and sometimes to generalization involving other stimuli [237]. Dishabituation is often reported nowadays in pathological studies, such as photic cephalalgia (headaches with photophobia *i.e.* migraine). A common background of these "dishabituated" patients is the presence of a magnesium depletion with hypofunction of the biological clock (hBC) [102]. Chemical odor intolerance and anxiety sensitivity in asthma patients were significant predictors of physical symptoms [51].

b) Cephalalgia mainly migraine: A frequent association between migraine and various allergic disorders have been reported [75, 213, 316]. Bronchial asthma is, like migraine, a paroxysmal disorder with attacks and symptom-free intervals which alter the quality of life [253]. In addition, both migraine and asthma are psychosomatic disorders [205, 366]. Finally, recent studies using anti-inflammatory drugs (montelukast, a leukotriene receptor antagonist or coxibs, inihibitors of cyclooxygenase) demonstrated consistent beneficial results in both asthma and migraine prevention [71, 77, 83, 117].

The prevalence of migraine is significantly higher in children with atopic disorders compared to those without [239]. Rhinitis in children was found to be associated with maternal migraine [145]. Among children whose mothers had neither migraine nor asthma/allergies, 3.2% had asthma while this incidence was found to be more than 6% for children whose mothers had migraine, but not asthma/allergies [60]. The risk of asthma among children born of women who had both migraine and asthma/allergies was greater than the risk associated with each maternal disease [316]. Headaches in adults were found to be more prevalent among those whose family members were reported to have allergy, asthma and migraine [160]. Genetic-epidemiological studies showed that migraine and asthma co-segregate in the family, indicating a possible common genetic background, involving some specific HLAs [60, 128, 222, 316]. The comorbidity asthma-migraine may rely on increased plasma levels of endothelin-1, a potent vasoconstrictor and a mediator in the inflammatory process (through matrix-metalloproteinase 9 (MMP-9) particularly [230, 323]. These disorders are inkeeping with the well-known similar disturbances due to magnesium deficit [99, 262].

c) Dyssomnia, mainly represented by delayed sleep phase syndrome. In asthma and COPD, the night sleep is delayed or shortened and deep sleep is often reduced or even absent [197]. A large study showed that asthma individuals are in addition at increased risk for complaints of difficulty with inducing sleep [224].

d) Anxiety. A strong and consistent link between asthma and anxiety disorders has been often reported. An important comorbidity of anxiety with asthma (40-53% of asthma patients) was shown in random and representative population samples and in clinical samples [4, 7, 135, 247, 260]. This relationships appear strongest among those with more severe disorders in terms of both asthma and anxiety disorders. The strongest links appear between lifetime severe asthma and generalized anxiety disorder (GAD), as well as panic attacks and panic disorder [5, 49, 58, 124, 133, 137-140, 247, 260, 269, 335, 357, 369]. An association between respiratory diseases and panic attacks was documented among adults [137, 260, 369] and youths [135, 260]. Several studies have also noted elevated rates of asthma among psychiatric inpatients and outpatients with anxiety disorders [44, 232].

II.2.2.2.2. Peripheral Manifestations

The ***central and peripheral manifestations*** are neuromuscular, mainly represented by photosensitive epilepsia, which may be either generalized or focal, authentified through EEG with intermittent light stimulation (ILS) with its corresponding form observed among TV viewers and video game players [99, 148, 265, 299]. Some migraine equivalents may be associated in this context.

Accessorily, the nervous form of chronopathological magnesium depletion with hBC may appear clinically as chronic fatigue syndrome (CFS) [93, 301] or as fibromyalgia [99, 363].

II.2.3. Indirect Evidences Suggesting the Possible Role of HBC in Asthma

Physiological and chronobiological factors for decrease in **melatonin production** are similarly deleterious factors for asthma with hBC.

a) For instance, in some mild or moderate asthma patients (about 12%) asthma improved during pregnancy. This results mirrors the worsening previously described in a majority of severe asthma with HBC and would indicate an increase in melatonin during pregnancy.

b) Aspirin sensitive asthma patients usually suffer from an active disease, despite the avoidance of aspirin and cross-reactive drugs, attributed to a decreased melatonin synthesis and an increased sensitivity of platelet to melatonin (and its metabolite) as compared to aspirin-tolerant asthma patients [109].

c) Diurnal, seasonal, climatic photostimulation must be at risk in those patients. A retrospective study, on a cohort of 108 cases of asthma death in 1-19-year-old in Denmark, showed that death occurred predominantly in summer in the 15-19-year age group [174]. The authors attributed the death to an insufficient medical survey But, we suggest that the decrease in melatonin levels at puberty aggravated by light exposure in summer could be also involved. Increased visits to hospital were also reported during the wet season in Trinidad, i.e. during summer, when the sunlight is obviously important [168].

d) Finally both corticotherapy and hormone replacement therapy cause a decrease in daily melatonin secretion without disturbing circadian rhythm [185]. This data must be taken into account by clinicians in those forms of asthma with hBC.

To sum up: The frequency of asthma linked to Mg depletion with HBC or hBC is presently unknown. It may be assumed that a number of nocturnal asthma are probably related to magnesium depletion with HBC, and conversely that some forms of non nocturnal asthma are linked to magnesium depletion with hBC. The response would be brought by appropriate measurements of both magnesium and melatonin levels in various fluids or tissues.

III. Treatment of Asthma with Dysfunctions of BC

The two opposite chronobiological forms of asthma would benefit from the same pharmacologic asthma treatment, the same balanced magnesium intake but the right opposite treatments of the chronobiological disorders.

III.1. Conventional Pharmacological Treatment

Asthma management guidelines recommend the use of preventive medication in sufficient amounts to control asthma symptoms [353]. Nonadherence to treatment is often implicated in the aggravation of asthma. According to current US guidelines, nocturnal symptoms of asthma occurring more often than once weekly may indicate inadequate control of asthma [249].

III.1.1.General Considerations

The therapeutic agents used for the management of **chronic asthma** are mainly inhaled long-acting beta-2 agonists and steroids. **Acute exacerbations** can occur and are challenging to manage. Supplemental oxygen, repeated doses of inhaled beta-2 agonists and systemic corticosteroids (oral if tolerated or inhaled) [40, 121, 313] are the mainstay therapies used to relieve bronchospasm and airway obstruction. Because all patients do not respond to maximal therapy, other strategies either older (theophylline, magnesium) or more recent (heliox, leukotriene modifiers) are being evaluated [329].

Understanding the kinetics of the different drug preparations allowed most effective timing of dose [225, 318]. Chronopharmacology should optimize the desired effects of medications and minimize undesired ones in asthmatic patients [114, 321].

However, the treatment of asthma is not under the scope of the present paper and will not be developed hereafter, with exception of beta-2 agonists and magnesium. We would only point out some informations on current asthma agents which may be important in chronopathological asthma.

Briefly, **beta-2 agonists** which are detailed below (cf III.1.2) are the first line of asthma therapy, but their safety is debated [101]. The mortality rate in patients with acute severe asthma is still rising and has been partly attributed to their adverse effects [11].

The anti-inflammatory properties of **corticosteroids** make them reference for the treatment of **acute asthma**. All of them (including prednisone, methylprednisolone, hydrocortisone and dexamethasone) are efficient in acute asthma whatever the administration route (oral, intravenous or intramuscular) [14]. However, controlled trials found that a single dose of dexamethasone suppressed melatonin production in eleven healthy volunteers [80] or in asthma patients [185, 203]. These observations may be of clinical relevance in chronobiological asthma. Finally, *in vitro*, in peripheral blood mononuclear cell from patients with nocturnal asthma, or *in vivo*, in glucocorticoid-resistant asthma, a reduced responsiveness to corticosteroids at night, requiring an increase dosing has been reported. This resistance to the effects of steroids was attributed to an inhibition of glucocorticoid receptor (GR) linked to a circadian increased expression of GRbeta, an endogeneous inhibitor of steroid action, mainly in macrophage [55, 120, 192, 208]. The dosing of corticosteroids in the morning optimally improve bronchial potency in asthma while the risks of adrenal suppression and of osteopenia observed with dosing at other times are significantly reduced or even suppressed [275]. A retrospective study showed that inhaled corticosteroid dispensing to adult asthmatics led to a reduced risk of intensive care unit admission for asthma, a surrogate for life threatening exacerbation (103). Finally, a large retrospective study showed that inhaled corticosteroids administered chronically and prudently within the recommended dose ranges do not endanger the functioning of the hypothalamic-pituitary-adrenal axis whereas the increasing tendency to use higher doses of inhaled corticosteroids is not supported by reliable published information [63].

Theophylline may have some interesting therapeutic effect, but given its toxicity profile, it is unclear whether it offers any advantage over maximal beta-2 agonist.

Ironically, different electrolyte disturbances are induced by acute asthma medications. Among them, hypomagnesemia which is attributed to an increased urinary magnesium excretion and/or to various indirect mechanisms including lipolysis and calcium redistribution [95] appears as a side effect of beta agonists, steroids and xanthines, used for the management of acute asthma [11, 37, 181, 284]. Hypomagnesemia, as the other electrolyte disturbances, may result in exacerbation of the overall condition. Consequently, nebulized beta-2 agonists and aminophylline which are the mainstay therapies for asthma exacerbation must be used carefully in subjects presenting abnormal electrolyte levels. In contrast to acute asthma, therapeutic agents used to treat patients with chronic asthma would not induce electrolyte disturbances [12]. In addition, the toxicity of theophylline, a phosphodiesterase inhibitor that lowers myocardial magnesium levels, is intensified by beta-adrenergic agonists and corticosteroids and may lead to severe nervous and cardiac effects with often fatal issue [309].

Newer therapies such as ventilation strategies with **heliox** (helium and oxygen) and intravenous **leukotriene modifiers** currently being evaluated may or may not prove to be beneficial in the future [329]. A substantial improvement has been observed with the combination of salbutamol and **ipratropium bromide** [280] and from the triple combination of salbutamol, ipratropium and flunosolide [47, 281].

The data evaluating the use of **magnesium** in asthmatic patients are scare and most are small trials or case reports. In addition the results are often conflicting (cf III.4.2.1.2.) In any case, our purpose is to focus mainly on beta-mimetics and magnesium, to take stoke on the possibility of magnesium therapies in asthma and to differentiate between cases where the therapeutic association of beta-2 mimetics and magnesium is beneficial and those where it is deleterious hence contraindicated.

III.1.2. Beta-2 Agonists

For acute asthma, repeated doses of nebulized beta-2 agonists and to a lesser extent IV aminophylline are the mainstays therapies used to relieve bronchospasm and airway obstruction [181, 365]. Beta-2 agonists are the first line of asthma therapy, but their safety is debated. Importantly, beta stimulation may have consequence on regulation of magnesium status. **Physiological** beta stimulation during magnesium deficiency may induce an homeostatic **increase** in magnesemia. In contrast, excessive beta stimulation, by use of **pharmacological** high doses of beta-2 agonists, may induce a **decrease** in magnesemia which could be deleterious for asthmatic patients [101].

III.1.2.1. Nature and Action of Beta-2 Adrenergic Receptors

Adrenergic receptors are classified as alpha (α-1, α-2) and beta (β-1, β-2, β-3) according to their responses to diverse adrenergic stimulations. Generally, adrenergic stimulations have an excitatory effect on alpha receptors and an inhibitory effect on beta receptors [9]. Beta-1 receptors mainly concern the heart. Beta-2 receptors are implicated in smooth muscle relaxation in pulmonary, vascular and uterine apparatus particularly. Beta-3 receptors are the main beta adrenoreceptors in adipocytes with some distinctive links with magnesium status. Beta adrenergic receptors belong to the very large family of seven transmembrane domain-containing stimulatory G protein-coupled membrane receptors. They interact with guanine nucleotide regulatory proteins and magnesium dependent adenylate cyclase. Their activation increases the intra-cellular concentration of cyclic AMP (cAMP) which induces phosphorylation of many key proteins of muscle contraction through activation of a cAMP dependent-Protein Kinase A (PKA) [10, 87, 141, 164, 223, 304, 362]. cAMP induces myorelaxation directly by inhibiting myosine-kinase through phosphorylation by PKA and indirectly (i) by decreasing cellular free Ca^{2+} resulting from Ca^{2+} reuptake by the sarcoplasmic reticulum (ii) by activating K+ channels by phosphorylation thus provoking cell hyperpolarization and inhibition of calcium inflow [364].

A genetic variation in beta adrenergic receptors influencing both susceptibility for asthma and therapeutic response was reported recently [106]. Indeed, A/J inbred mice bound less dihydroalprenolol (beta-antagonist) than C57/BL/6J inbred mice in the absence but not in the presence of magnesium. The gene responsible for the Mg^{2+}-sensitive dihydroalprenolol binding was named “Badm” for beta-adrenergic magnesium effect.

Two main genetic variations in beta 2 receptor itself were reported in a group of asthma patients [273]. The more frequent polymorphism (arginine16→ glycine) identified a subset of asthmatic patients likely to be steroid-dependent and to require immunization therapy. This severe phenotype, frequent in nocturnal asthma patients, was found only in homozygous patients [349]. It corresponds to an increase in agonist-promoted down-regulation of beta-2 receptor expression [143, 273, 339] resulting in an inefficiency of beta-2 agonist treatment [187, 209, 228]. This mutation could have a role in NA [349]. Indeed, the beta2-adrenergic receptors in circulating white blood cells are down regulated at 4AM in patients with NA, which does not happens in normal subjects [337]. The other polyporphism (Glutamine 27→ glutamic acid) was resistant to agonist-promoted down-regulation of receptor expression [143] and was found to be associated with elevated levels of IgE in subjects from asthmatic families [82], supporting previous data relating increased levels of cAMP to increased IgE synthesis [113]. These studies allowed highly significant associations with a number of phenotypes related to asthma, including steroid dependence and bronchodilator responsiveness.

Beta adrenergic receptors play a major role in the regulation of the magnesium status since they can modify exchanges between intra-cellular and extra-cellular magnesium. Activation and modulation of beta-adrenergic receptors might intervene among the neurohormonal factors of the physiological regulation of magnesium status [37, 38, 89-91, 95, 102, 288-290, 177, 361]. Beta receptor physiological stimulation may induce hypermagnesemia through an efflux of magnesium out of the cell via a Na^+-dependent mechanism. But the regulating feedback mechanism of magnesium status through beta-adrenergic receptors may become ineffective when an excessive beta stimulation occurs. These last beta-adrenergic effects are coupled to **lipolysis which reduces magnesemia** mainly through (i) chelation of magnesium by non esterified fatty acids, (ii) increased magnesium uptake by adipocytes, and (iii) at least partly, enhanced urinary excretion of magnesium [37, 38, 89-91, 95, 102, 288-290, 177, 361].

To sum up, the **physiological beta stimulation** may be involved in the regulation of magnesium status by an homeostatic increase in magnesemia during magnesium deficiency. Reversely, **excessive beta stimulation by pharmacological high doses of beta 2 agonists** may induce a deleterious decrease in magnesemia. Reversely, magnesium homeostasis is required for beta receptor function .

III.1.2. 2. Beta-2 Agonists and Obstructive Disorders

The short acting beta-2 agonists (salbutamol, fenoterol, terbutaline, pirbuterol) are essential in emergency treatment of severe asthma and have an important prophylactic role in the prevention of exercise-induced bronchoconstriction. Different routes of administration may be used including inhalation, nebulisation, subcutaneous or intravenous injection. Inhaled beta-2 agonists are initially used. In absence of response, intravenous associated beta-2-agonists are generally useful. The therapeutic response should be evaluated mainly by using the peak expiratory flow (PEF) determination [199, 308].

Long acting beta-2-agonists (salmeterol, formeterol, bambuterol), used in inhalation or *per os*, have provided advantages on short acting beta-2 agonists such as prolonged bronchodilation, reduced diurnal and nocturnal symptoms, improved sleep quality and reduced requirement for short acting beta-2-agonists. When added to inhaled corticosteroids, they produce greater improvement in lung function than increased steroid dose alone [199, 308].

Their mechanism of action is pharmacodynamic. Through stimulation of beta-2 receptor, these drugs lead to bronchorelaxation either directly by enzymatic stimulation or indirectly through Ca^{2+} redistribution (cf above). These mechanisms agree with the beta-adrenergic theory of atopic abnormality in bronchial asthma [338] and with the « calcium hypothesis of asthma » [101, 136].

III.1.2. 3. Side Effects of Beta-2 Agonists

Little if any benefit seems to be derived from regular use of short acting beta-2 agonists. Regular or frequent use can increase the severity of the pathological status. There has been controversy about the possible relationship between use of beta-2 agonists and morbidity or mortality related to asthma and COPD. For instance, the relatively non beta-2 selective agonist, **fenoterol** doubled the risk of asthma [324]. However results from a cohort study including 12.301 patients suggested that increased asthma deaths and near-deaths would be better **a class effect of beta agonists** and would not be reduced to a specific molecule such as fenoterol [324]. Various authors pointed out the severity of asthma as a potential confounding factor. However, a stratified analysis utilizing markers of chronic asthma severity showed, after adjustment by available markers of asthma severity, that the increased risk of death either persisted or disappeared. This discrepancy was attributed to differences in the populations studied [2, 23, 24, 107, 125, 207, 267, 324].

Beta-2 agonists used in COPD treatment can induce numerous side-effects including consequences on cardiac function. They increase heart rate, prolong the electrical action potential duration, induce abnormal myocardial repolarisation. They may cause hyperglycemia, hypokaliemia and hypomagnesaemia with low potassium and magnesium concentrations in skeletal muscles. These biochemical changes may induce at the cardiac level alterations of the conduction pathways, arrhythmias leading to an increased risk of cardiac death [29, 146, 207, 210, 331, 351].

To sum up, beta-2 adrenergic receptor agonists are first-line of asthma therapy but their safety is debated. Fixed combination seems particularly indicated for severe asthma. Free combination appears as first-line therapy for patients with mild to moderate asthma [2, 29, 146, 207, 210, 331].

III.2. Indirect Asthma Therapies

Eviction of allergens, psychotherapic and alternative therapies will be also considered.

III.2.1. Environmental Control Measures

Environmental control measures are essential and should focus on limiting the patient's exposure to allergens. Removal of pets from the bedroom, use of mattress and pillow covers, and carpet-free floors are some examples of helpful changes [318]. Food allergy and intolerance can have a major part to play . Identification and elimination of certain foods or additives can have a major benefit.

III.2.2. All the Pathological Entities Accompanying Asthma Should be Diagnosed and Treated Appropriately [318]

a) Allergic rhinitis should be treated with anti-inflammatory medications;
b) Obstructive sleep apnea syndrome and snoring may be improved by continuous positive airway pressure;
c) Classical pharmacotherapy using psychoanaleptics (HBC) or psycholeptics (hBC) may be successful.

III.2.3. Asthma Education Programs

Asthma education programs that teach about the nature of the disease, medications, and trigger avoidance tend to reduce asthma morbidity. Other promising psychological interventions as adjuncts to medical treatment include training in symptom perception, stress management, hypnose, yoga and several biofeedback-assisted relaxation and breathing exercises are beneficial for stress reduction in general and may be helful in further controlling asthma [169, 206]. The need for ongoing education of the patient's family, the patient and doctors on long-term management and management of acute attacks has be underlined (Jorgensen et al, 2003).

III.2.4. Herbal Medicine

Herbal Medicine has been shown in a number of trials to be beneficial in the treatment of asthma [162]. Safe herbs such as Boswellia and Ginkgo may be used as adjuncts to comprehensive plan of care while staying alert for drug-herb interactions [32, 169].

III.2.5. Needle Acupuncture

Needle Acupuncture is also useful if used regularly. Initially weekly treatments are reduced to, possibly monthly, enabling reduction of conventional medication in many cases. [32, 169, 320].

III.2.6. Homeopathic Remedies

Homeopathic remedies based on extreme dilutions of the allergen may be beneficial in allergic rhinitis but requires collaboration with an experienced homeopath. But they have not been yet validated.

III.2.7. Diet Is Important.

Asthmatics may benefit from hydration and a diet low in sodium and in omega-6 fatty acids and transfatty acids, but high in omega-3 fatty acids, in antioxidant vitamins and magnesium [32, 169, 320].

III.3. Balanced Magnesium Intake

As previously reported, about half the asthma are accompanied by symptoms of latent tetany due to primary Mg deficiency. Reversely, the frequency of allergic antecedents is high in cases of neural forms of primary magnesium deficit (39%). Today the main form of magnesium therapy is oral physiological magnesium supplementation. These palliative nutritional magnesium doses needed to balance magnesium deficiency are obviously devoid of any toxicity since their purpose is to normalize the insufficient magnesium intake [90, 91, 95, 98-102, 134]. It evenly can cause mild side-effects like diarrhea and abdominal cramps [303].

A large epidemiological study carried out in 2633 subjects showed that a high dietary magnesium intake was associated with better lung function and reduced risk of airway hyperreactivity and wheezing [41, 42]. In another study on 20 asthmatics, it was associated with significant improvement of asthma symptom scores whereas FEV1, PEF variables or decrease in use of a bronchodilator was not improved. But, the duration of Mg supplementation may have been too short to detect any improvement in their pulmonary function [158]. A decrease in airway responsiveness was observed in hyperresponsive asthmatics after 6 weeks of nutritional Mg supplementation [24]. Long lasting Mg supplementation (200 mg/day to 7-year old and 290 mg/day to older children) was clearly of benefit in moderate asthma children and was recommended as a concomitant drug in stable asthma [25]. As a whole, nutritional magnesium therapy for pulmonary obstructive diseases physiologically palliates the coexistent primary Mg deficiency. The atoxic adjuvant therapy is always beneficial without side effects [100, 101].

But, when different stress transform the Mg deficiency into Mg depletion related to a dysregulation of the control mechanisms of magnesium status, nutritional physiological magnesium supplementation alone is ineffective. Mg depletion needs not only a balanced Mg intake but also and mainly the correction of its causal dysregulation. In the case of chronobiological forms of asthma treatment must include either "phototherapies" or "darkness therapies".

III.4. Chronobiological Treatments

III.4.1. Asthma with HBC

The different forms of HBC may be treated by various **phototherapies**. It is obvious that in chronobiological asthma with HBC, supplemental over-the-counter melatonin must be carefully avoided since it is yet present in large excess .

III.4.1.1. Bright Light Phototherapy

As for the other diseases based upon Mg depletion with HBC, BLT may be beneficial in this clinical form of NA. Even though not yet evaluated in proper clinical trials, three studies reported on a small number of patients the beneficial effects of BLT in asthma [193, 215, 216]. Therapeutic effect of the method occurs because of correction of internal asynchronism, stimulation of endogeneous synthesis of corticosteroids and antidepressive action [216]. The aim of bright light phototherapy is to lengthen the photoperiod, the marker of its efficiency being the decrease in plasma MT. BLT protective effect may result not only from melatonin suppression but also from multiple other mechanisms *i.e.* depression of immune response with suppression of inflammatory leukotrienes and cytokines [98, 270].

Classically, bright light phototherapy used in seasonal affective disorder requires full spectrum light with an intensity higher than 2000 lux, the best timing being early morning, optimally about 8.5 hours after melatonin onset [341, 342]. Conventional therapy uses full spectrum light without infrared nor ultraviolet rays. The circadian resetting response in humans, as measured by the pineal melatonin rhythm, is wavelength dependent, the peak of sensitivity of the human circadian pacemaker to light being blue-shifted (460 nm) relative to the three cone visual photopic system, the sensitivity of which peaks at approximately 555 nm [211, 317]. Since the 1980s numerous studies have shown that light therapy has beneficial effects when applied in certain types of sleep and mood disorders [292, 343]. Early clinical studies exposed subjects to 2,500 lux for 2-6 hours daily. These lengthy daily treatments induced two serious difficulties: compliance to treatment and side effects (headaches or vision problems) in some users. Shorter exposure (30 min) to brighter 10,000 lux light therapy produced a 75% rate of improvement in SAD without increasing side effects [341, 343]. However the treatment must be applied for the whole winter duration, since SAD symptoms rapidly reappear after treatment has ceased [201]. If conventional BLT constitutes now the therapeutic tool considered as inseparably linked to SAD, it has been also used in non seasonal depressions, senile dementia and sleep disorders in the elderly. In those indications, bright light therapy appears as a non specific antidepressant agent and constitutes a speedy and efficient adjuvant to antidepressant medication [194, 234]. Non migrainous headaches, without photophobia, may be also an indication for bright light therapy through this antidepressant action [102]. We consequently think that BLT must be efficient in asthma with HBC, by improving chronobiolocal dysfunction of the BC and consequently both biological and clinical consequences.

Bright light therapy is operative through various neural and perhaps humoral mechanisms. Today, the mean central neural mechanisms of phototherapy seem to be increased serotoninergy, hypoactivity of inhibitory modulators such as taurine and kappa opioid receptors, and finally stimulation of inflammatory and oxidative processes [98]. An evolutive perspective suggests that heme moieties and bile pigments in animals mediate some non visual influence of light upon neuroactive gases (including CO and NO) and upon biorythms [259] through humoral phototransduction. Bright light can break the carboxyhemoglobin (HbCO) bond releasing CO and stimulate nitric oxide synthase to produce NO. If one considers hemoglobin not only as a scavenger but also as a transporter, it may convey photic information to all tissues, notably the brain, through the neuroactive gases: CO and NO in blood [119, 198, 259, 356]. Bright light is also able to reduce circulating levels of bilirubin and biliverdin, thus removing their vasoconstrictive and sedative effects [259]. The fall in bile pigments may result *in vivo* from the absorption of photons by the photo-sensitizer riboflavin [186] and from an effect of light on plasma albumin [6, 255].

III.4.1.2. Chromatotherapy

According to Agrapart's theory, the physical energy brought by one wavelength could act like the energy brought by the corresponding oligoelement [7, 8]. For instance, purple for 4-8 minutes would bring the same energy as magnesium ions. Chromatotherapy uses a short exposure to a specific wavelength once a week and like other energetic therapies carefully takes into account the nocturnal or diurnal prevalence of clinical symptoms. In asthma with nocturnal prevalence, purple irradiation of the chest for 4 minutes followed by 20 min of darkness once a week would be beneficial. More specific treatment of asthma using chromatotherapy on acupuncture points would give better result but may be used only by specialists. Even though successfully used in clinical practice, this method has not yet been validated [98, 102]. However, we could show the neuroprotective effects of one wavelength used in chromatotherapia on a validated neuropharmacological nutritional model, in DBA2 mice [261, 263].

III.4.1.3. Low Power Laser Biostimulation

A prospective analysis including 50 asthmatics showed that daily laser irradiation of acupuncture points for 10 days lead to a significant improvement of bronchial asthma which was achieved in a short time and last for several weeks, even months [235].

III.4.1.4. Pharmacotherapy of the Clinical Manifestations of HBC

The many studies demonstrating the efficacy of pharmacotherapy in mood disorders have supported the use of conventional, first-line antidepressant pharmacotherapy (i.e. amitryptilline, fluoxetin, d-fenfluramine) [297, 343]. Analeptics such as psychostimulants (including caffeine) have also been found effective in other diseases with HBC [98, 102].

III.4.2. Asthma with hBC

The best physiologic stimulation of the BC is induced by light deprivation.

III.4.2.1. Stimulating "Darkness Therapies":

They may be physiologic, psychotherapic, physiotherapic or pharmacologic.

III.4.2.1.1. Physiological Darkness Therapies:

Darkness therapy per se and chromatotherapy

III.4.2.1.1.1. Darkness Therapy Per Se

Light deprivation may be obtained by placing the patient in a closed room, in a totally dark environment, with an eye mask on. This **genuine darkness therapy** may be used in acute indications, but should be of short duration. It is not compatible with any activity and is frequently associated with induction of bed rest, inactivity and sleep [13, 98].

Relative darkness therapy may be obtained by wearing dark goggles or dark sun glasses but the number of lux passing through is not negligible. This relative darkness therapy may be used as an accessory treatment in the restoration of a light dark schedule: a transition before a totally dark environment [98, 259].

III.4.2.1.1.2. Chromatotherapy

The diurnal forms of asthma may be benefit from a 4-min exposure of the chest once a week to yellow wavelength, the complementary color of purple indicated in the treatment of asthma with HBC. It must be followed by 20 minutes of darkness. Chromatotherapy on acupuncture points would be even more efficient. This method, although successfully used in practice, has not been validated yet [7, 8, 98-102, 104].

III.4.2.1.2. Psychotherapeutic Darkness Therapies

Asthma education programs are important (cf. III.2.3.). Cognitive behavioral strategies have been efficient for the treatment of photosensitivity. The treatment was to gradually increase exposure to computer monitor and television screen photostimulation. This desensitization procedure resulted in a complete removal of the patient's phobic anxiety from photostimulation and of avoidant behavior. This behavioral therapy has been used in photo-sensitive epilepsy and in migraine [204, 252]. Psychological therapies of migraine in childhood, such as relaxation training and biofeedback, were potentially superior to pharmacological treatment [153, 316].

III.4.2.1.3. Physiotherapic Darkness Therapy

Magnetic fields may be used to stimulate the BC in a variety of ways to treatment using very weak (picotesla), extremely low frequency (2 to 7 Hz) electromagnetic fields. Transcranial treatment with alternative currents pulsed electromagnetic fields of picotesla flux density may stimulate various brain areas (hypothalamus particularly) and the pineal gland (which functions as a magneto-receptor). Clinical studies showed an improvement in both FEV1, PEF and other variables of lung function by pulsatile electromagnetic fields in both asthma children and in adults with asthma or COPD [295, 296].

III.4.2.1.4. Pharmacological Darkness Therapy

Three agents may stimulate the BC: magnesium, L-tryptophan and taurine but their efficiency seems limited.

III.4.2.1.4.1. Magnesium Treatment for Obstructive Disorders: A Reappraisal

As previously reported in this paper, two different types of magnesium therapy must be distinguished: nutritional physiological oral magnesium supplementation (cf III.3) and pharmacological magnesium therapy. Their nature and action are basically different. It is a real scientific fraud and an ethical misconduct to fail to differentiate between the safety of a nutritional physiological oral magnesium supplementation and the potentially dangerous effects of high pharmacological doses [90, 91, 95]. But this basic distinction between the two types of magnesium treatments is too often overlooked in papers on magnesium therapy. To discriminate between the two types of magnesium therapy it is necessary to kept in mind that the only indication for nutritional magnesium therapy is the disorder related to **magnesium deficiency** *i.e* to an insufficient magnesium intake, whereas pharmacological magnesium therapy is indicated whatever the magnesium status.

III.4.2.1.4.1.1. Pharmacological Magnesium Therapy

Pharmacodynamic effects of pharmacological magnesium therapy in obstructive pulmonary disorders are mainly **bronchodilatation** and antiinflammatory properties. In order to use the pharmacological properties of magnesium, *whatever the magnesium status*, it is necessary to over pass the magnesium homeostasis mechanisms and to induce a therapeutic magnesium overload *i.e.* a genuine iatrogenic hypermagnesemia. The parenteral route is suitable for acute applications whereas large doses of magnesium orally given are advisable for chronic indications. Both types of pharmacological magnesium treatments may induce magnesium toxicity [90, 91, 95, 102]. Early signs of Mg toxicity during intravenous treatment include vomiting, nausea, feeling of warmth, flushing, hypotension, bradycardia and other cardiac arrythmias, somnolence, double vision, slurred speech and weakness [303]. These side effects usually occur at total plasma Mg of 3.5-5 mmol/l. Hyporeflexia (loss of patella reflex), muscular paralysis, respiratory or cardiac arrest develop only at extremely high plasma Mg concentration (5-15 mmol/l). Magnesium toxicity is exaggerated in presence of hypocalcemia, hyperkalemia and uremia [303].

Indications for pharmacological magnesium therapy are of 3 types including **purely pharmacodynamic**, **etiopathogenic** [in three particular situations *i.e.* emergency, necessity (when the oral form is impossible) and sometimes after failure of nutritional oral physiological therapy] and **mixed** when the pharmacological magnesium treatment combines its useful *pharmacodynamic* effects and a *etiopathogenic* treatment for magnesium deficiency [90, 91, 95].

Obstructive pulmonary diseases *per se* constitute pure pharmacodynamic indications of pharmacological magnesium therapy, irrespective to the magnesium status. But their frequent association with concomitant primary magnesium deficiency [41, 90, 97, 102, 157, 294] constitutes a mixed indication of magnesium pharmacological treatment. The **efficiency** of such pharmacological magnesium therapy **is dubious,** the results being conflicting and sometimes negative [34, 36, 45, 59, 72, 88, 142, 144, 151, 170, 218, 254, 256, 279, 282, 305, 325].

III.4.2.1.4.1.2. Use of Magnesium Sulfate in Acute Asthma

A. Intravenous administration

The initial clinical use of intravenous $MgSO_4$ in bronchial asthma, in 1936, by Rosello and Pla [291] relieved dyspnea and stridor in an asthmatic patient. Subsequent observations (cf above) led to progressive partial disinterest [303]. In the last decade, the potential role of IV Mg in acute asthma has gained renewed interest [34, 65, 81, 256, 312, 313, 314]. The main effects of magnesium sulfate include decrease in airway resistance, increase in FEV1, increased in forced vital capacity and decrease in dyspnea and respiratory frequency [81, 249, 254, 256, 311, 319, 302]. There have been a number of case reports and uncontrolled studies indicating its effectiveness in relieving bronchospasm [34, 45, 64, 65, 81, 131, 195, 256, 282, 306, 312, 313, 314, 319, 344]. Generally, magnesium sulfate is administered intravenously to patients either children or adults with severe exacerbations of asthma. An intravenous administration of 2 g magnesium sulphate, as an adjunct to standard therapy, led to a significant improvement in pulmonary function [47]. However, recent controlled clinical trials have nor agreed on its efficacy [34, 36, 142, 254, 344]. Nevertheless, it seems in FEV_1 did not significantly improved in the moderate-group (FEV_1 >25% on presentation) of patients receiving as an adjunct to standardized emergency procedure 2 g of $MgSO_4$. In contrast, in the severe group (FEV_1 <25% on admission), there was a significant improvement in FEV_1 at 120 and 204 min and a decrease admission rate as compared to the placebo-treated group [34, 293].

In any case, this mode of administration requires careful monitoring for prevention of local and mainly systemic symptoms of magnesium overload, since peripheral vasodilatation and systolic hypotension can occur and patients sometimes have unpleasant flushing, nausea, and venous phlebitis from the infusion [94, 96, 98, 11, 161].

Monitoring of pulse, arterial pressure, deep tendon reflexes, hourly diuresis, electrocardiogram and respiratory rhythm recording is necessary [34, 36, 45, 72, 94, 96, 98, 101, 142, 144, 150, 151, 170, 254, 257, 311, 319, 325].

The possible role of the **anion** SO_4^{--} as regards toxicity must be discussed. The selection of a particular magnesium salt among others should take into account reliable pharmacological and toxicological data. It seems necessary to determine **the therapeutic index** (LD50 / ED50) of the various available magnesium salts before any pharmacological use.

Finally, the combination of intravenous relatively high doses of magnesium (pharmacological magnesium therapy) and beta-2 mimetics may be toxic, more often in obstetrical indications than in pulmonary diseases since the doses are clearly lower in pulmonary indications. Contra-indications of this latter form of pharmacological magnesium treatment combined with beta-2 mimetics for pulmonary indications are less imperative than for tocolysis [101, 199, 219, 285].

B. Nebulized administration

Eventhough intravenous $MgSO_4$ has been shown to increase the bronchodilating response and to improve lung functions in treatment of severe asthma, however, its effect by the nebulized route is uncertain [161] (table I).

Table I – Pharmacological effects of nebulized magnesium ($MgSO_4$) in obstructive pulmonary disorders [47, 161]

Patients	Response	Reference
Magnesium alone before challenge testing in provocation tests		
Direct stimuli using either histamine or methacholine.	Dose-dependent decrease in bronchial hyperresponsiveness	286, 287
Indirect stimulus using indirect bronchostrictor (sodium metabisulfite)	Dose-dependent decrease in bronchial hyperresponsiveness	246
Provocation test using histamine	No effect **on bronchial hyperresponsiveness**	157
Magnesium alone		
Acute exacerbation of asthma (adults)	Bronchodilatation (magnitude similar in to salbutamol)	218
Acute exacerbation of asthma (children)	Bronchodilatation (magnitude and duration of the effect were less than due to salbutamol)	233
Stable asthma	**No effect** on bronchodilatation	156
Magnesium as an adjunct to nebulized salbutamol or albuterol		
Severe Asthma	Improvement in PEF *vs* salbutamol in isotonic saline*	246
Severe asthma; 30 min after 2-5 mg nebulized salbutamol	Increase in bronchodilator response (twice the increase in FEV_1) *vs* salbutamol in isotonic saline*	161
Mild to Moderate asthma exacerbations	**No benefits** *vs* salbutamol therapy alone	31, 305

*according to Kurtaran et al. [196] nebulized saline is not a placebo since it may trigger asthma [15, 307]

Beta-2-mimetic and magnesium therapies have common pulmonary indications. The specific beta-2-agonists represent the priority treatment. Combination with corticosteroids is useful and efficient. Other associated treatments failed to demonstrate their efficiency as adjunctive treatments but magnesium use may be of interest. Indeed, the possible additive bronchodilating effects of magnesium and salbutamol has shown that a mild sustained increase in serum magnesium concentration caused a significant leftward shift of the dose response curve to inhaled salbutamol in asthmatic patients, with no change in the maximum response. This finding suggests that magnesium increased beta2-receptor affinity [47].

When isotonic magnesium sulfate was used as a vehicle for nebulized salbutamol for patients with acute asthma, it increases the peak flow response to treatment in comparison with salbutamol plus normal saline in severe asthma [161, 246] but failed in mild to moderate asthma exacerbations [31]. It seems that bronchodilator effectiveness of adjuvant Mg is seen in life-threatening, rather than less severe exacerbations of asthma [34]. The increase in peak expiratory flow (PEF) is inversely related to the baseline value, which supports the observation that magnesium is particularly effective in the most severe asthma exacerbations [314]. However, nebulized saline used as a vehicle for salbutamol is not a placebo since it may trigger asthma [15, 196, 307].

Nebulisation of three 2.5 mg doses of salbutamol at 30 min intervals is within the therapeutic range recommended for treatment of severe asthma in emergency department. They can be mixed with 2.5 mL isotonic magnesium sulphate [161].

Inhaled magnesium seems well tolerated [59, 218, 282]. However, according to Hughes et al. [282] most crucial in terms of use of magnesium as an adjuvant was its formulation as an isotonic solution (250 mmol/L, resulting in a tonicity of 289 mosmol). Both hypotonic and hypertonic nebulizer solutions cause bronchostriction in patients with asthma.

III.4.2.1.4.1.3. Oral Administration of Magnesium in Stable Asthma

Long term Mg repletion may be achieved by the daily administration of 300-600 mg of Mg orally [1, 25]. A randomized, double blind placebo-controlled, prospective study showed that long lasting Mg supplementation (200 mg in children < 7 years old and 290 mg magnesium citrate in older children) is clearly benefit (lower requirement of short term inhaled beta-2 mimetics, higher FIV_1) in mild-moderate asthmatic children and is recommended as a concomitant drug in stable asthma [25]. Similarly, a daily magnesium intake of 400 mg/day can improve clinical symptoms in adults [158].

Beta-2 mimetics and palliating **nutritional magnesium** therapies may be associated in the COPD treatment. This combination may be beneficial and remains atoxic. In asthmatic patients, the coexistence of other clinical manifestations of magnesium deficiency such as neuromuscular hyperexcitability must be investigated: Chvostek sign click, iterative EMG tracings, idiopathic mitral valve prolapse. But the dynamic oral physiological magnesium load test (5mg/kg/day) constitutes the best evidence of magnesium deficiency [41, 42, 90, 91, 94, 95, 97, 101, 157, 158, 294].

III.4.2.1.4.2. *L Tryptophan* or 5-OH Tryptophan

L tryptophan or 5-OH tryptophan may stimulate the tryptophan pathway but they are unspecific as they do not only concern melatonin production but also serotonin synthesis. They may induce toxicity: eosinophilia-myalgia syndrome particularly [1, 98-102, 231, 328].

III.4.2.1.4.3. *Taurine*

Taurine is a sulfonated aminoacid which is present in the whole body in high concentration, mainly in the brain. It is the most abundant free aminoacid in many tissues mainly in proinflammatory cells such as polymorphonuclear leukocytes and tissues exposed to elevated levels of oxidants [326]. It has multiple function in cell homeostasis such as membrane stabilization, buffering, osmoregulation and antioxidant activities together with effects on neurotransmitter release and receptor modulation. Taurine may act as a protective inhibitory neuromodulator which participates in the functional quality of the neural apparatus and in melatonin production and action. Taurine plays a role in the maintenance of homeostasis in the central nervous system, during central nervous hyperexcitability particularly. This volume-regulating aminoacid is released upon excitotoxicity induced cell swelling. It has an established function as an osmolyte in the central nervous system. In the course of Mg deficit, the organism appears to stimulate taurine mobilization to play a role of a "magnesium vicariant agent". But this compensatory action is rather limited [94-100, 102, 163, 200, 212, 266]. In addition, taurine either intracellularly or released into the extracellular medium, may protect cells against attack by oxidants either directly or via the formation of its chlorinated derivatives taurine-chloramine [69, 326]. It decreases the release of inflammatory mediators by neutrophils and macrophages and modulate T-cell activation *in vitro* [220, 345]. It reduces *in vivo* lung oxidant damages induced by a number of chemicals including ozone, nitrogen dioxide, paraquat, amiodarone and bleomycin [69]. At a daily oral dose of 1-3 mmol/Kg for 7 days before challenge, taurine did not reduce the bronchospasm produced by antigen challenge in an experimental model of asthma using sensitized Brown-Norway rats, but it prevented airway hyperreactivity, reduced the number of eosinophils and of lipid hydroperoxides and prevented dye extravasation in bronchoalveolar fluid [69]. This means that taurine, in addition to reducing the number of inflammatory cells, may lessen the oxidant burden by diminishing the generation by these cells of superoxide anion and other cytotoxic mediators [69]. Finally, taurine levels in bronchoalveolar fluid from antigen-challenged rats were higher than control values but treatment with taurine fails to further increase this levels [69]. This is of importance, since taurine levels in bronchoalveolar lavage fluid and airway secretions were increased in asthma patients [159]. The same results were obtained while replacing taurine by a daily dose of the antioxidant N-acetylcysteine (1 mmol/Kg for 7 days) [33].

III.4.2.2. "Substitutive Darkness Therapy" or Darkness Mimicking Agents

Because of the limited efficiency of the previous chemical agents, palliative treatments of hBC may be necessary.

III.4.2.2.1. Mechanisms of the Action of Darkness

The mechanisms of action of the darkness appear as the reverse of those obtained with bright light where direct cellular and neural effects intervene. Increased melatonin production is the best marker of darkness but it is only an accessory mechanism in the darkness effect. The main central neural mechanisms of darkness therapy associate decreased serotoninergy together with stimulation of the inhibitory neuromodulators (GABA, taurine) and stimulation of anti-inflammatory and anti-oxidative processes, which may lead to neural hypoexcitability (sedative and anticonvulsant). Humoral transduction may reinforce these last effects by decreasing neuroactive gases (CO and NO) through binding of CO with haemoglobin and by increasing melatonin, bilirubin and biliverdin, three antioxidants which have the capacity to quench NO. Apart from the exception of decreased serotoninergy, these effects of darkness are similar to those of magnesium.

Substitutive darkness therapy should palliate all the mechanisms of the action of darkness. The only available darkness mimicking agents are melatonin (its analogous and its precursors, L-tryptophan, 5-hydroxytryptophan) [98, 102].

III.4.2.2.2. Melatonin, an Accessory Darkness Mimicking Agent

Melatonin is the prototype of darkness mimicking agents. But, although the production of melatonin is the best marker of photoperiod, it appears to be only an accessory factor among the mechanisms of photoperiod actions. Most of the other mechanisms of the effects of darkness have been overlooked, which may account for the controversy around the therapeutic efficiency of MT. Its dosage varies from physiological doses (around 0,3 mg) to pharmacological doses: usually 3 mg/per dose and per day and even up to 300 mg as a contraceptive (testifying to the weak toxicity of the hormone). In case of chronopathology, with decreased MT production, MT constitutes a substitutive treatment of its deficiency [43, 68, 98, 99, 102, 348, 367, 368, 371]. Melatonin (3 mg for 4 weeks) was shown to improve subjective sleep quality in asthma whereas it did not induce significant difference in asthma symptoms [57]. Further studies looking into long-term effects of melatonin on airway inflammation and bronchial hyperresponsiveness are needed before melatonin can be recommended in patients with asthma [57]. Our paper indicates that it would be at least avoided in asthma forms with HBC.

Conclusion

Asthma prevalence and severity are increasing over the world besides effective treatments and may led in some cases to fatal death. Many factors may interact in the physiopathology of the disease and contribute to the severity of asthma. Nocturnal asthma seem very frequent and represent a severe form of asthma leading to the idea that asthma is chronopathological.

We recently suggested that various pathologies, including asthma would be linked to a magnesium depletion with chronopathological dysfunction of the BC either HBC or hBC. These forms are characterized mainly by variations of their biological marker, melatonin and by well identified clinical symptoms of either hypo- or hyper-nervous excitability respectively. This led us to suggest the measurement of plasma or salivary melatonin and plasma or erythrocyte magnesium levels in asthma patients. This would allow first to identify the possible presence of a chronopathological form of asthma thus justifying, in addition to conventional treatments, a complementary beneficial treatment including a balanced magnesium intake and either phototherapies or darkness therapies in asthma with either HBC or hBC.

References

[1] Abbott, L.G., Rude, R.K. (1993) Clinical manifestations of magnesium deficiency. *Miner. Electrolyte Metab.,19,* 314-22.

[2] Abramson, M.J., Bayley, M.J., Couper, F.J., Driver, J.S., Drummer, O.H., Forbes, A.B., McNeill, J.J., and Haydn Walters, E. (2001) The Victorian Asthma Mortality Study Group. Are asthma medications and management related to deaths from asthma? *Am. J. Resp. Crit. Care Med., 163*, 12-18.

[3] Acuña-Castroviejo, D., Escames, G., Muñoz, M.M., Hoyos, A., Molina Carballo, A., Arauzo, M., Montes, R. and Vives, F. (1995) Cell protective role of melatonin in the brain. *J. Pineal. Res., 19*, 57-63.

[4] Adams, R.J., Wilson, D.H., Taylor, A.W., Daly, A., Tursan d'Espaignet, E., Dal Grande E. and Ruffin, R.E. (2004) Psychological factors and quality of life: a population based study. *Thorax, 59*, 930-935.

[5] Afari, N., Schmaling, K.B., Barnhart, S. and Buchwald, D. (2001) Psychiatric comorbidity and functional status in adult patients with asthma. *J. Clin. Psychol. Med., 8*, 245-252.

[6] Agati, G. and McDonagh, A.F. (1995) Chiroptical switch based on photoisomerization on bilirubin-like bound to human serum albumin. *J. Am. Chem. Soc., 117*, 4425-4426.

[7] Agrapart C and Agrapart-Delmas, M. (1989) Guide thérapeutique des couleurs. Dangles ed., St Jean de Braye, France.

[8] Agrapart, C. Oligoéléments et couleurs. Guide pratique de Chromatothérapie*. Sully ed. 2000

[9] Ahlquist R.P. (1948) A study of adrenotropic receptors. *Am. J. Physiol., 153*, 586-600.

[10] Ahmed M., Hanaoka Y., Nagatomo T., Kiso T., Kurose H., Nagao T. (2003) Binding and functional activity of some newly synthetised phenethylamine and phenoxypropanolamine derivatives for their agonistic activity at recombinent human beta-3-adrenoreceptor. *J. Pharm. Pharmacol., 51*: 95-101.

[11] Alamoudi, O.S.B. (2000) Hypomagnesemia in chronic stable asthmatics: prevalence, correlation with severity and hospitalization. *Eur. Resp. J., 16*, 427-431.

[12] Alamoudi, O.S.B. (2001) Electrolytes disturbances in patients with chronic stable asthma. *Chest, 120*, 431-436.

[13] Allen, C., Glasziou, P. and Del Mar, C. (1999) Bed rest: a potentially harmful treatment needing more careful evaluation. *Lancet, 354*, 1229-1233.

[14] Amantea SL, Sanchez I, Piva JP and Garcia PC. (2002) Controversies in the pharmacological management of acute asthma in children. *J. Pediatr. (Rio J), 78 Suppl 2*, S151-60.

[15] Anderson, S.D., Schoeffel, R.E. and Finney, M. (1983) Evaluation of ultrasonically nebulised solutions for provocation testing in patients with asthma. *Thorax, 38*, 284-291.

[16] Arnouts, P.J., Colemont, L.J., van Outryve, M.J. and van Moer, E.M. (1991) L-Tryptophan-induced eosinophilia-myalgia syndrome. *J. Intern. Med., 230,* 83-86.

[17] Baker, J.C., Tunnicliffe W.S., Duncanson, R.C. and Ayres, J.G. (1999) Dietary antioxidants and magnesium in type 1 brittleasthma: a case control study. *Thorax, 54*, 115-118.

[18] Baker, J.C., Ayres, J.G. (2000) Diet and asthma. *Respir. Med., 94*, 925-934.

[19] Barnes, P.J. (1977) A new approach to the treatment of asthma. *N. Engl. J. Med., 297*, 476-482.

[20] Barnes, P., Fitzgerald, G., Brown, M. and Dollery, C. (1980) Nocturnal asthma and changes in circulating epinephrine, histamine, and cortisol. *N. Engl. J. Med., 303*, 263–267.

[21] Barriga, C., Martin, M.I., Tabla, E., Ortega, E. and Rodriguez, A.B. (2001) Circadian rhtythm of melatonin, corticosterone and phagocytosis: effect of stress. *J. Pineal Res., 30*, 180-187.

[22] Bates, M.E., Clayton, M., Calhoun, W., Jarjour, N., Schrader., L, Geiger., K, Schultz, T., Sedgwick, J., Swenson, C. and Busse, W. (1994) Relationship of plasma epinephrine and circulating eosinophils to nocturnal asthma. *Am. J. Respir. Crit. Care Med., 149*, 667–672.

[23] Beasley, R., Burgess, C., Pearce, N., Woodman, K. and Crane, J. (1994) Confounding by severity does not explain the association between fenoterol and asthma death. *Clin. Exp. Allergy, 24,* 660-668.

[24] Beasley, R., Pearce, N., Crane, J. and Burgess, C. (1999) Beta agonists: what is the evidence that their use increases the risk of asthma morbidity and mortality? *J. Allergy Clin. Immunol.,104*, S18-S30.

[25] Bede, O., Surany, A., Slavik, M. and Gyurkovits, K. (2003) Urinary magnesium excretion in asthmatic children receiving magnesium supplementation: a randomized, placebo-controlled, double-blind study. *Magnes. Res., 16,* 262-270.

[26] Bednarek, A., Pasternak, K., Karsha, M. (2003) Evaluation of blood serum, erythrocyte and urine magnesium concentrations in babies with pneumonia or bronchial obstructive bronchitis. *Magnes. Res., 16,* 271-280.

[27] Bellia, V., Catalano, F., Scichilone, N., Incalzi, R.A., Spatafora, M., Vergani and C., Rengo, F. (2003) Sleep disorders in the elderly with and without chronic airflow obstruction: the SARA study. *Sleep, 26,* 318-323.

[28] Bender, B.G. and Annett, R.D. (1999) Neuropsychological outcomes of nocturnal asthma. *Chronobiol. Int., 16*, 695-710.

[29] Bennett, A. and Tattersfield, A.E. (1997) Time course and relative dose potency of systemic effects from salmeterol and salbutamol in healthy subjects *Thorax,* 52, 458-464.

[30] Bergholtz, B. (1989) Nocturnal asthma. Causes and treatment. *Tidsskr Nor Laegeforen.,109*, 17961-17967.

[31] Bessmertny, O., DiGregorio, R.V., Cohen, H., Becker, E., Looney, D., Golden, J., Kohl, L. and Johnson, T. (2002) A randomized clinical trial of nebulized magnesium sulfate in addition to albuterol in the treatment of acute mild-to-moderate asthma exacerbations in adults. *Ann. Emerg. Med., 39*, 585-591.

[32] Bielory, L., Chiaramonte, L., Ehrlich, P. and Field, J. (2003) Alternative treatment for allergy and asthma. *J. Asthma, 40,* 47-53.

[33] Blesa, S., Cortijo, J., Martinez-Losa, M., Mata, M., Seda, E., Santangelo, F. and Morcillo, E.J. (2002) Effectiveness of oral N -acetylcysteine in a rat experimental model of asthma. *Pharmacol. Res., 45*, 135-140.

[34] Bloch, H., Silverman, R., Mancherje, N., Grant, S., Jagminas, L. and Scharf, S.M. (1995) Intravenous magnesium sulphate as an adjunct in the treatment of acute asthma. *Chest, 107*, 1576-1581.

[35] Bohadana, A.B., Hannhart, B. and Teculescu, D.B. (2002) Nocturnal worsening of asthma and sleep disorders breathing. *J. Asthma, 39*, 85-100.

[36] Boonyavorakul, C., Thakkinstian, A. and Charoenpan, P. (2000) Intravenous $MgSO_4$ in acute severe asthma. *Respirology*, 5, 221-225.

[37] Bos, W.J.W., Postma, D.S. and Van Doormaal, J.J. (1988) Magnesiuric and calcium effects of terbutaline in man. *Clin Sci* (Lond), 74, 595-597.

[38] Bremme, K., Eneroth, P., Nordström, L. and Nilsson, B. (1986) Effects of infusion of the beta-adrenoreceptor agonist terbutaline on serum Mg in pregnant women. *Magnesium*, *5*, 85-94.

[39] Brenner, B.E., Chavda, K.K., Karakurum, M.B., Karras, D.J. and Camargo, C.A. (2001) Circadian differences among 4,096 emergency department patients with acute asthma. *Crit. Care Med. 29*, 1124-1129.

[40] British Thoracic Society (2003) Guidelines of the management of asthma: management of acute asthma. *Thorax, 58*, i32-i50.

[41] Britton J. Dietary magnesium, lung function, wheezing and airway hyperreactivity in a random population sample. *Lancet* 1994; 344: 357-362.

[42] Britton, J.R., Pavord, I.D., Richards, K.A., Wisniewski, A.F., Knox, A.J., Lewis, S.A., Tattersfield, A.E. and Weiss, S.T. (1994) Dietary magnesium, lung function, wheezing, and airway hyperreactivity in a random adult population sample. *Lancet, 344*, 357-362.

[43] Brown, G.M. (1995) Melatonin in psychiatric and sleep disorders. Therapeutic implications. *CNS Drugs, 3*, 209-226.

[44] Brown, E.S., Khan, D.A. and Maleaedi, S. (2000) Psychiatric diagnosis in inner-city outpatients with moderate to severe asthma. *Int. J. Psychiatry Med., 30*, 319-327.

[45] Brunner, E.H., Delabroise, A.M. and Haddad, J.H. (1985) Effect of parenteral magnesium on pulmonary function, plasma cAMP, and histamine in bronchial asthma. *J. Asthma, 23*, 3-11,

[46] Bubenik, G.A., Blask, D.E., Brown, G.M., Maestroni, G.J.M., Pang, S.F., Reiter, R.J., Visvanathan, M. and Zisapel, N. (1998) Prospects of the clinical utilization of melatonin. *Biol. Signals Recept., 7*, 195-219.

[47] Bucca, C. and Rolla, G. (2003) Nebulised salbutamol in asthma: the right solution for an old remedy? *Lancet, 361*, 9375, 2095-2096.

[48] Burney, P.G.J., Chinn, S. and Rhona, R.J. (1990) Has the prevalence of asthma increased in children? Evidence from the national study of health and growth. *B.M.J., 300*, 1306-1310.

[49] Bussing, R., Burket, R.C. and Kelleher, E.T. (1996) Prevalence of anxiety disorders in a clinic-based sample of pediatric asthma patients. *Psychosomatics, 37*, 108-115.

[50] Butland, B.K., Fehily, A.M. and Elwood, P.C. (2000) Diet, lung function and lung function decline in a cohort of 2512 middle aged men. *Thorax, 55,* 102-108,

[51] Caccappolo-Van Vliet, E., Kelly-McNeil, K., Natelson, B., Kipen, H. and Fiedler, N. (2002) Anxiety sensitivity and depression in multiple chemical sensitivities and asthma. *J. Occup. Environ. Med., 44*, 890-901.

[52] Cairns, C.B. and Kraft, M. (1996) Magnesium attenuates the neutrophil respiratory burst in adult asthmatic patients. *Acad. Emerg. Med., 3*, 1093-1097.

[53] Calhoun, W.J. (1999) Asthma entities. *Drugs Today, 35*, 595-603.

[54] Calhoun, W.J. (2003) Nocturnal asthma. *Chest, 123*, 399S-405S.

[55] Calhoun, WJ, Bates, ME, Schrader, L, Sedgwick, JB and Busse, WW. (1992) Characteristics of peripheral blood eosinophils in patients with nocturnal asthma. *Am. Rev. Respir. Dis., 145*, 577–581.

[56] Calvo, J.R., Guerrero, J.M., Osuna, C., Molinero, P. and Carrillo-Vico, A. (2002) Melatonin triggers Crohn's disease symptoms. *J. Pineal Res., 32*, 277-278.

[57] Campos, F.L., da Silva-Junior F.P., de Bruin, P.F. (2004) Melatonin improves sleep in asthma: a randomized, double-blind, placebo-controlled study. *Am. J. Respir. Crit. Care Med., 170*, 947-951.

[58] Carr, R.E., Lehrer, P.M., Rausch, L.L. and Hochron, S.M. (1994) Anxiety sensitivity and panic attacks in an asthmatic population. *Behav. Res. Ther., 32*, 411-418.

[59] Chande, V.T. and Skoner, D.P. (1992) A trial of nebulized MgSO4 to reverse bronchospasm in asthmatic patients. *Ann. Emerg. Med., 21*, 1111-1115.

[60] Chen, TC and Leviton, A. (1990) Asthma and eczema in children born to women with migraine. *Arch. Neurol., 47*, 1227-1230.

[61] Chen, L.D., Tan, D.X., Reiter, R.J., Poeggeler, B., Kumar, P., Manchester, L.C. and Chambers, J.P. (1993) *In vivo* and *in vitro* effects of the pineal gland and melatonin on Ca and Mg-dependent ATP-ase in cardiac sarcolemna. *J. Pineal Res., 14*, 178-183.

[62] Chewin, R.D., Zalleck, S.N., Lin, X., Hall, J.M., Sharma, N. and Hedjer, K.M. (2000) Timing pattern of cluster headaches and association with symptoms of obstructive sleep apnea. *Sleep Res. Online, 3*, 107-112.

[63] Chrousos, G.P. and Harris, A.G. (1998) Hypothalamic-pituitary-adrenal axis suppression and inhaled corticosteroid therapy. *Neuro Immuno Modulation, 5,* 288-308.

[64] Ciarallo, L., Brousseau, D. and Reinert, S. (2000) Higher-dose intravenous magnesium therapy for children with moderate to severe asthma. *Arch. Pediatr. Adolesc. Med., 154*, 979-983.

[65] Ciarallo, L., Sauer, A.H. and Shanon, M.W. (1996) Intravenous magnesium therapy for moderate to severe pediatric asthma: results of a randomized placebo-controlled trial. *J. Pediatr., 129*, 809-814.

[66] Clark, T.J. and Hetzel, M.R. (1977) Diurnal variation of asthma. *Br. J. Dis. Chest, 71*, 87-92.

[67] Clark, T.J. (1987) Diurnal rhythm of asthma. *Chest, 91 (6 Suppl)*, 137S-141S.

[68] Copinski, G., Van Reeth, D and Van Cauter, E. (1999c) Etudes du vieillissement et de la desynchronisation entre la rythmicité endogène et les conditions d'environnement. *Presse Méd., 28,* 942-946.

[69] Cortijo, J., Blesa, S., Martinez-Losa, M., Mata, M., Seda, E., Santangelo, F. and Morcillo, E.J. (2001) Effects of taurine on pulmonary responses to antigen in sensitized Brown-Norway rats. *Eur. J. Pharmacol., 431*, 111-117.

[70] Crighton, E.J., Mamdani, M.M. and Upshur, R.E. (2001) A population based time series analysis of asthma hospitalizations in Ontario, Canada: 1988 to 2000. *B.M.C. Health Serv. Res., 1,* 7-13.

[71] Currie, G.P., Lee, D.K.C., Dempsey, O.J., Fowler, S.J., Cowan, L.M. and Lipworth, B.J. (2003) A proof of concept study to evaluate putative benefits of montelukast in moderate persistent asthmatics. *Brit. J. Clin. Pharmacol., 55*, 609-615.

[72] Cydulka, R.K. (1996) Why magnesium for asthma? *Acad. Emerg. Med., 3*, 1084-1085.

[73] Czaba, G. and Bokay, J. (1977) The effects of melatonin and corpus pineal extract on serum electrolytes in the rat. *Acta Biol. Acad. Sci. Hung., 28*, 143-144.

[74] D'Angelo, E.K., Singer, H.A. and Rembold, C.M. (1992) Magnesium relaxes arterial smooth muscle by decreasing intracellular Ca^{2+} without changing intracellular Mg^{2+}. *J. Clin. Invest., 89*, 1988-1994.

[75] Davey, G., Sedwick, P., Maier, W., Visick, G., Strachan, D.P. and Anderson, H.R. (2002) Association between migraine and asthma: matched case-control. *Br. J. Gen. Pract., 52*, 723-727.

[76] Davis, T.M., Ross, C.J. and Mac Donald, G.F. (2002) Screening and assessing adult asthmatics for anxiety disorders. *Clin. Nurs. Res., 11*, 173-189.

[77] De Souza Carvalho, D., Fragoso, YD, Coelho, FM and Pereira, MM. (2002) Asthma plus migraine in childhood and adolescence: prophylactic benefits with leukotriene receptor antagonist. *Headache, 42,* 1044-1047.

[78] de Walk, H.W., Kok, P.T.M., Struyvenberg, A., Van Rijn, H.J.M., Halboom, J.R.E., Kreukniet, J. and Lammers, J.W.J. (1993) Extracellular and intracellular magnesium concentrations in asthmatic patients. *Eur. Respir. J., 6*, 1122-1125.

[79] Del Castillo, J. and Engbaek, L. (1954) The nature of the neuromuscular block produced by magnesium. *J. Physiol., 124*, 370-384.

[80] Demisch, L., Demisch, K. and Nickelsen T. (1987) Influence of dexamethasone on nocturnal melatonin production in healthy adult subjects. *J Pineal Res*, *5*, 317–322.

[81] Devi, P.R., Kumar, L., Singh, S.C., Prasad, R. and Singh, M. (1997) Intravenous magnesium sulphate in acute sever asthma not responding to conventional therapy. *Indian Pediatr., 34*, 389-397.

[82] Dewar, J.C., Wilkinson, J., Wheatley, A., Thomas, N.S., Doull, I., Morton, N., Lio, P., Harvey, J.F., Liggett, S.B., Holgate, S.T. and Hall, I.P. (1997) The glutamine 27 beta2-adrenoceptor polymorphism is associated with elevated IgE levels in asthmatic families. *J. Allergy Clin. Immunol., 100*, 261-265.

[83] Dahlen, S.E., Malmstrom, K., Nizankowska, E., Dahlen, B., Kuna, P., Kowalski, M., Lumry, W.R., Picado, C., Stevenson, D.D., Bousquet, J., Pauwels, R., Holgate, S.T., Shahane, A., Zhang, J., Reiss, T.F. and Szczeklik, A. (2002) Improvement of aspirin-intolerant asthma by montelukast, a leukotriene antagonist: a randomized, double-blind, placebo-controlled trial. *Am. J. Respir. Crit. Care Med., 165*, 9-14.

[84] Dhingra, S., Solven, F., Wilson, A. and McCarthy, D. (1984) Hypomagnesemia and respiratory muscle power. *Am. Rev. Respir. Dis., 129*, 497-498.

[85] Dominguez, L.J., Barbagallo, M. and Di Lorenzo, G. (1998) Bronchial reactivity and intracellular magnesium: a possible mechanism for the bronchodilating effects of magnesium in asthma. *Clin. Sci., 95*, 137-142.

[86] Duffy, D .L., Mitchell, C.A. and Martin N. G. (1998) Genetics and environmental risk factors for asthma. *Am. J. Respir. Crit. Care Med., 157*, 840-845.

[87] Dunnett, J. and Nayler, W.G. (1978) Calcium efflux from cardiac reticulum: Effects of Ca and Mg. *J. Molec. Cell Cardiol., 10,* 487-498.

[88] Durlach J. (1975) Rapports expérimentaux et cliniques entre magnésium et hypersensibilité. *Rev. Franç. Allerg., 15,* 133-146.

[89] Durlach, J., Durlach, V. (1984) Speculations on hormonal controls of magnesium homeostasis: a hypothesis. *Magnesium, 3*, 109-131.

[90] Durlach, J. (1985) Le magnésium en pratique clinique. J.B. Baillère ed. EMI Paris, p. 412.

[91] Durlach, J. (1988) Magnesium in clinical practice, London-Paris John Libbey, pp.369.

[92] Durlach, J., Durlach, V., Rayssiguier, Y., Ricquier, D., Goubern, M., Bertin, R., Bara, M., Guiet-Bara, A., Olive, G. and Mettey, R. (1991) Magnesium and thermoregulation. I. Newborn and infant. Is sudden infant death syndrome a magnesium-dependent disease of the transition from chemical to physical thermoregulation? *Magnes. Res., 4,* 137-152.

[93] Durlach, J. (1992) Chronic fatigue syndrome and chronic primary magnesium deficiency. *Magnes. Res., 5,* 68.

[94] Durlach, J. (1995) Magnesium depletion, magnesium deficiency and asthma. *Magnes. Res., 8*, 403-406.

[95] Durlach, J. and Bara, M. (2000): Le Magnésium en biologie et en médecine, Paris, Tec et Doc ed EMI, Cachan, 403 p. see p.23, 26-28, 37, 44 ; for excessive stimulation of beta mimetics p.27, 198

[96] Durlach, J., Bac, P., Bara, M. and Guiet-Bara, A. (2000) Physiopathology of symptomatic and latent forms of central nervous hyperexcitability due to magnesium deficiency: a current general scheme. *Magnes. Res., 13*, 293-302.

[97] Durlach J. Importance and clinical forms of chronic primary magnesium deficiency in human beings. In: Advances in Magnesium Research Nutrition and Health. *Y. Rayssiguier, A. Mazur, J. Durlach eds* John Libbey Compagny LTD 2001; chapter 2: 13-20.

[98] Durlach, J, Pagès, N., Bac, P., Bara M. and Guiet-Bara A. (2002). Biorhythms and possible central regulation of Mg status, phototherapy, darkness therapy and chronopathological forms of Mg depletion. *Magnes. Res., 15*, 49-66.

[99] Durlach, J., Pagès, N., Bac, P., Bara, M., Guiet-Bara, A. and Agrapart, C. (2002) Chronopathological forms of magnesium depletion with hypofunction or with hyperfunction of the biological clock. *Magnes. Res., 15*, 263-268.

[100] Durlach, J., Pagès, N., Bac, P., Bara, M. and Guiet-Bara, A. (2002) Magnesium deficit and sudden infant death syndrome (SIDS): SIDS due to magnesium deficiency and SIDS due to various forms of magnesium depletion: possible importance of the chronopathological form. *Magnes. Res. 15*, 269-278.

[101] Durlach, J., Pagès, N., Bac, P., Bara, M. and Guiet-Bara, A. (2003) Beta-2 mimetics and magnesium: true or false friends? *Magnes. Res.,16*, 218-233.

[102] Durlach, J., Pagès, N., Bac, P., Guiet-Bara, A. and Bara, M. (2004) Importance of magnesium depletion with hypofunction of the biological clock in the pathophysiology of headaches with photophobia, sudden infant death and some clinical forms of multiple sclerosis. *Magnes. Res., 17*, 314-326.

[103] Eisner, M.D., Lieu, T.A., Chi, F., Capra, A.M., Mendoza, G.R., Selby, J.V. and Blanc, P.D. (2001) Beta agonists, inhaled steroids, and the risk of intensive care unit admission for asthma. *Eur. Respir. J., 2*, 233-240.

[104] Emelyanov, A., Fedoseev, G. and Barnes, P.J. (1999) Reduced intracellular magnesium concentrations in asthmatic patients. *Eur. Respir., 13*, 38-40.

[105] Engst, R. and Vocks, E. (2000) High mountain climatotherapy for dermatological and allergic diseases. Results, Impacts and influence on immunity. *Rehabilitation, 39*, 215-222.

[106] Erickson, R.P. and Graves, P.E. (2004) Genetic variation in beta-adrenergic receptors and their relationship to susceptibility for asthma and therapeutic response. *Drug Metab. Dispos., 29*, 557-561.

[107] Ernst, P., Habbick, B., Suissa, S., Hemmelgarn, B., Cockcroft, D., Buist, A.S., Horwitz, R.I., McNutt M. and Spitzer W.O. (1993) Is the association between inhaled beta agonist use and life threatening asthma because of confounding by severity? *Am. Rev. Respir. Dis.,148*, 75-79.

[108] Escames, G., Acuña-Castroviejo, D., Leon, J.and Vives, F. (1998) Melatonin interaction with Mg and Zn in the response to the striatum to sensitivomotor cortical stimulation in the rat. *J. Pineal Res., 24*, 123-129.

[109] Evsyukova, HV. (1999) The role of melatonin in pathogenesis of aspirine-sensitive asthma. *Eur. J. Clin. Invest., 29*, 563-567.

[110] Falkner, D., Glauser, J. and Allen, M. (1992) Serum Mg levels in asthmatic patients during acute exacerbation of asthma. *Am. J. Emerg. Med.,10,* 1-3.

[111] Fantidis, P., Ruiz Cacho, J., Marin, M., Madera Jarabo, R., Solera, J. and Herrero, E. (1995) Intracellular (polymorphonuclear) magnesium content in patients with bronchial asthma between attacks. *J. R. Soc. Med., 88*, 441-445.

[112] Fauteck, J.D., Bockmann, J., Böckers, T.M., Wittkowski, W., Köhling, R., Lücke, A., Straub, H., Speckmann, E.J., Tuxhorn, L., Wolf, P., Pannek, H. and Oppel, F. (1995) Melatonin reduces low Mg^{2+} epileptiform activity in human temporal slices. *Exp. Brain Res., 107*, 321-325.

[113] Fedyk, E.R., Adawi, A., Looney, R.J. and Phipps, R.P. (1996) Regulation of IgE and cytokine production by cAMP: implications for extrinsic asthma. *Clin. Immunol. Immunopathol., 81*, 101-13.

[114] Fei, G.H., Liu, R.V., Zhang, Z.H. and Zhou, J.N. (2004) Alterations in circadian rhythms of melatonin and cortisol in patients with bronchial asthma. *Acta Pharmacol. Sin., 25*, 651-656.

[115] Finocchiaro, L.M., Nahmod, V.E. and Launay, J.M. (1991) Melatonin biosynthesis and metabolism in peripheral blood mononuclear leukocytes. *Biochem. J., 280*, 727-731.

[116] Fitzpatrick, M.F., Engelman, H., Whyte, K.F., Deary, I.J., Shapiro, C.M. and Douglas, N.J. (1991) Morbidity in nocturnal asthma: sleep quality and daytime cognitive performance. *Thorax, 46*, 569-573.

[117] Freitag, F.G., Diamond, S., Diamond, M.L., Urban, G.J. and Pepper, B.J. (2001) Preventive treatment of migraine headache with rofecoxib and montelukast. *Headache, 12*, 237-239.

[118] Frick, W.E., Sedgwick, J.B. and Busse, W.W. (1989) The appearance of hypodense eosinophils in antigen-dependent late phase asthma. *Am. Rev. Respir. Dis., 139*, 1401–1406.

[119] Furchgott, R.F. and Jothianandan, D. (1991) Endothelium dependent and independent vasodilatation involving cyclic GMP relaxation induced by nitric oxide, carbon monoxide and light. *Blood vessels*, *28,* 52-61.

[120] Gagliardo, R., Vignola, A.M. and Mathieu, M. (2001) Is there a role for glucocorticoid reeceptor B in asthma? *Respir. Res., 2*, 1-4.

[121] Garcia Martinez, J.M. (1999) Severe asthma in pediatrics: treatment of acute crises. *Allergol. Immunopathol., 27*, 53-62.

[122] Garcia-Maurino, S., Gonzalez-Haba, M.G., Calvo, J.R., Rafii-El-Idrissi, M., Sanchez-Margalet, V., Goberna, R. and Guerrero, J.M. (1997) Melatonin enhances IL-2, IL-6, and IFN-γ production by human circulating $CD4^+$ cells: a possible nuclear receptor-mediated mechanism involving T helper type 1 lymphocytes and monocytes. *J. Immunol., 159*, 574–581.

[123] Garcia-Maurino, S., Pozo, D., Carrillo-Vico, A., Calvo, J.R., Guerrero, J.M. (1999) Melatonin activates Th1 lymphocytes by increasing IL-12 production. *Life Sci.,65*, 2143–2150.

[124] Garden, G.M.F. and Ayres J.G. (1993) Psychiatric and social aspects of brittle asthma. *Thorax*, *48*, 501-505.

[125] Garrett, J.E., Lanes, S.F., Kolbe, J. and Rea, H.H. (1996) Risk of severe life threatening asthma and beta agonist type: an example of confounding by severity. *Thorax, 51,*1093-1099.

[126] Gergen, P.J., Mitchell H. and Lynn H. (2002) Understanding the seasonal pattern of childhood asthma: results from the National Cooperative Inner-City Asthma Study (NCICAS). *J. Pediatr., 141*, 631-636.

[127] Georges, G., Bartelson, B.B., Martin, R.J. and Silkoff, P.E. (1999) Circadian variation in exhaled nitric oxide in nocturnal asthma. *J. Asthma., 36*, 467-73.

[128] Giacovazzo, M., Valeri, M., Piazza, A., Torlone, N., Bernoni, R.M., Martelletti, P. and Adorno, D. (1987) Elevated frequency of HLA shared-haplotypes in migraine families. *Headache, 27*, 575-577.

[129] Gilad, E., Wong, H.R., Zingarelli, B., Virag, L., O'Connor, M., Salzman, L. and Szabo, C. (1998) Melatonin inhibits expression of the inducible isoform of nitric oxide synthase in murine macrophages: role of inhibition of NFKB activation. *FASEB J., 12*, 685-693.

[130] Giron-Caro, F., Muñoz-Hoyos, A., Ruz-Cosano, C., Bonillo-Perales, A., Molina-Carballo, A., Escames G., Macias M. and Acuña-Castroviejo D. (2001) Melatonin and β-endorphin changes in children sensitized to olive and grass pollen after treatment with specific immunotherapy. *Int. Arch. Allergy Immunol., 126*, 91-96.

[131] Glover, M.L., Machado, C. and Totapally, B.R. (2002) Magnesium sulfate administered via continuous intravenous infusion in pediatric patients with refractory wheezing. *J. Crit. Care, 17*, 255-258.

[132] Gluck, J.C. (2004) The change of asthma course during pregnancy. *Clin. Rev. Allergy Immunol., 26*, 171-180.

[133] Goethe, J.W., Maljanian, R., Wolf, S., Hernandez, P. and Cabrera, Y. (2001) The impact of depressive symptoms on the functional status of inner-city patients with asthma. *Ann. Allergy Asthma Immunol., 87*, 205-210.

[134] Goldberg, P., Fleming, M.C. and Picard, E.H. (1986) Decreased relapse rate through dietary supplementation with Ca, Mg and vitamin D. *Med. Hypotheses, 21*, 193-200.

[135] Goldney, R.D., Ruffin, R.., Fisher, L.J. and Wilson, D.H. (2003) Asthma symptoms associated with depression and lower quality of life: a population survey. *Med. J. Aust., 178*, 437-441.

[136] Golf, S.W., Enzinger, D., Temme, H., Graef, V., Katz, N., Roka, L., Friemann, E., Lascha, G., Friemann, S., Tross, H. and Morr, H. (1991) Effects of magnesium in theophylline treatment of chronic obstructive lung disease. In: B. Lasserrc and J. Durlach eds *Mg: a relevant ion.* (John Libbey publ., London): p 443-451.

[137] Goodwin, R.D. and Pine, D.S. (2002) Respiratory disease and panic attacks among adults in the United States. *Chest., 122*, 645-650.

[138] Goodwin, R.D. and Pine, D.S., Hoven C.W. (2003) Asthma and panic attacks among youth. *J Asthma., 40*, 139-145.

[139] Goodwin, R.D. (2003)Asthma and anxiety disorders. *Adv. Psychosom. Med., 24*, 51-71.

[140] Goodwin, R.D., Jacobi F., Thefeld W. (2003) Mental disorders and asthma in the community. *Arch. Gen. Psychiatry, 60*, 1125-1130.

[141] Goubern, M., Rayssiguier, Y., Miroux, B. Chapey, M.F., Ricquier, D. and Durlach, J. (1993) Effect of acute magnesium deficiency on the masking and unmasking of the proton channel of the uncoupling protein in rat brown fat. *Magnes Res., 6*, 135-143.

[142] Green, S.M. and Rothrock, S.G. (1992) Intravenous magnesium for acute asthma: failure to decrease emergency treatment duration or need for hospitalization. *Ann. Emerg. Med., 21*, 260-265.

[143] Green, S.A., Turki, J., Innis, M. and Liggett, S.B. (1994) Amino-terminal polymorphisms of the human beta 2-adrenergic receptor impart distinct agonist-promoted regulatory properties. *Biochemistry, 33*, 9414-9419.

[144] Gürkan, F., Haspolat, K., Bosnak, M., Dikici, B., Derman, O. and Ece, A. (1999) Intravenous $MgSO_4$ in the management of moderate to severe acute asthmatic children non responding to conventional therapy. *Eur. J. Emerg. Med., 6*, 201-205.

[145] Gürkan, F., Ece, A., Haspolat, K. and Dikici, B. (2000) Parental history of migraine and bronchial asthma in children. *Allergol. Immunopathol., 28*, 15-17.

[146] Gustafson, T., Boman, K., Rosenhall, L., Sandström, T., Wester, P.O. (1996) Skeletal muscle magnesium and potassium in asthmatics treated with oral beta2 agonists. *Eur. Resp. J., 9*, 237-240.

[147] Guy, E.S., Kirumaki, A. and Hanania, N.A. (2004) Acute asthma in pregnancy. *Crit. Care Clin. 20*, 731-745.

[148] Harding, G.F.A. (1998) TV can be bad for your health. *Nature Med., 4*, 265-267.

[149] Hashimoto, Y., Nishimura, Y., Maeda, H. and Yokoyama, M. (2000) Assessment of magnesium status in patients with bronchial asthma. *J. Asthma, 37*, 489-496.

[150] Haury, V.G. (1938) The bronchodilator action of magnesium and its antagonistic (dilator action) against pilocarpine, histamine and barium chloride. *J. Pharmacol.* , *64,* 58-64.

[151] Hauser, S.P. (1991) Magnesium bei Asthmapatienten. *Magn. Bull., 13*, 3-5.

[152] Heiman-Patterson, T.D., Bird, S.J., Parry, G.J., Varga, J., Shy, M.E., Culligan, N.W., Edelsohn, L., Tatarian, G.T., Heyes, M.P. and Garcia, C.A. (1990) Peripheral neuropathy associated with eosinophilia-myalgia syndrome. *Ann. Neurol., 28*, 522-528.

[153] Herman, C., Kim, M. and Blanchard, E.B. (1995) Behavioral and prophylactic pharmacological intervention studies of paediatric migraine: an exploratory meta-analysis. *Pain, 60*, 239-255.

[154] Hetzel, M.R. and Clark, T.J. (1979) Does sleep cause nocturnal asthma? *Thorax, 34,* 749-754.

[155] Hijazi, N., Abalkhail, B. and Seaton, A. (2000) Diet and childhood asthma in a society in transition: a study in urban and rural Saudi Arabia. *Thorax, 55*, 775-779.

[156] Hill, J. and Britton, J. (1995) Dose-response relationship and time-course of the effect of inhaled magnesium sulfate on airflow in normal and asthmatic subjects. *Br. J. Clin. Pharmacol., 40*, 539-544.

[157] Hill, J., Lewis, S. and Britton, J. (1997) Studies on inhaled magnesium on airway reactivity to histamine and adenosine monophosphate in asthmatic subjects. *Clin. Exp. Allergy, 27*, 546-551.

[158] Hill, J., Micklewright, A., Lewis, S. and Britton, J. (1997) Investigations of the effect of short-term change in dietary magnesium intake in asthma. *Eur. Respir. J., 10*, 2225-2229.

[159] Hofford, J.M., Milakofsky, L., Pell, S., Fish, J.E., Peters, S.P., Pollice, M. and Vogel, W.H. (1997) Levels of amino acids and related compounds in bronchoalveolar lavage fluids of asthmatic patients. *Am. J. Respir. Crit. Care Med., 155*, 432-435.

[160] Hoyos, MD. (1998) Headaches in persons attending polyclinics in Barbados. *West Indian Med. J., 47*, 59-63.

[161] Hughes, R., Goldkorn, A., Masoli, M., Weatherall, M., Burgess, C. and Beasley, R. (2003) Use of isotonic nebulised magnesium as an adjuvant to salbutamol in treatment of severe asthma in adults: randomised placebo-controlled trial. *Lancet, 361*, 9375, 2114-2117.

[162] Huntley, H. and Ernst, E. (2000) Herbal remedies for asthma: a systematic review. *Thorax, 55*: 925-929.

[163] Husy, N., Deleuze, C., Bres, V. and Moos, F.C. (2000) New role of taurine as an osmomediator between glial cells and neurons in the rat supraoptic nucleus. In: Taurine 4. Della Corte L., Huxtable R.J., Sgaragli G. and Tipton K.F. eds. (Kluwer Ac. and Plenum Publ., New-York) *Adv. Exp. Med. Biol., 483,* 227-237.

[164] Huszar, G. and Roberts, J.M. (1982) Biochemistry and pharmacology of the myometrium and labor: Regulation at the cellular and molecular levels. *Am. J. Obstet. Gynecol.,142*, 225-237.

[165] Ianello, S., Spina, M. and Leotta, P. (1998) Hypomagnesemia and smooth muscle contractility: diffuse oesophageal spasm in an old female patient. *Miner. Electrol. Metab., 24*, 348-356.

[166] International Study of Asthma and Allergies in Childhood (ISAAC) steering Committee. (1998) Worldwide variations in the prevalence of asthma symptoms: the International Study of Asthma in Childhood (ISAAC). *Eur. Respir. J, 12*, 315-335.

[167] Irie, M., Nagata, S., Endo, Y. and Kobayashi F. (2003) Effect of rapid eye movement sleep deprivation on allergen-induced airway responses in a rat model of asthma. *Int. Arch. Allergy Immunol., 130*, 300-306.

[168] Ivey, M.A., Simeon, D.T. and Monteil, M.A. (2003) Climatic variables are associated with seasonal acute asthma admissions to accident and emergency room facilities in Trinidad, West Indies. *Clin. Exp Allergy, 33*, 1526-1530.

[169] Jaber, R. (2002) Respiratory and allergic diseases: from upper respiratory tract infections to asthma. *Prim. Care, 29*, 231-261.

[170] Jagoda, A., Shepperd, S.M., Spevitz, A. and Joseph M. (1997) Refractory asthma. Part 1: epidemiology, pathophysiology, pharmacologic interventions. *Ann. Emerg. Med., 29*, 262-274.

[171] Janson, C., Gislason, T., Boman, G., Hetta, J. and Roos, B.E. (1990) Sleep disturbances in patients with asthma. *Respir. Med., 84*, 37-42.

[172] Jatakanon, A., Uasuf, C., Maziak, W., Lim, S., Chung, K.F. and Barnes, P.J. (1999) Neutrophilic inflammation in severe persistent asthma. *Am. J. Respir. Crit. Care Med., 160*, 1532-1539.

[173] Joborn, H., Akerström, G. and Ljunghall, S. (1985) Effects of exogenous catecholamines and exercise on plasma Mg concentrations. *Clin. Endocrinol., 23*, 219-227.

[174] Jorgensen, I.M., Jensen, V.B, Bulow, S, Dahm, T.L., Prahl, P. and Juel, K. (2003) Asthma mortality in the Danish child population: risk factors and causes of asthma death. *Pediatr. Pulmonol., 36*, 142-147.

[175] Kakish, K.S. (2001) Serum magnesium levels in asthmatic children during and between exacerbations. *Arch. Pediatr. Adolesc. Med., 155*, 181-183.

[176] Kashiwabara, K., Itonaga, K. and Moroi, T. (2003) Airborne water droplets in mist or fog may affect nocturnal attacks in asthmatic children. *J. Asthma, 40*, 405-411.

[177] Keenan, D., Romani, A. and Scarpa, A. (1995) Diffferential regulation of circulating Mg^{2+} in the rat by beta-1 and beta-2 adrenergic receptor stimulation. *Circ. Res., 77*, 973-983.

[178] Khilnani, G., Parchani, H. and Toshnival, G. (1992) Hypomagnesemia due to beta 2-agonist in bronchial asthma. *J. Assoc. Physician India, 40*, 346.

[179] Kleijnen, J., ter Riet, G. and Knipschild, P. (1991) Acupuncture and asthma: a review of controlled trials. *Thorax*, *46*, 799–802.

[180] Knook, L., Kavelaars, A., Sinnema, G., Kuis, W. and Heijnen, C.J. (2000) High nocturnal melatonin in adolescents with chronic fatigue syndrome. *J. Clin. Endocrinol. Metab., 85*, 3690-3692.

[181] Knutsen, R., Bohmer, T. and Falch, J. (1994) Intravenous theophylline-induced excretion of calcium, magnesium and sodium in patients with recurrent asthmatic attacks. *Scand. J. Clin. Lab. Invest., 54*, 119-125.

[182] Koltek, M., Wilkes, T.C. and Atkinson, M. (1998) The prevalence of posttraumatic stress disorder in an adolescent inpatient unit. *Can. J. Psychiatry, 43*, 64-68.

[183] Korszun, A., Sackett-Lundeen L., Papadopoulos, E., Brucksch, C., Masterson, L., Engelberg, N.C., Haus, E., Demitrack, M.A. and Crofford, L. (1999) Melatonin levels in women with fibromyalgia and chronic fatigue syndrome. *J. Rheumatol., 26*, 2975-2980.

[184] Kos-Kudla, B., Ostrowska, Z., Marek, B., Ciesielska-Kopacz, N., Kajdaniuk, D., Kudla, M. and Buntner, B. (1997) Diurnal rhythm of serum melatonin, ACTH and cortisol in asthma patients with long term glucocorticoid treatment. *Endocr Regul, 31*, 47-54.

[185] Kos-Kudla, B., Ostrowska, Z., Marek, B., , Kajdaniuk, D., Ciesielska-Kopacz, N., Kudla, M., Mazur, B., Glogowska-Szelag, J. and Nasiek, M. (2002). Circadian rhythm of melatonin in postmenopausal asthmatic women with hormone replacement therapy. *Neuro. Endocrinol. Lett., 23*, 243-248.

[186] Kostenbauder, H.B. and Sanvordeker, D.R. (1973) Riboflavin enhancement of bilirubin photocatabolism *in vivo*. *Experientia, 3,* 282-283.

[187] Kotani, Y., Nishimura, Y., Maeda, H. and Yokoyama, M. (1999) Beta2-adrenergic receptor polymorphisms affect airway responsiveness to salbutamol in asthmatics. *J. Asthma, 36,* 583-590.

[188] Kraft, M. and Martin, R.J. (1995) Chronobiology and chronotherapy in medicine. *Dis. Mon., 41,* 501-575.

[189] Kraft, M., Djukanovic, R., Wilson, S, Holgate, S.T. and Martin, R.J. (1996) Alveolar tissue inflammation in asthma. *Am. J. Respir. Crit. Care Med., 154*, 1505–1510.

[190] Kraft, M., Martin, R.J., Wilson, S., Djukanovic, R. and Holgate, S.T. (1999) Lymphocyte and eosinophil influx into alveolar tissue in nocturnal asthma. *Am. J. Respir. Crit. Care Med., 159*, 228–234.

[191] Kraft, M., Vianna, E., Martin, R.J. and Leung, D.Y.M. (1999) Nocturnal asthma is associated with reduced glucocorticoid receptor binding affinity and decreased steroid responsiveness at night. *J. Allergy Clin. Immunol., 103*, 66–71.

[192] Kraft, M., Pak, J., Martin, R.J., Kaminsky, D. and Irvin, C.G. (2001) Distal lung dysfunction at night in nocturnal asthma. *Am. J. Resp. Care Med., 163*, 1551-1556.

[193] Kravchenko, O.V. (2002) Effect of polarized light on the immune status and cytokine levels of patients with bronchial asthma during immunotherapy with bronchomunal. *Fiziol. Zh., 48*, 87-94.

[194] Kripke, D.F. (1998) Light treatment for non seasonal depression: speed, efficacy and combined treatment. *J. Affect. Disord., 49*, 109-117.

[195] Kuitert, L.M. and Kletchko, S.L. (1991) Intravenous magnesium sulphate in acute, life threatening asthma. *Ann. Emerg. Med., 20*, 1243-1245.

[196] Kurtaran, H., Karadag, A., Catal, F., Isik, B. and Uras, N. (2003) Nebulised salbutamol and magnesium sulphate in acute asthma. *Lancet, 362*, 1079-1080.

[197] Kurtz, D. (1990) Changes in sleep and night respiration in asthma and obstructive or restrictive lung diseases. *Presse Med., 28*, 1857-1861.

[198] Kutty, R.K., Kutty, G., Wiggert, B., Chader, G.J., Darrow, R.M. and Organisciak, D.T. (1995) Induction of heme oxygenase 1 in the retina by intense visible light: suppression by the antioxidant dimethylthiourea. *Proc. Natl. Acad. Sci. USA, 92,* 1177-1181.

[199] L'Her, E. (2002) Revision of the 3rd Consensus Conference in Intensive Care and Emergency Medicine in 1988: management of acute asthmatic crisis in adults and children (excluding infants). *Rev. Mal. Respir., 19*, 658-665.

[200] Labiner, D.M., Yan, C.C., Weinand, M.E and Huxtable, R.J. (1999) Disturbances of aminoacids from temporal lobe synaptosomes in human complex partial epilepsy. *Neurochem. Res., 24,* 1379-1383.

[201] Lahmeyer, H.W. (1991) Seasonal affective disorders. *Psychiatr. Med., 9,* 105-114.

[202] Landon, R.A. and Young, E.A. (1993) Role of magnesium in regulation of lung function. *J. Am. Diet Assoc., 93*, 674-678.

[203] Lang, U., Theintz, G., Rivest, R.W., Sizonenko, P.C. (1986) Nocturnal urinary melatonin excretion and plasma cortisol levels in children and adolescents after a single oral dose of dexamethasone. *Clin. Endocrinol. (Oxf), 25*, 165-172.

[204] Langs, G., Fabisch, K. and Fabisch, H. (2000) A case of comorbidity between panic disorder and photosensitive epilepsy. *Psychopathology, 33*, 271-4.

[205] Lehrer, P.M., Isenberg, S. and Hochron, S.M. (1993) Asthma and emotion: a review. *J. Asthma, 30*, 5-21.

[206] Lehrer, P., Feldman, J., Giardino, N., Song, H.S., Schmaling, K. (2002) Psychological aspects of asthma. *J. Consult. Clin. Psychol., 70*, 691-711.

[207] Lemaitre, R.N., Siscovick, D.S., Psaty, B.M., Pearce, R.M., Rhagunathan, T.E., Whitsel, E.A., Weinmann, S.A., Anderson, G.D. and Lin, D. (2002) Inhaled beta-2 adrenergic receptor agonists and primary cardiac arrest. *Am. J. Med.,113*, 711-716.

[208] Leung, D.Y.M. and Chrousos, G.P. (2000) Is there a role for glucocorticoid receptor beat in glucocorticoid-dependent asthmatics? Am. J. Respir. Crit. Care Med., 162, 1-3

[209] Lima, J.J., Thomason, D.B., Mohamed, M.H., Eberle, L.V., Self, T.H., and Johnson, J. A. (1999) Impact of genetic polymorphisms of the beta2-adrenergic receptor on albuterol bronchodilator pharmacodynamics. *Clin. Pharmacol. Ther., 65*, 519-25.

[210] Lipworth, B.J., Clark, R.A., Fraser, C.G. and McDevitt, D.G. (1989) The biochemical effects of high dose inhaled salbutamol in patients with asthma. *Eur. J. Clin. Pharmacol., 36*, 357-360.

[211] Lockley, S.W., Brainard, G.C. and Czeisler, C.A. (2003) High sensitivity of the human circadian melatonin rhythm to resetting by short wavelength light. *J. Clin. Endocrinol. Metab., 88*,4502-4505.

[212] Lopez-Colome, A., Erlig, D. and Pasantes-Morales, H. (1976) Different effects of Ca flux blocking agents on light and K stimulated release of taurine from retina. *Brain Res., 113,* 527-534.

[213] Low, N.C. and Merikangas, K.R. (2003) The comorbidity of migraine. *CNS. Spectr., 8*, 437-444.

[214] Maestroni, G.J. (1999) MLT and the immune–hematopoietic system. *Adv. Exp. Med. Biol.,* 460, 395-405.

[215] Maevskii, A.A. (1991) Phototherapy and sleep deprivation as additional methods of treating bronchial asthma patients. *Vrach. Delo., 5*, 8-90.

[216] Maevskii, A.A. (1995) The circadian phototherapy of bronchial asthma. *Klin. Med., 73*, 43-44.

[217] Main, A., Dawson, A. and Gross M. (1997) Photophobia and phonophobia in migraineurs betwen attacks. *Headache, 37*, 492-495.

[218] Mangat, H.S., D'Souza, G.A. and Jacob M.S. (1998) Nebulized magnesium sulphate versus nebulized salbutamol in acute bronchial asthma: a clinical trial. *Eur. Respir. J., 12*, 341-344.

[219] Manzke, H., Thiemeier, M., Elster, P. and Lemke, J. (1990) $MgSO_4$ as adjuvant in beta-2 sympathomimetic inhalation therapy of bronchial asthma. *Pneumologie, 44*, 1190-1192.

[220] Marcinkiewicz, J., Grabowska, A. and Chain, B.M. (1998) Modulation of antigen-specific T-cell activation in vitro by taurine chloramine. *Immunology., 94*, 325-30.

[221] Marek W. (1997) Chronobiology of the bronchial system. *Pneumologie, 51*, 430-439.

[222] Marsh, DG. Genetic factors of allergy. Michel FB, Bousquet J., Godard P.H., eds. *Highlights in Asthmology*. New York: Springer Verlag Inc; 1987. p. 31-6.

[223] Marthan, R. (1998) Polymorphisme génétique des récepteurs β-2-adrénergiques. *Asthme, Allergie, Environnement Respiratoire, 1*, 56-58.

[224] Martin, R.J. and Banks-Schlegel, S. (1998) Chronobiology of asthma. *Am. J. Resp. Crit. Care Med., 158*, 1002-1007.

[225] Martin, R.J. (1993) Nocturnal asthma: circadian rhythms and therapeutic interventions. *Am. Rev. Respir. Dis., 147*, S25-S28.

[226] Martin, R.J. (1999) Location of airway inflammation in asthma and the relationship to circadian change in lung function. *Chronobiol. Int.,16,* 623–630.

[227] Martin, R.J., Cicutto, L.C. and Ballard, R.D. (1990) Factors related to the nocturnal worsening of asthma. *Am. Rev. Respir. Dis., 141*, 33–38.

[228] Martinez, F.D., Graves, P.E., Baldini, M., Solomon, S. and Erickson, R. (1997) Association between genetic polymorphisms on the β2-adrenoreceptor and response to albuterol in children with and without a history of wheezing. *J. Clin. Invest., 100*, 3184-3188.

[229] Martins, E. Jr., Ligeiro de Oliveira, A.P., Fialho de Araujo, A.M., Tavares de Lima, W., Cipolla-Neto, J. and Costa Rosa, L.F. (2001) Melatonin modulates allergic lung inflammation. *J. Pineal Res., 31*, 363-369

[230] Mattos, W., Lim, S., Russel, R., Jatakanon, A., Chung, F. and Barnes, P.J. (2002) Matrix metalloproteinase-9 expression in asthma. *Chest, 122*, 1543-1552.

[231] Mayeno, AN and Gleich, GJ. (1994) Eosinophilia-myalgia syndrome and tryptophan production: a cautionary tale. *Trends Biotechnol., 12*, 346-352.

[232] McLaughlin, T., Geissler, E.C. and Wan, G.J. (2003) Comorbidities and associated treatment charges in patients with anxiety disorders. *Pharmacotherapy, 23*, 1251-1256.

[233] Meral A, Coker M and Tanac R. (1996) Inhalation therapy with magnesium sulfate and salbutamol sulfate in bronchial asthma. *Turk J Pediatr., 38*, 169-75. Metzger, J.Y., Berthou, V., Perrin, P. and Sichel, J.P. (1998) Photothérapie: bilan clinique et thérapeutique d'une experience de 2 ans. *L'encéphale 24*, 480-485.

[234] Metzger, J.Y., Berthou, V. and Sichel, J.P. (1999) Approche critique du concept de dépression saisonnière et du traitement par photothérapie. *Ann. Méd-Psychol., 157*, 1-11.

[235] Milojevic, M. and Kuruk, V. (2003) Low power laser biostimulation in the treatment of bronchial asthma. *Med. Pregl., 56*, 413-418.

[236] Moldofsky, H. (1993) A chronopathological theory of fibromyalgia. *J. Musculoskeletal Pain, 1,* 49-59.

[237] Monnier, M., Boehmer, A. and Scholer, A. (1976) Early habituation, dishabituation and generalization induced in the visual centers by colour stimuli. *Vision Res., 16*, 1497-1504.

[238] Montealegre, F., Bayona, M., Chardon, D. and Trevino F. (2002) Age, gender and seasonal patterns of asthma in emergency departments of southern Puerto Rico. *P.R. Health Sci. J., 21*, 207-212.

[239] Mortimer, M.J., Kay, J., Gawkrodger, D.J., Jaron, A. and Barker, D.C. (1993) The prevalence of headache and migraine in atopic children: an epidemiological study in general practice. *Headache, 33*, 427-431.

[240] Morton, D.J. and James, M.F.M. (1985) Effect of Mg ions on rat pineal N-acetyltransferase (E.C. 2.3.1.5) activity. *J. Pineal Res., 2*, 387-391.

[241] Morton, D.J. (1989) Possible mechanisms of inhibition and activation of rat N-acetyltransferase (E.C. 2.3.1.5) by cations. *J. Neural Transmission, 75*, 51-64.

[242] Mrazek, D.A. (2003) Psychiatric symptoms in patients with asthma causality, comorbidity, or shared genetic etiology. *Child Adolesc. Psychiatr. Clin. N. Am., 12*, 459-471.

[243] Nadler, J.L., Goodson, S. and Rude, R.K. (1987) Evidence that prostcyclin mediates the vascular action of magnesium in humans. *Hypertension, 9*, 379-383.

[244] Nakagawa, H., Oomura, J. and Nagai, K. (eds) (1993) *New functional aspects of the suprachismatic nucleus of the hypothalamus*. London: John Libbey.

[245] Nannini, L.J. and Hofer, D. (1997) Effect of inhaled magnesium sulfate on sodium metabisulfite-induced bronchostriction in asthma. *Chest, 111*, 858-861.

[246] Nannini, L.J. Jr., Pendino, J.C., Corna, R.A., Mannarino, S. and Quispe, R. (2000) Magnesium sulfate as a vehicle for nebulized salbutamol in acute asthma. *Am. J. Med., 108*, 193-197.

[247] Nascimento, I., Nardi, A.E., Valenca, A.M., Lopes, F.L., Messasalma, M.A., Nascentes, R., Zin, W.A. (2002) Psychiatric disorders in asthmatic outpatients. *Psychiatry Res., 110*, 73-80.

[248] Nathan, C., Xie, Q.W. (1994) Nitric oxide synthases: roles, tolls and controls. *Cell, 78,* 915-917.

[249] National Heart, Lung and Blood Institute. Expert panel report 2: Guidelines for the diagnosis and prevention of asthma. Bethesda, MD: National Institutes of Health, April 1997; Publication n°97-4051.

[250] National Research Council (NRC), Recommended dietary allowances, 10th ed. Washington, DC, National Academic Press, 1989

[251] Nicolai, T., Illi, S., Tenbörg, J., Kiess, W. and Mutius, V. (2001) Puberty and prognosis of asthma and bronchial hyper-reactivity. *Pediatr. Allergy Immunol., 12*, 142-149.

[252] Noeker, M., Haverkamp, F. (2001) Successful cognitive-behavioral habituation training towrd phtophobia in photiogenic partial seizures. *Epilepsia, 42*, 689-691.

[253] Nolte, D. Asthma. Verlauf, Ursachen, Behandlung. Stuttgart: TRIAS Thieme Hippokrates Enke, 1995.

[254] Noppen, M., Vanmaele, L., Impens, N. and Schandevyl, W. (1990) Bronchodilating effects of intravenous magnesium sulfate in bronchial asthma. *Chest, 97*, 373-376.

[255] O'Dell, G., Brown, R. and Holtzman, N. (1970) Dye-sensitized photooxidation of albumin associated with a decreased capacity for protein-binding of bilirubin. *Symposium on Bilirubin Metabolism 6/2,* 31-36.

[256] Okayama, H., Aikawa, T., Okayama, M., Sasaki, H., Mue, S. and Takishima, T. (1987) Bronchodilating effects of intravenous magnesium sulfate in bronchial asthma. *JAMA, 257*, 1076-1078

[257] Oladipo, O.O., Chukwu, C.C., Ajala, M.O., Adewole, T.A. and Afonja, O.A. (2003) Plasma magnesium in adult asthmatics at the Lagos University Teaching Hospital. *East Afr. Med. J., 80*, 488-491.

[258] Omran, M. and Russell, G. (1996) Continuing increase in respiratory symptoms and atopy in Aberdeen school children. *B.M.J., 312*, 34.

[259] Oren, DA. (1996) Humoral phototransduction: blood is a messenger. *Neuroscientist, 2*, 207-210.

[260] Ortega, A.N., Huertas, S.E., Canino, G., Ramirez, R. and Rubio-Stipec, M. (2002) Childhood asthma, chronic illness, and psychiatric disorders. *J. Nerv. Ment. Dis., 190*, 275-281.

[261] Pagès, N., Bac, P., Maurois, P., Vamecq, J. and Agrapart, C. (2001) Effect of chromatotherapia audiogenic seizure magnesium deficient adult DBA/2 mice: preliminary results. Nutrition and Health. J. RAYSSIGUIER, A. MAZUR, J. DURLACH (eds) John Libbey and compagny, Londres, Chapitre 73, pp 427-430.

[262] Pagès, N., Gogly, B., Godeau, G., Igondjo-Tchen, S., Maurois, P., Durlach, J. and Bac, P. (2003) Structural alterations of the vascular wall in magnesium-deficient mice. A possible role of gelatinases A (MMP-2) and B (MMP-9). *Magnes. Res., 16*, 1, 43-48.

[263] Pagès, N., Bac, P., Maurois, P. and Agrapart, C. (2003) Effect of different wavelengths of the visible spectrum for a short period (50 sec) on audiogenic seizures in mice. *Magnes. Res., 16,* 29-34.

[264] Pang, C.S., Brown, G.M., Tang, P.L. and Pang, S.F. (1993) G-protein linked melatonin binding sites in the chicken lung. *Neurosci. Lett., 162*, 17-20.

[265] Parain, D. (2000) Les epilepsies photosensibles généralisées ou focales. *Rev. Neurol., 154,* 757-761.

[266] Pasantes-Morales, H., Quesada, O. and Moran, J. (1998) Taurine: an osmolyte in mammalian tissue. In: Taurine 3. Schaffer S., Lombardini J.B. and Huxtable R.J. eds. (Plenum publ., New-York). *Adv. In Exp. Med. Biol., 442*, 209-217.

[267] Pearce, N. and Hensley, N.J. (1998) Epidemiologic studies of beta agonists and asthma deaths. *Epidemiol. Rev*., 20, 173-186.

[268] Peat, J.K., Van den Berg, R.H., Green, W.F., Mellis, C.M., Leeder, S.R. and Woolcock, A.J. (1994) Changing prevalence of asthma in Australian children. *B.M.J., 308*, 1591-1596.

[269] Perna, G., Bertani, A., Politi, E., Columbo, G. and Bellodi, L. (1997) Asthma and panic attacks. *Biol Psychiatry., 42*, 625-630.

[270] Ponsonby, A.L., McMichael, A. and Van der Mei I. (2002) UV radiation and autoimmune disease: insights from epidemiological research. *Toxicology, 181-182*, 71-78.

[271] Ravn, H.B. and Dorup, I. (1997) The concentration of Na, K pumps in **C**hronic **O**bstructive **L**ung **D**isease (COLD) patients: the impact of magnesium depletion and steroid treatment. *J. Intern. Med., 241,* 23-29.

[272] Rehaminoff, R. and Bruderman, I. (1965) Changes in pulmonary mechanics induced by melatonin. *Life Sci., 4*, 183-189.

[273] Reihsaus, E., Innis, M., MacIntyre, N. and Liggett, S.B. (1993) Mutations in the gene encoding for the beta 2-adrenergic receptor in normal and asthmatic subjects. *Am. J. Respir. Cell Mol. Biol., 8*, 334-9.

[274] Reilly, P.A. and Littlejohn, G.O. (1993) Diurnal variation in the symptoms and signs of the Fibromyalgia Syndrome (F.S.). *J. Musculoskeletal Pain, 3/4,* 237-239.

[275] Reinberg, A., Smolensky, M.H., D'Alonzo, G.E. and McGovern, J.P. (1988) Chronobiology and asthma. III. Timing corticotherapy to biological rhythms to optimize treatment goals. *J. Asthma, 25*, 219-48.

[276] Reiter R.J. (1991a) Pineal gland. Interface between the photoperiodic environment and the endocrine system. *Trends Endocrinol. Metab., 2,* 13-29.

[277] Reiter R.J. (1991b) Melatonin: the chemical expression of darkness. *Mol. Cell Endocrinol., 79*, C153-C158.

[278] Reiter R.J. (1993) The melatonin rhythm: both a clock and a calendar. *Experientia 49,* 654-664.

[279] Rodrigo, G., Rodrigo, C. and Burschtin, O. (2000) Efficacy of magnesium sulfate in acute adult asthma: a meta-analysis of randomized trials. *Amer. J. Emerg. Med., 18*, 216-221.

[280] Rodrigo, G.J., and Rodrigo, C. (2002) The role of anticholinergics in acute asthma treatment: an evidence-based evaluation. *Chest, 121*, 1977-1987.

[281] Rodrigo, G.J., and Rodrigo, C. (2003) Triple inhaled drug protocol for the treatment of acute severe asthma. *Chest, 123*, 1908-1915.

[282] Rolla, G., Bucca, C. and Carla, E. (1988) Acute effect of intravenous magnesium sulphate on airway obstruction of asthmatic patients. *Ann. Allergy, 61*, 388-391.

[283] Rolla G. and Bucca C. (1989) Hypomagnesemia and bronchial hyperreactivity. A case report. *Allergy, 44*, 519-521.

[284] Rolla G., Bucca C., Buggiani, M., Oliva, A. and Branciforte, L. (1990) Hypomagnesemia in chronic obstructive lung disease: effect of therapy. *Mg Trace Elem., 9*, 132-136.

[285] Rolla, G., Bucca, C., Brussino, L. and Colagrande, P. (1994) Effect of intravenous magnesium infusion on salbutamol-induced bronchodilation in patients with asthma. *Magnes. Res.,7*, 129-133.

[286] Rolla, G., Bucca, C., Arossa, W. and Buggiani, M. (1997a) Magnesium attenuates methacholine-induced bronchostriction in asthmatics. *Magnesium, 6940*, 201-204.

[287] Rolla, G., Bucca, C., Buggiani, M., Arossa, W. and Spinaci, S. (1997b) Reduction of histamine-induced bronchostriction by magnesium in asthmatic subjects. *Allergy, 42*, 186-188.

[288] Romani, A. and Scarpa, A. (1992a) Regulation of cell magnesium. *Arch. Bichem. Biophys., 298*, 1-12.

[289] Romani, A. and Scarpa, A. (1992b) cAMP control of Mg^{2+} homeostasis in heart and liver cells. *Magnes. Res.*, 5, 131-137.

[290] Romani, A. and Scarpa, A. (2000) Regulation of cellular magnesium. *Frontiers Biosci., 5*, 720-734.

[291] Rosello, H.J. and Pla, J.C. (1936) Sulfato de magnesio en la crisis de asma. *Prensa Med. Argentina, 29*, 1677-1680.

[292] Rosenthal, N.E., Sack, D.A., Gillin, J.C., Lewy A.J., Goodwin, F.K., Davenport, Y., Mueller, P.S., Newsome, D.A. and Wehr, T.A. (1984) Seasonal affective disorder: a description of the syndrome and preliminary findings with light therapy. *Arch. Gen. Psychiatry, 41*, 72-80.

[293] Rowe, B.H., Bretzlaff, J.A., Bourdon, C., Bota, G.W. and Camargo, C.A. Jr. (2000) Intravenous magnesium sulfate treatment for acute asthma in the emergency department: a systematic review of the literature. *Ann. Emerg. Med., 36*, 181-190.

[294] Rylander, R., Dahlberg, C. and Rubenowitz, E. (1997) Magnesium supplementation decreases airway responsiveness among hyperreactivity subjects. *Mg-Bull., 19*, 4-6.

[295] Sadlonova, J., Korpas, J., Salat, D., Miko, L. and Kudlicka, J. (2003) The effect of the pulsatile electromagnetic field in children suffering from bronchial asthma. *Acta Physiol. Hung., 90*, 327-334.

[296] Sadlonova, J., Korpas, J., Vrabec, M., Salat, D., Buchancova, J. and Kudlicka, J. (2002) The effect of the pulsatile electromagnetic field in patients suffering from chronic obstructive pulmonary disease and bronchial asthma. *Bratisl. Lek. Listy, 103,* 260-265.

[297] Saeed S.A., Bruce T.J. (1998) Seasonal affective disorders. *Amer. Fam. Physician, 15*, 1340-1346.

[298] Sakamoto, K., Nagata, M., Houya, I., Inoue, K., Kiuchi, H., Sakamoto, Y., Yamamoto, K. and Dohi, Y. (1993) Improvement of intractable nocturnal asthma treated by therapeutic awakening. *Arerugi., 42*, 840-845.

[299] Salas-Puig, J., Parra J. and Fernandez-Torre, J.L. (2000) Photogenic epilepsy. *Rev. Neurol., 30,* S81-S84.

[300] Salvesen, R. and Bekkelund S.I. (2000) Migraine as compared to other headaches is worse during midnight-sun summer than during polar night. A questionnaire study in an Arctic population. *Headache, 40*, 824-829.

[301] Sandrini, G., Proietti-Ceccini, A. and Nappi, G. (2002) Chronic fatigue syndrome: a borderline disorder (abst.). *Functional Neurol., 17*, 51-52.

[302] Santana, J.C., Barreto, S.S., Piva, J.P. and Garcia, P.C. (2001) Randomized clinical trial of intravenous magnesium sulfate versus salbutamol in early management of severe acute asthma in children. *J. Pediatr., 77*, 279-287.

[303] Saris, N.E., Mervaala, E., Karppanen, H., Khawaja, J.A. and Lewenstam, A. (2000) Magnesium. An update on physiological, clinical and analytical aspects. *Clin. Chim. Acta, 294*, 1-26.

[304] Savineau, J.P. and Marthan, R. (1997) Modulation of the calcium sensitivity of the smooth muscle contractile apparatus: molecular mechanisms, pharmacological and pathophysiological implications. *Fundam. Clin. Pharmacol.,* 11, 289-299.

[305] Scarfone, R.J., Loiselle, J.M., Joffe, M.D., Mull, C.C., Stiller, S., Thompson, K. and Gracely, E.J. (2000) A randomized trial of magnesium in the emercency department treatment of children with asthma. *Ann. Emerg. Med., 36,* 572-578.

[306] Schenk, P., Vonbank, K., Schnack, B., Haber, P., Lehr, S. and Smetana, R. (2001) Intravenous magnesium sulfate for bronchial hyperreactivity: a randomized, controlled, double blind study. *Clin. Pharmacol. Ther., 69*, 365-3371.

[307] Schoni, M.H. and Brueder, K. (1988) The effect of hyperosmolar mixed solution of sodium chloride and beta 2 sympathomimetics on lung function in ashtmatic children and adolescents. *Schweiz Med. Woschenschr., 118*, 1377-1381.

[308] Sears, M.R. (2001) The evolution of beta-2 agonists. *Respir. Med., 95* (Suppl. B), 52-56.

[309] Seelig, M.S. (1994) Consequences of magnesium deficiency on the enhancement of stress reactions; preventive and therapeutic implications. *J. Am. Coll. Nutr., 5*, 429-446.

[310] Shapiro, C.M., Catterall, J.R., Montgomery, I., Raab G.M. and Douglas, N.J. (1986) Do asthmatics suffer bronchostriction during rapid eye movement sleep? *Br. Med. J., 292*, 1161-1164.

[311] Sidow, M., Crozier, T.A., Zielmann, S., Radke, J. and Burchardi, H. (1993) High-dose intravenous $MgSO_4$ in the management of life threatening status asthmaticus. *Intensive Care Med., 19*, 467-471.

[312] Silverman, R., Osborn, H., Runge, J. et al. (1996) Magnesium sulphate as an adjunct to standard therapy in acute severe asthma. *Acad. Emerg. Med., 3*, 467-468.

[313] Silverman, R. (2000) Treatment of acute asthma. A new look at the old and at the new. *Clin. Chest Med., 21*, 361-379.

[314] Silverman, R., Osborn, H., Runge, J., Gallagher, E.J., Chiang, W., Feldman, J., Gaeta, T., Freeman, K., Levin, B., Mancherje, N. and Scharf, S. Acute Asthma/Magnesium Study Group (2002) IV magnesium sulphate in the treatment of acute severe asthma: a multicenter randomized controlled trial. *Chest, 122*, 489-497.

[315] Sinaii, N., Cleary, S.D., Ballweg, M.L., Nieman, L.K. and Stratton, P. (2002) High rate of autoimmune and endocrine disorders, fibromyalgia, chronic fatigue syndrome and atopic diseases among women with endometriosis: a survey analysis. *Hum. Reprod., 17*, 2715-2724,

[316] Siniatchkin, M., Kirsch, E., Arslan, S., Stegemann, S., Gerber, W-D. and Stephani, U. (2003) Migraine and asthma in childhood: evidence for specific asymmetric parent-child interactions in migraine and asthma families. *Cephalalgia, 23*, 790-802.

[317] Skene, D.J., Lockley, S.W., Thapan, K. and Arendt, J. (1999) Effects of light on human circadian rhythms. *Reprod. Nutr. Dev., 39*, 295-304.

[318] Skloot, G.S. (2002) Nocturnal asthma: mechanisms and management. *Mt Sinai J. Med., 69*, 140-7.

[319] Skobeloff, E.M., Sperey, W.H., McNamara, R.M. and Greenspon, L. (1989) Intravenous magnesium sulphate for the treatment of acute asthma in the emergency department. *JAMA, 262*, 1210-1213.

[320] Smitt, H.A. (2001) Chronic obstructive pulmonary disease, asthma and protective effects of food intake: from hypothesis to evidence? *Respir. Res., 2*, 261-264.

[321] Smolensky, M.H., Reinberg, A.E., Martin, R.J. and Haus E. (1999) Clinical chronobiology and chronotherapeutics with applications to asthma. *Chronobiol. Int., 16*, 539-563.

[322] Soutar, A., Seaton, A. and Brown, K. (1997) Bronchial reactivity and dietary antioxidants. *Thorax, 52*, 166-170.

[323] Spiropoulos, K., Trakada, G., Nikolaou, E., Prodromakis, E., Efremidis, G., Pouli, A. and Koniavitou, A. (2003) Endothelin-1 levels in the pathophysiology of chronic obstructive pulmonary disease and bronchial asthma. *Respir. Med., 97*, 983-989.

[324] Spitzer, W.O., Suissa, S., Ernst, P., Horwitz, R.I., Habbick, B., Cockcroft, D., Boivin, J.F., McNutt, M., Buist, A.S. and Rebuck, A.S. (1992) The use of beta agonists and the risk of death and near death from asthma. *N. Engl. J. Med., 326*, 501-506.

[325] Spivey, W.H., Skobeloff, E.M. and Levin, R.M. (1990) Effect of magnesium chloride on rabbit bronchial smooth muscle. *Amer. Emerg. Med., 19*, 1107-1112.

[326] Stapleton, P.P., O'Flaherty, L., Redmon, H.P. and Bouchier-Hayes, D.J. (1998) Host defense. A role for the amino acid taurine? *J. Parenteral. Enteral Nutr., 23*, 366-367.

[327] Stenius-Aarniala, B., Piirila, P. and Teramo, K. (1988) Asthma and pregnancy: a prospective study of 198 pregnancies. *Thorax, 43*, 12-18.

[328] Sternberg, E.M. (1996) Pathogenesis of L-tryptophan eosinophilia-myalgia syndrome. *Adv. Exp. Med. Biol., 398,* 325-330.

[329] Streetman, D.D., Bhatt-Mehta, V. and Johnson, C.E. (2002) Management of acute, severe asthma in children. *Ann. Pharmacother., 36*, 1287-1289.

[330] Sturman, J.A., Lu, P., Xu, Y.X. and Imaki, H. (1994) Feline maternal taurine deficiency: effects on visual cortex of the offspring. A morphometric and immunohistochemical study. In: Taurine in Health and Disease. Huxtable R. and Michalk D.V. eds. (Plenum Publ., New-York) *Adv. Exp. Med. Biol., 359,* 369-392.

[331] Suissa, S., Assimes, T. and Ernst, P. (2003) Inhaled short acting beta agonist use in COPD and the risk of acute myocardial infarction. *Thorax, 58,* 43-46.

[332] Sutherland, ER, Martin, RJ, Ellison, M.C. and Kraft, M. (2002) Immunomodulatory effects of melatonin in asthma. *Amer. J. Respir. Crit. Care Med.,* 166, 1055-1061.

[333] Sutherland, E.R., Ellison, M.C., Kraft, M. and Martin, R.J. (2003) Elevated serum melatonin is associated with nocturnal worsening of asthma. *J. Allergy Clin. Immunol., 112*, 513-517.

[334] Sutherland, ER, Kraft, M., Rex, M.D., Ellison, M.C. and Martin, R.J. (2003) Hypothalamic-Pituitary-adrenal axis dysfunction during sleep in nocturnal asthma. *Chest, 123*, 405S.

[335] Swadi H. (2001) Psychiatric morbidity in a community sample of Arab children with asthma. *J. Trop. Pediatr., 47*, 106-107.

[336] Syabbalo, N. (1997) Chronobiology and chronopathophysiology of nocturnal asthma.. *Int. J. Clin. Pract., 51*,455-462.

[337] Szefler, S.J., Ando, R., Cicutto, L.C., Surs, W., Hill, M.R. and Martin, R.J. (1991) Plasma histamine, epinephrine, cortisol, and leukocyte beta-adrenergic receptors in nocturnal asthma. *Clin. Pharmacol. Ther., 49*, 59-68.

[338] Szentivanyi, A. (1968) The beta adrenergic theory of the atopic abnormality in bronchial asthma. *J. Allergy, 42,* 203-232.

[339] Tan, S., Hall, I.P., Dewar, J. and Lipworth, B. (1997) Association between β2-adrenoreceptor polymorphism and susceptibility to bronchodilator desensitisation in moderately severe stable asthmatics. *Lancet, 350*, 995-999.

[340] Tattersfield, A.E., Knox A.J, Britton J.R. and Hall I.P. (2002) Asthma. *Lancet, 360*, 1313-1322.

[341] Terman, J.S., Terman, M., Schlager, D., Rafferty, B., Rosofsky, M., Link, M.J., Gallin, F.F. and Quitkin, F.M. (1990) Efficacy of brief intense light exposure for treatment of winter depression. *Psychopharmacol. Bull. 26*, 3-11.

[342] Terman, M., Levine, S.M., Terman, J.S. and Doherty, S. (1998) Chronic fatigue syndrome and seasonal affective disorders: comorbidity, diagnostic overlap and implications for treatment. *Am. J. Med., 105* (3A), 115S-124S.

[343] Terman, M. and Terman, J.S. (2000) Light therapy. In: Principles and practice of sleep Medicine (3rd edit.). M.H. Kryger, T. Roth, W.W. Dement eds. Philadelphia, W.B. Saunders publ., 1258-1274.

[344] Tiffany, B.R., William, A.B., Todd, I.K. and White, S.R. (1993) Magnesium bolus or infusion fails to improve expiratory flow in acute asthma exacerbations. *Chest, 104*, 831-834.

[345] Timbrell, J.A., Seabra, V. and Waterfield, C.J. (1995) The *in vivo* and *in vitro* protective properties of taurine. *Gen. Pharmacol., 26*, 453-462.

[346] Touitou, Y. and Haus, E. (eds) (1994) Biologic rhythms in clinical and laboratory medicine. Paris: Springer Verlag.

[347] Touitou, Y., Bogdan, A., Auzéby, A. and Selmaoui, B. (1998) Mélatonine et vieillissement. *Thérapie, 53*, 473-478.

[348] Touitou, Y. (1998) La mélatonine: hormone et medicament. *C.R. Soc. Biol., 192*, 643-657.

[349] Turki, J., Pak, J., Green, S.A., Martin, R.J. and Liggett, S.B. (1995) Genetic polymorphisms of the β_2-adrenergic receptor in nocturnal and nonnocturnal asthma: evidence that Gly16 correlates with the nocturnal phenotype. *J. Clin. Invest., 95*, 1635–1641.

[350] Turner-Warwick, M. (1988) Epidemiology of nocturnal asthma. *Am. J. Med., 85*, 6-8.

[351] Tveskov, C., Djurhuus, M.S., Klitgaard, N.A.H., Egstrup, K. (1994) K and Mg distribution, ECG changes and ventricular ectopic beats during beta-2 adrenergic stimulation with terbutaline in healthy subjects. *Chest, 106*: 1654-1659.

[352] Ulrik, C.S. (1995) Peripheral eosinophil counts as a marker of disease activity in intrinsic and extrinsic asthma. *Clin. Exp. Allergy, 25*, 820–827.

[353] Ungar, W.J., Chapman, K.R. and Santos, M. (2002) Assessment of a medication-based asthma index for population research. *Am. J. Respir. Crit. Care Med., 165*, 190-194.

[354] Van Keimpema, A.R., Ariaansz, M., Tamminga, J.J., Nauta, J.J. and Postmus, P.E. (1997) Nocturnal waking and morning dip of peak expiratory flow in clinically stable asthma patients during treatment: occurrence and patient characteristics. *Respiration, 64*, 29–34.

[355] Van Keimpema, A.R., Ariaansz, M., Tamminga, J.J., Nauta, J.J. and Postmus, P.E. (1995) Subjective sleep quality and mental fitness in asthmatic patients. *J. Asthma, 32*, 69-74.

[356] Venturini, C.M., Palmer, R.M.and Moncada, S. (1993) Vascular smooth muscle contains a depletable store of a vasodilator which is light-activated and restored by donor of nitric oxide. *J Pharmacol Exp Ther, 266*, 1497-1500.

[357] Vila, G., Nollet-Clemencon, C., de Blic, J., Mouren-Simeoni, M.C. and Scheinmann, P. (2000) Prevalence of DSM-IV anxiety and affective disorders in a pediatric population of asthmatic children and adolescents. *J. Affect. Disord., 58*, 223-233.

[358] Voultsios, A., Kennaway, D.J. and Dawson, D. Salivary melatonin as a circadian phase marker. Validation and comparison to plasma melatonin. *J. Biol. Rhythms, 187*, 457-466.

[359] Weekley, L.B. (1993) Influence of melatonin on bovine pulmonary vascular and bronchial airway smooth muscle tone. *Clin. Auton. Res., 5*, 53-56.

[360] Weiland, S.K., Von Mutius, E., Husing, A. and Asher M.I. (1999) Intake of trans fatty acids and prevalence of childhood asthma and allergies in Europe. *Lancet, 353*, 2040-2041.

[361] Whyte, K.F., Addis, G.J., Whitesmith, R., Reid, J.L. (1987) Adrenergic control of plasma Mg in man. *Clin. Sci. (Lond), 72,*135-138.

[362] Wikberg G.E. Adrenergic receptors: classification, ligand binding and molecular properties. *Acta Med Scand. (Suppl)* 1982 ; 665: 19-36.

[363] Wikner, J., Hirsh, U., Nettenberg, L. and Röjdmark, S. (1998) Fibromyalgia: a syndrome associated with decreased nocturnal MT secretion. *Clin. Endocrinol. (Oxford), 49*, 179-183.

[364] Wong C.S., Pavord, I.D., Williams, J., Britton, J.R. and Tattersfield, A.E. (1990) Bronchodilator, cardiovascular, and hypokalaemic effects of fenoterol, salbutamol, and terbutaline in asthma. *Lancet, 336*, 1396-1399.

[365] Woodcock, A.A., Johnson, M.A. and Geddes, D.M. (1983) Theophylline prescribing, serum concentrations, and toxicity. *Lancet, 2*, 610-613.

[366] Wright, R.J., Rodriguez, M. and Cohen, S. (1998) Review of psychosocial stress and asthma: an integrated biopsychosocial approach. *Thorax, 53*, 1066-1074.

[367] Wurtman, R.J., Lynch, H.J. and Sturner, W.Q. (1991) Melatonin in humans: possible involvement in SIDS and use in contraceptives. *Adv. Pineal Res. 5,* 319-327.

[368] Wurtman, R.J. (2000) Editorial: Age-related decreases in melatonin secretion. Clinical consequences. *J. Clin. Endocr. Metab., 85*, 2135-2136.

[369] Yellowless, P.M., Haynes, S., Potts, N. and Ruffin, R.E. (1988) Psychiatric morbidity in patients with life-threatening asthma: initial report of a controlled study. *Med. J. Aust.,149*, 246-249.

[370] Yigla, M., Tov, N., Solomonov, A., Rubin, AH., Harlev, D. (2003) Difficult-to-control asthma and obstructive sleep apnea. *J. Asthma, 40*, 865-871.

[371] Zaidan, R., Geoffriau, M., Brun, J., Taillard, J., Bureau, C., Chazot, G. and Claustrat, B. (1994) Melatonin is able to influence its secretion in humans: description of a phase-response curve. *Neuroendocrinol., 60*, 105-112.

[372] Zannolli, R. and Morgese G. (1997) Does puberty interfere with asthma? *Med. Hypotheses, 48*, 27-32.

[373] Zervas, E., Loukides, S. and Papatheodorou, G. (2000) Magnesium levels in plasma and erythrocytes before and after histamine challenge. *Eur. Resp. J., 16*, 621-625.

[374] Zervas, E., Papatheodorou, G., Psathzkis, K., Panagou, P., Georgatou, N. and Loukides, S. (2003) Reduced intracellular Mg concentrations in patients with acute asthma. *Chest, 123*, 113-118.

[375] Zhou, J.N., Liu, R.Y., Heerikhuize, J., Hofman, M.A. and Swaab, D.F. (2003) Alterations in the circadian rhythm of salivary melatonin begin during the middle-age. *J. Pineal Res., 34*, 11-16.

[376] Ziem, G. and McTamney, J. (1997) Profile of patients with chemical injury and sensitivity. *Environ. Health Perspect., 105* Suppl, 417-36.

In: Dietary Magnezium: New Research
Editor: Andrew W. Yardley

ISBN 978-1-60692-109-8

Chapter III

Low Birth Weight and Magnesium: From the Standpoint of "Fetal Origin" Hypothesis

Junji Takaya
Department of pediatrics, Kansai Medical University,
10-15 Fumizonocho, Moriguchi, Osaka, Japan

Abstract

Magnesium deficiency in pregnant women is frequently seen because of inadequate or low intake of magnesium. Magnesium deficiency during pregnancy can induce not only maternal and fetal nutritional problems, but also consequences that might last in offspring throughout life. Many epidemiological studies have disclosed that restricted fetal growth, i.e. intrauterine growth retardation (IUGR), is associated with an increased risk of insulin resistance in adult life.

We previously postulated that intracellular magnesium of cord blood platelets is lower in the small for gestational age group than in the appropriate for gestational age group, suggesting that intrauterine magnesium deficiency may result in IUGR.

Taken together, intrauterine magnesium deficiency in the fetus may lead to or program the insulin resistance after birth.

We hypothesize that intrauterine magnesium deficiency may induce metabolic syndrome in later life. Intracellular magnesium of the cord blood platelet may be a marker of early fetal growth, and can be used as a novel predictor of adult diseases. Low intracellular magnesium may represent the prenatal programming of insulin resistance and may have lifelong effects on metabolic regulation.

Introduction

Exposure of the fetus to maternal malnutrition is a well-known causal factor for intrauterine growth retardation, both in humans and other animals. Several studies have shown the association of size at birth or indices in poor fetal growth with later development of metabolic syndrome in adulthood characterized by insulin resistance such as type 2 diabetes, hypertension, dyslipidemia and coronary heart disease [1, 2]. Barker and Hales [2] proposed that impaired glucose tolerance and type 2 diabetes may arise as a result of programming, a term used to describe persistent changes in organ structure and function caused by exposure to adverse environmental influences during critical periods of development [3]. Because size at birth is determined largely by non-genetic factors, these findings have led to the "fetal origin" hypothesis, which proposes that fetal adaptation to an adverse intrauterine environment affecting fetal growth may program lifelong physiological changes [4].

As magnesium (Mg) is an important cofactor for the enzymes involved in carbohydrate metabolism, an important role of Mg in insulin action has been reported (5). Mg deficiency occurs in patients with diabetes and vascular diseases [6,7,8,9]. Taken together, these experimental and epidemiological results suggest that the correlation between Mg and birth weight are important determinants of insulin resistance.

In this review, we hypothesize that intrauterine Mg deficiency may induce metabolic syndrome in later life, and discuss the potential contribution of aberrant Mg regulation to low birth weight and to the pathogenesis metabolic syndrome.

Magnesium Deficiency in Pregnant Woman

It is reported that the amount of maternal Mg intake is not only associated with pregnancy outcome but also with infant [10]. Based on the cohort study consisting of 912 people, aged 50 years, born as term singletons around the time of the 1944-1945 Dutch famine, coronary heart disease, raised lipids, altered clotting and obesity were more frequently observed after exposure to famine in early gestation compared to those not exposed to famine, and decreased glucose tolerance was more frequently found in people exposed to famine in later gestation [11]. These findings show that maternal under-nutrition during gestation has serious effects on health in later life. Another study demonstrated that a risk of having very low birth weight infants (less than 1,500g of birth weight) is reduced in mothers' drinking water containing higher amount of Mg [12]. By the end of normal pregnancy, the fetus is believed to acquire approximately 28g of calcium (Ca), 16g of phosphorous and 0.7g of Mg, mostly during the third trimester: 80 % of fetal accretion of Mg occurs during the third trimester (Figure 1) [13].

From these findings, maternal under-nutrition including Mg deficiency during gestation obviously affects health of the fetus in adult life, while the timing of the nutritional insult on the mother is an important determinant. Barker speculated that fetal undernutrition in middle to late gestation, which leads to disproportionate fetal growth, programmed later metabolic disease [4].

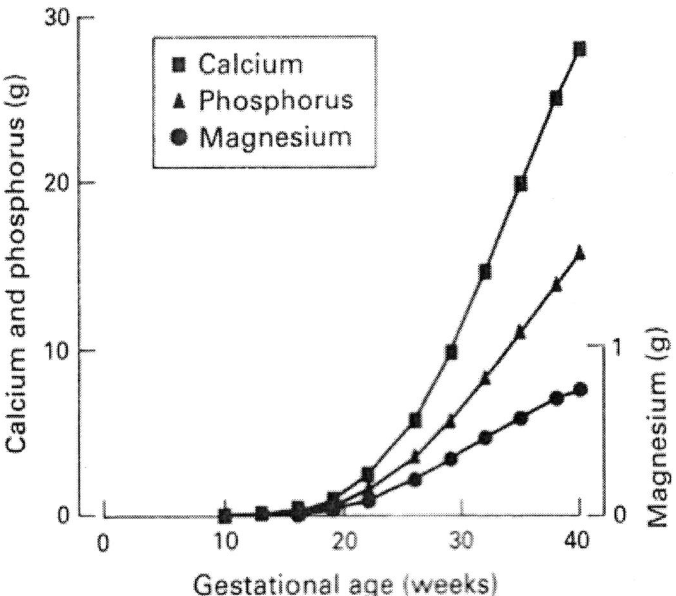

Figure 1. Total fetal content of calcium, phosphorus, and magnesium with increasing gestational age (adapted from Widdowson (Reference [13]).

Mineral Concentration of Meconia

The mineral concentration of meconia of small for gestational age (SGA) newborns were compared with those of appropriate for gestational age (AGA) newborns of similar gestational ages to determine whether differences may provide clues of possible nutritional deficits of SGA infants, given that levels of meconium minerals could indicate the use of minerals by the fetus and the sufficiency of the maternal supply of minerals [14]. In the less than 35-week subgroups, the SGA infants had lower meconium iron and manganese concentrations than that of the AGA. Among more than 36-week newborns, SGA infants had a higher birthweight-adjusted copper concentration than AGA infants, but no differences were observed for the zinc, Ca, Mg, and phosphorus. These results may reflect either a greater use or a decreased maternal supply [14].

Placental Transport of Magnesium

The levels of total Ca, ionized Ca, and Mg are higher in the fetal circulation compared to those in the maternal blood [15]. Copper and selenium share the same transport pathway in the placental membrane along a concentration gradient in maternal-fetal direction, while an active transport plays a predominant role for Mg and iron [16]. In fact, the existence of an active transport mechanism for Mg in the placenta was suggested by using cultured trophoblast cells, i.e. a functional Na^+/Mg^{2+} exchanger that functions to maintain low intracellular Mg in the cells [17]. The activity of this exchanger might be influenced by maternal plasma sodium concentration because acute maternal hyponatremia in experimental rats reduced the maternal-fetal transfer of Mg via placenta [18], while there may be other pathways of Mg transport in the placenta. Whereas mean levels of ionized Ca do not change during labor, the mean maternal serum levels of ionized Mg and total Mg fall at delivery, which suggests the presence of homeostatic mechanisms in the fetus and placenta, indicating that free Mg in umbilical venous blood may enhance Mg transport to the fetus [19].

In mammals, the nutrient exchange process takes place across the placenta, a highly developed organ with numerous functions throughout the most of gestational period, and maternal-fetal homeostasis depends on a properly functioning placenta. Maternal Mg deficiency obviously affects health of the fetus.

Placental Vascular Flow and Magnesium

Calcium and Mg are co-factors in the synthetic activity of a variety of enzymes. A variety of hormones, cytokines and growth factors produced by fetal membranes and placenta can act locally on the myometrium [20]. The ability of the uterine artery to dilate during pregnancy may be specifically related to upregulation of multiple pathways for production of nitric oxide (NO) [21].

The activity of constitutive NO synthase is dependent on Ca and is inhibited by a reduction in the concentration of Mg [22]. Markedly reduced permeability to Ca and Mg of fetal membranes in preterm labor suggests that this abnormality could be an important factor for the activation of the myometrium in preterm labor [23]. Placental insufficiency as well as maternal malnutrition is also an important cause for intrauterine growth retardation (IUGR) (Figure 2). Model experiments of IUGR have been conducted by the reduced uterine blood flow. One of these IUGR models is prepared by uterine artery ligation in pregnant dams and their offspring were studied: Jansson and Lambert reported that this IUGR model was associated with impaired glucose tolerance in adult life only in female rats [24].

Mg has an immediate effect on placental vascular flow as well as Ca and NO. Reduced placental vascular flow is at least, in part, responsible for placental insufficiency and IUGR.

Experimental Consequences of Gestational Magnesium Deficiency in Animal Studies

Maternal Mg restriction that continued through lactation and weaning decreased the pup's body weight at weaning and thereafter, indicating the importance of neonatal and postnatal Mg nutrition in developing rat pups [25,26].

In rat experiment, Venu et al reported that maternal Mg restriction irreversibly increases body fat and induces insulin resistance in pups by 6 months of age [27]. Additional perinatal Mg deficiency impairs glucose tolerance.

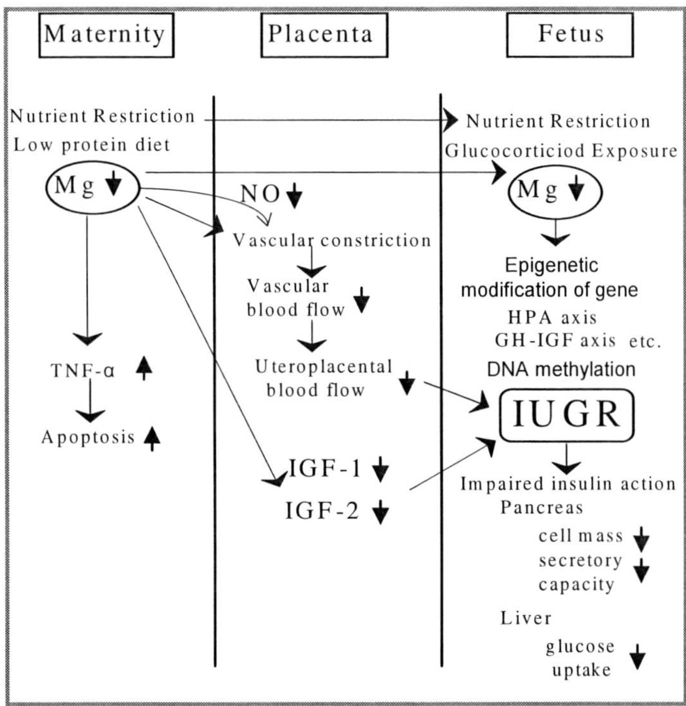

Figure 2. A placenta possesses an active transport mechanism for magnesium. A variety of hormones, cytokines and growth factors produced by fetal membranes and placenta can act on the myometrium. The ability of the uterine artery to dilate may be related to nitric oxide. There are several candidates for explaining gestational programming, i.e. epigenetic modification of gene. (adapted from Takaya, J., Yamato, F., and Kaneko, K. (2006): Possible relationship between low birth weight and magnesium status: from the standpoint of "fetal origin" hypothesis. Magnes. Res. 19, 63-9).

Mg Supplement and Pregnancy Outcome

It is well known that plasma Mg falls in pregnancy because of accumulation of ions in the placenta and fetus. Many women, especially those from disadvantaged backgrounds, have lower Mg intakes than recommended doses [28]. Mg is therefore widely given as a supplement during pregnancy, particularly in cases of preterm labor. There are several reports that oral Mg supplementation in pregnancy is safe and that it has a positive effect on the fetal morbidity [29]. Patients in preterm labor have significantly depressed serum Mg levels, while in patients with pre-eclampsia Mg levels were not significantly different from controls (30). Several papers reported that Mg supplementation during pregnancy could reduce fetal growth retardation and pre-eclampsia and increase birth weight [29,31,32]. Mg therapy decreased the rate of IUGR, premature rupture of membranes and premature delivery in risk pregnancies treated with betamimetics [31]. Oral Mg treatment from before the 25th week of gestation was associated with a lower frequency of preterm birth, a lower frequency of low birth weight and fewer SGA infants compared with a placebo [32]. Mg intake of 513 women towards the end of the first trimester of pregnancy was calculated from a record of food consumption. Mg intake was correlated with weight, length, and head circumference at birth as well as length of gestation up to a threshold of around 3,200g birth weight [33]. In addition, the supplement of Mg (100mg/day) during the second and third trimesters had no effect on the outcome of pregnancy.

Mg supplementation is beneficial in the management of pregnancy-induced hypertension. The effect of Mg was compared with that of placebo in a randomized double-blind controlled study of patients with pregnancy-induced hypertension [34]. Mg supplementation reduced maternal mean arterial blood pressure.

On the other hand, some papers reported that Mg supplementation during pregnancy did not improve pregnancy outcome. Between 13 and 24 weeks' gestation, 400 young normotensive primigravid women randomly received oral Mg (365mg/day) or a placebo. The Mg-supplemented group had significantly higher Mg levels at delivery. However, between the groups there were no differences in either systolic or diastolic blood pressure, incidence of pre-eclampsia, fetal growth retardation, preterm labor, birth weight, gestational age at delivery, or number of infants admitted to the special care unit [10].

Any influence of Mg is confined to the first trimester or before. However, the timing and dose of Mg supplementation may alter the pregnancy outcome.

Intracellular Mg in Cord Blood Platelets

Human platelets are often used for the study of cellular cation metabolism in various diseases [35] because they are readily available and are thought to share a number of features with vascular smooth muscle cells. In addition, they have been shown to have insulin receptors with similar characteristics as those in other cells [36].

We and other investigators reported that insulin action could be mediated by intracellular Mg^{2+} ($[Mg^{2+}]_i$) in platelets [37,38]. In fact, Mg deficiency occurs in adult patients with diabetes mellitus and vascular diseases [7,8,9] and children with diabetes and obesity have been reported to have $[Mg^{2+}]_i$ deficiency [39].

Taken together, we hypothesized that decreased $[Mg^{2+}]_i$ might underlie the initial pathophysiologic events leading to insulin resistance and further tested whether the origin of $[Mg^{2+}]_i$ deficiency may start from fetal life in SGA caused by genetic factors or intrauterine environment.

(A) Intracellular Mg and Small for Gestational Age

By using a fluorescent probe, mag-fura-2, we examined $[Mg^{2+}]_i$ of platelets in the cord blood of infants with SGA and with AGA [40]. Mean $[Mg^{2+}]_i$, but not plasma Mg, was lower in the SGA than in the AGA group (291±149 μmol/L vs 468±132 μmol/L, $p<0.001$). $[Mg^{2+}]_i$ was significantly correlated with the birth weight ($p<0.001$) and birth length ($p<0.001$). (Figure 3, 4)

As $[Mg^{2+}]_i$ plays a promotive role in fetal growth, low $[Mg^{2+}]_i$ may partly be responsible for SGA. In regard to fetal life, it has been postulated that nutritional and environmental factors during pregnancy, as well as hormonal factors such as insulin and IGF-1 [41] play important roles in addition to genetic predisposition.

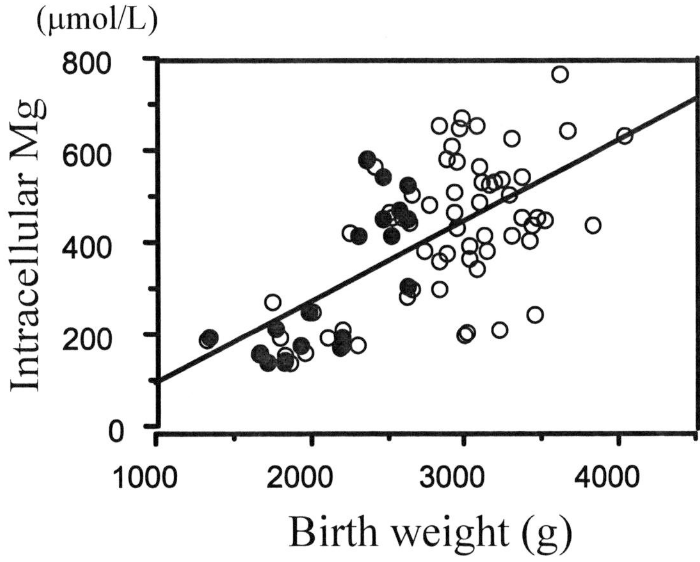

Figure 3. The correlation between intracellular Mg2+ and birth weight. The basal level of intracellular Mg2+ of cord blood platelets is significantly correlated with birth weight ($p<0.001$, $r=0.61$). O, AGA; ●, SGA. (adapted from Reference [40]).

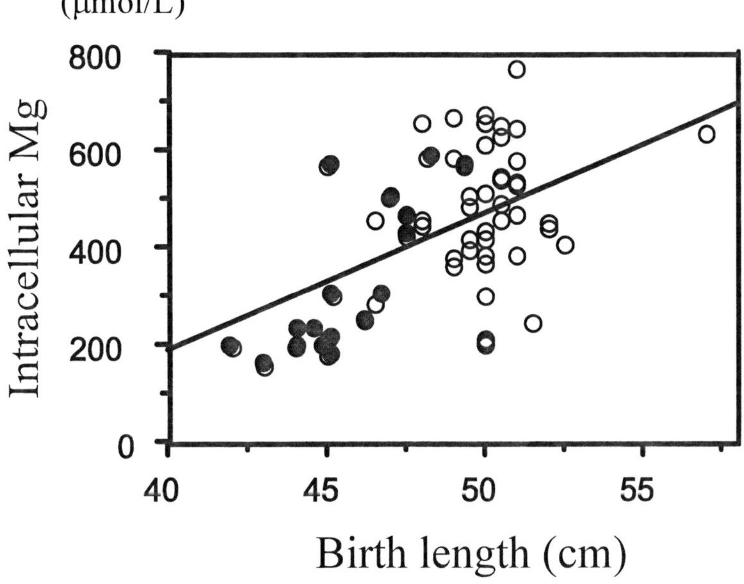

Figure 4. The correlation between intracellular Mg2+ and birth length. The basal level of intracellular Mg2+ of cord blood platelets is significantly correlated with birth length ($p<0.001$, $r=0.48$). O, AGA; ●, SGA. (adapted from Reference [42]).

(B) Correlation of $[Mg^{2+}]_i$ and Insulin Resistance

Adiponectin and IGF-1 were lower in SGA than in AGA, while plasminogen activator inhibitor (PAI)-1 and ghrelin were higher in SGA (Table 1). Quantitative insulin sensitivity check index (QUICKI) was lower in the SGA than in the AGA (Table 1). Birth weight was correlated with cord plasma IGF-1 ($p<0.001$), adiponectin ($p<0.001$) and leptin ($p<0.005$). $[Mg^{2+}]_i$ and adiponectin were correlated with QUICKI in all subjects (Figure 5) [42].

Table 1. A comparison of the metabolic hormones between SGA and AGA

	SGA (n=20)	AGA (n=45)
$[Mg^{2+}]i$ (μmol/L)	284±33***	468±132
Plasma Mg(mg/dL)	1.45±0.07	1.48±0.04
Adiponectin(μg/mL)	11.4±1.8**	17.1±1.0
IGF-1(ng/mL)	14.3±2.1**	30.3±2.2
Leptin(pg/mL)	845±215	1,260±137
Ghrelin(fmol/mL)	76.8±11.0*	53.7±5.1
PAI-1(ng/mL)	13.20±2.52*	7.97±0.94
QUICKI	0.35±0.02***	0.41±0.01

*p<0.05, **p<0.005, ***p<0.0001.

Table 2. Correlation between [Mg2+]i and anthropometric indices and other metabolic hormones

	Parameters	r	P values
$[Mg^{2+}]i$	Gestational age	0.485	<0.0001
	Birth weight	0.618	<0.0001
	Length	0.476	<0.0001
	Ponderal Index	0.053	0.691
	Glucose	0.014	0.908
	Insulin	-0.138	0.253
	IGF-1	0.272	0.030
	QUICKI	0.592	<0.0001
	Leptin	0.073	0.547
	Ghrelin	-0.227	0.064
	Adiponectin	0.246	0.040
	PAI-1	-0.180	0.138

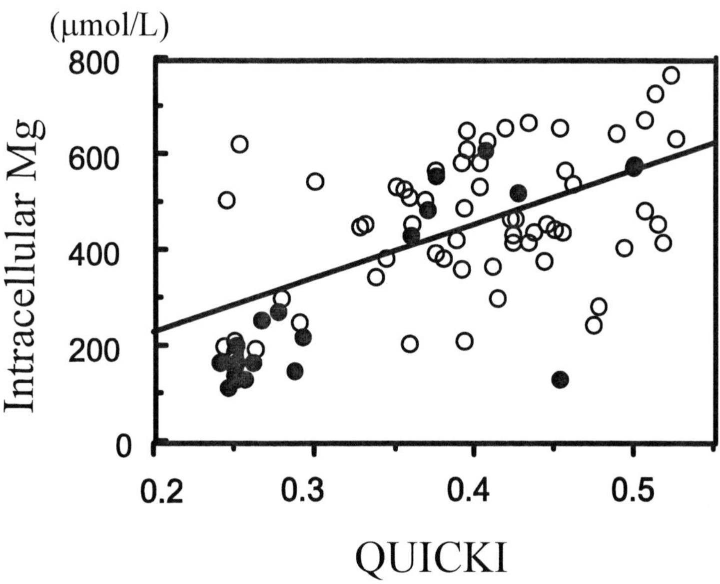

Figure 5. The correlation between intracellular Mg2+ and QUICKI. The basal level of intracellular Mg2+ of cord blood platelets is significantly correlated with QUICKI ($p<0.001$, $r=0.59$). O, AGA; ●, SGA. (adapted from Reference [42]).

These results show that SGA has the tendency of insulin resistance. $[Mg^{2+}]_i$ was significantly associated with adiponectin ($r=0.246$, $p=0.04$), IGF-1($r=0.272$, $p<0.03$), QUICKI ($r=0.592$, $p<0.0001$) (Table 2). From these findings, $[Mg^{2+}]_i$ as well as leptin and IGF-1 reflects the extent of fetal growth. Decreased $[Mg^{2+}]_i$ may be involved in the underlying processes to insulin resistance.

Thus, $[Mg^{2+}]_i$ of the cord blood platelet may be a marker of early fetal growth, and can be used as a novel predictor of adult diseases. Low $[Mg^{2+}]_i$, may represent the prenatal programming of insulin resistance, and may have lifelong effects on metabolic regulation. Our results indicate a possible role of $[Mg^{2+}]_i$ in fetal life for future disorders characterized by insulin resistance.

Fetal / Early Childhood Antecedents and Adult Chronic Diseases

Epidemiological studies in humans have shown that impaired intrauterine growth is associated with an increased incidence of cardiovascular, metabolic, and other diseases in later life [43,44]. Low birth weight is often followed by accelerated postnatal growth, and this may be important for risk of metabolic syndrome in adult life. People who had low birth weight or who subsequently showed catch-up growth have higher susceptibility for central obesity, type 2 diabetes, and cardiovascular disease in later life [45].

(A) Fetal Programming

Fetal programming is the phenomenon whereby alteration in fetal growth and development in response to the prenatal environment has long-term or permanent effects. The mechanisms are supposed to be as a direct effect on cell number, altered stem cell function and resetting of regulatory hormonal axes (Figure 2).

There are several candidates for explaining gestational programming as follows: [1] a potential role for the hypothalamic-pituitary-adrenal (HPA) axis has been suggested, as the mediators of the fetal response to nutrient stress, i.e. maternal low protein diet, were profoundly suppressed [46,47]; [2] fetal programming of the growth hormone insulin-like growth factor (GH-IGF) axis also has been proposed to serve as a link between fetal growth and adult-onset disease [48].

(B) Thrifty Phenotype Hypothesis

The "thrifty phenotype hypothesis", which postulates that fetal programming for adaptation to an adverse intrauterine environment results in lower insulin sensitivity in utero, is one of the hypotheses to explain the association between low birth weight and insulin resistance in later life [49].

Decreased in $[Mg^{2+}]_i$ in infants with SGA can be the initial pathophysiologic events of fetal programming. In fact, a recent animal study supported our data demonstrating that the maternal Mg restriction irreversibly increases body fat and induces insulin resistance in pups by 6 months of age [27].

(C) Epigenetic Modification of Gene

It is intriguing in clinical practice that the intrauterine environment can program adult disease susceptibility by altering the epigenetic state of the fetal genome, hence affecting the phenotype without changing the DNA sequence [50]. The changes in the intrauterine environment may ultimately lead to altered gene expression via alterations in DNA methylation and other epigenetic mechanisms, resulting in an increased susceptibility to chronic disease in adulthood [51]. Biological methylation reaction is dependent on dietary methyl donors and on cofactors. Mg acts as a cofactor for the binding of protein to its specific site in DNA by inducing conformational changes in the protein [52]. Mg also changes the conformation to a more helical structure which could provide specific geometrical constraints complementary to those of DNA helix.

Conclusion

The fetal origin hypothesis by Barker et al. states that fetal under-nutrition in middle to late gestation leading to disproportionate fetal growth programs later metabolic diseases. As low $[Mg^{2+}]_i$ is an intrinsic abnormality seen in infants with low birth weight, it is considered that the fetal Mg deficiency resulting in low birth weight is an important determinant of insulin resistance in later life. Further exploration is, however, obviously needed to investigate the pathophysiological mechanism underlying the development of metabolic syndrome in the light of the unknown developmental abnormalities during the fetal period.

References

[1] Barker, D.J., Hales, C.N., Fall, C.H., Osmond, C., Phipps, K. and Clark, P.M. (1993): Type 2 (non-insulin-dependent) diabetes mellitus, hypertension and hyperlipidaemia (syndrome X):relation to reduced fetal growth. *Diabetologia.* 36, 62-67.

[2] Hales, C.N., Barker, D.J., Clark, P.M. et al. (1991): Fetal and infant growth and impaired glucose tolerance at age 64. *B.M.J.* 303,1019-1022.

[3] Lucas, A. (1994): Programming in determing adult morbidity. *Arch. Dis. Child.* 71, 288-290.

[4] Barker, D.J.P. (1995): Fetal origin of coronary heart disease. *B.M.J.* 311, 171-174.

[5] Paolisso, G., Scheen, A., D'Onofrio, F. and Lefebvre, P. (1990): Magnesium and glucose homeostasis. *Diabetologia.* 33, 511-514.

[6] Rosolova, H., Mayer, O. Jr. and Reaven, G.M. (2000): Insulin-mediated glucose disposal is decreased in normal subjects with relatively low plasma magnesium concentrations. *Metabolism.* 49,418-420.

[7] Resnick, L.M., Gupta, R.K., Gruenspan, H., Alderman, M.H., and Laragh, J.H. (1990): Hypertension and peripheral insulin resitance: possible mediating role of intracellular free magnesium. *Am. J. Hypertens.* 3,373-379.

[8] Nadler, J.L,, Buchanan, T., Natarajan, R. et al. (1993): Magnesium deficiency produces insulin resistance and increased thromboxane synthesis. *Hypertension.* 21,1024-1029.

[9] Huerta, M.G., Roemmich, J.N., Kington, M.L. et al. (2005): Magnesium deficiency is associated with insulin resistance in obese children. *Diabetes. Care.* 28,1175-1181.

[10] Sibal, B.M., Villar, M.A. and Bray, E.A. (1989): Magnesium supplementation during pregnancy: a double blind randomized controlled clinical trial. *J. Obstet. Gynecol.* 161, 115-119.

[11] Painter, R.C., Roseboom, T.J. and Bleker, O.P. (2005): Prenatal exposure to the Dutch famine and disease in later life: an overview. *Reprod. Toxicol.* 20, 345-352.

[12] Yang, C.Y., Chiu, H.F., Tsai, S.S., Chang, C.C. and Sung, F.C. (2002): Magnesium in drinking water and the risk of delivering a child of very low birth weight. *Magnes. Res.* 15, 207-213.

[13] Widdowson, E.M. (1981): Changes in body composition during growth. In: Davis, J.A., Dobbing, J., eds. *Scientific foundations of paediatrics*. London: William Heinemann Medical Books Ltd, 330-42.

[14] Lall R, Wapnir RA. Meconium mineral content in small for gestational age neonates. (2005): *Am. J. Perinatol.* 22, 259-63.

[15] Husain., M.E. and Mughal, M.Z. (1992): Mineral transport across the placenta. *Arch. Dis. Child.* 67, 874-878.

[16] Nandakumaran, M., Dashti, H.M. and Al-Zaid, N.S. (2002): Maternal-fetal transport kinetics of copper, selenium, magnesium and iron in perfused human placental lobule: in vitro study. *Mol. Cell Biochem*. 231, 9-14.

[17] Standley, P.R. and Standley, C.A. (2002): Identification of a functional Na+/Mg2+ exchanger in human trophoblast cells. *Am. J. Hypertension*. 15, 565-570.

[18] Husain, S.M., Mughal, M.Z. and Sibley,C.P. (2000): Effects of acute maternal hyperglycaemia and hyperosmolarity on maternofetal transfer of calcium and magnesium across the in situ perfused rat placenta. *Magnes. Res*.13, 239-47.

[19] Handwerker, S.M., Altura, B.T., Jones, K.Y. and Altura, B.M. (1995): Maternal-fetal transfer of ionized serum magnesium during the stress of labor and delivery: a human study. *J. Am. Coll. Nutr*. 14. 376-381.

[20] Bischof, P., Meisser, A., and Campana, A. (2000): Paracrine and autocrine regulators of trophoblast invasion—a review. Placenta 21, Suppl A, *Trophoblast Research*. 14, S55-S60.

[21] Yi, F.X., Magness, R.R. and Bird, I.M. (2005): Simultaneous imaging of $[Ca^{2+}]_i$ and intracellular NO prodiuction in freshly isolated uterine artery endothelial cells: effect of ovarian cycle and pregnancy. *Am. J. Physiol. Regul. Integr. Comp. Physiol*. 288, R140-R148.

[22] Pearson, P.J. Evora, P.R.B., Seccombe, J.F. et al. (1998): Hypomagnesemia inhibits nitric oxide release from coronary endothelium: protective role of magnesium infusion after cardiac operations. *Ann. Thorac. Surg*. 65, 967-972.

[23] Lemancewicz, A., Laudanska, H., Laudanski, T., Karpiuk, A. and Barta, S. (2000): Permeability of fetal membranes to calcium and magnesium:possible role in preterm labour. *Human Reproduction*. 15, 2018-2022.

[24] Jasson, T. and Lambert, G.W. (1999): Effect of intrauterine growth restriction on blood pressure, glucose tolerance and sympathetic nervous system activity in the rat at 3-4 months of age. *J. Hypertens*. 17, 1239-1248.

[25] Kubena, K.S., Edgar, S.E., and Veltmann, J.R. (1988): Growth and development in rats and deficiency of magnesium and pyridoxine. *J. Am. Coll. Nutr*. 7, 317-24.

[26] Buck D.R., and Bales, J. (1983): Maternal dietary magnesium effects on lactation success and on milk yield and composition in the rat. *J. Nutr*. 113, 2421-31.

[27] Venu, L., Kishore, D.K., and Raghnath, M. (2005): Maternal and perinatal magnesium restriction predisposes rat pups to insulin resistance and glucose intolerance. *J. Nutr*. 135,1353-8.

[28] USDA. (1990): Continuing survey of food intake by individuals 1989 and 1990, USDA Public Use Data Tape, Washington, DC: USDA

[29] Spatling, L. and Spatling, G. (1988): Magnesium supplementation in pregnancy. A double-blind study. *Br. J. Obstet .Gynaecol.* 95, 120-125.

[30] Kurzel, R. B. (1991): Serum magnesium levels in pregnancy and preterm labor. *Am. J. Perinatol.* 8, 119-127.

[31] Conradt, A., Weidinger, H. and Algayer, H. (1985): Magnesium therapy with betamimetics decreased the rate of intrauterine fetal retardation, premature rupture of membranes and premature delivery in risk pregnancies treated with betamimetics. *Magnesium.* 4,20-28.

[32] Makrides, M. and Crowther, C.A. (2002): Magnesium supplementation in pregnancy. Cochrane Database Syst Rev.In: *The Cochrane Library*, Issue 4: CD 000937. Update Software, Oxford.

[33] Doyle, W., Crawford, M.A., Wynn, A.H. and Wynn, S.W. (1989): Maternal magnesium intake and pregnancy outcome. *Magnes. Res.* 2, 205-210.

[34] Rudnicki, M., Frolich, A., Rasmussen, W.F. and McNair, P. (1991): The effect of magnesium on maternal blood pressure in pregnancy-induced hypertension. A randomized double-blind placebo-controlled trial. *Acta. Obstet. Gynecol. Scand.* 70, 445-450.

[35] Resnick, L.M., Gupta, R.K., Bhargava, K.K., Gruenspan, H., Alderman, M.H., and Laragh, J.H. (1991): Cellular ions in hypertension, diabetes, and obesity. *Hypertension.* 17, 951-957.

[36] Trovati, M., Anfossi, G., Cavalot, F., Massucco, P., and Emanuelli, G. (1988): Insulin directly reduces platelet sensitivity to aggregating agents. *Diabetes.* 37, 780-786.

[37] Takaya, J., Higashino, H., Miyazaki, R., and Kobayashi, Y. (1998): Effects of insulin and insulin-like growth factor-1 on intracellular magnesium of platelets. *Exp. Mol. Pathol.* 65, 104-109.

[38] Wang, D.L., Yen, C.F., and Nadler, J.L. (1993): Insulin increases intracellular magnesium transport in human platelets. *J. Clin. Endocrinol. Metab.* 76, 549-553.

[39] Takaya, J., Higashino, H., Kotera, F. and Kobayashi, Y. (2003): Intracellular magnesium of platelets in children with diabetes and obesity. *Metabolism.* 52, 468-471.

[40] Takaya, J., Yamato, F., Higashino, H. and Kobayashi, Y. (2004) relationship of intracellular magnesium of cord blood platelets to birth weight. *Metabolism.* 53, 1544-1547.

[41] Chiesa, C., Osborn, J.F., Haass, C., Natale, F., Spinelli, M. et al. (2008): Ghrelin, Leptin, IGF-1, IGFBP-3, and Insulin Concentrations at Birth: Is There a Relationship with Fetal Growth and Neonatal Anthropometry? *Clin. Chem.* 54, 550-8.

[42] Takaya, J., Yamato, F., Higashino, H., and Kaneko, K. (2007): Intracellular magnesium and adipokines in umbilical cord plasma and infant birth size. *Pediatr. Res.* 62, 700-703

[43] Barker, D.J.P. (1994): Mothers, babies and disease in later life. London: *B. M. J.* Publishing group.

[44] Phillips, D.I., Barker, D.J., Hales, C.N., Hirst, S. and Osmond, C. (1994): Thinness at birth and insulin resistance in adult life. *Diabetologia.* 37, 150-154.

[45] Hales, C.N., and Barker, D.J. (2001): The thrifty phenotype hypothesis. *Br. Med. Bull.* 60, 5-20.

[46] Phillips, I.D., Simonetta, G., Owens, J.A., Robinson, J.S., Clarke, I.J. and McMillen, I.C. (1996): Placental restriction alters has functional development of the pituitary-adrenal axis in the sheep fetus during late gestation. *Pediatr. Res.* 40, 861-866.

[47] Ozanne, S.E., Smith, G.D., Tikerpae, J. and Hales, C.N. (1996): Altered regulation of hepatic glucose output in the male offspring of protein-malnourished rat dams. *Am. J. Physiol.* 270, E559-E564.

[48] Holt, R.I. (2002): Fetal programming of the growth hormone insulin-like growth factor axis. *Trends. Endocrionol. Metab.* 13, 392-397.

[49] Hales, C.N., and Barker, D.J. (1992):Type 2 (non-insulin-dependent) diabetes mellitus: the thrifty phenotype hypothesis. *Diabetologia.* 35, 595-601.

[50] Reok, W., Dean, W., and Walter, J. (2001): Epigenetic reprogramming in mammalian development. *Science.* 293,1089-1093.

[51] Waterland, R.A., and Jirtle, R.L. (2004): Early nutrition, epigenetic changes at transposons and imprinted genes, and enhanced susceptibility to adult chronic diseases. *Nutrition.* 20,63-68.

[52] De, A., Ramesh, V., Mahadevan, S., and Nagaraja, V. (1998): Mg^{2+} mediated sequence-specific binding of transcriptional activator protein C. *Biochemistry.* 37, 3831-38.

In: Dietary Magnezium: New Research
Editor: Andrew W. Yardley

ISBN 978-1-60692-109-8

Chapter IV

Dietary Magnesium and Metabolic Syndrome

Fernando Guerrero-Romero* and Martha Rodríguez-Morán
Biomedical Research Unit, Mexican Social Security Institute
Nucleus of Research and Clinical Diagnosis (NIDIAC)
Durango, Mexico

Abstract

People with metabolic syndrome, a cluster of obesity, high blood pressure, dyslipidemia, and hyperglycemia, have at increased risk for cardiovascular disease and diabetes. Although components of the metabolic syndrome are related with inappropriate dietary patterns, the role of dietary constituents in the pathogenesis of the syndrome is poorly understood.

Evidence show that low dietary intakes of magnesium contributes to development of insulin resistance, a major component of the metabolic syndrome, supporting the hypothesis that suboptimal intake of magnesium might play a significant role in the development of the syndrome. On the other hand, recently has been reported that magnesium depletion is independently associated to low chronic inflammatory syndrome, suggesting that hypomagnesemia and low-grade inflammation are interactive risk factors for the metabolic syndrome and chronic disease.

Cross-sectional analyses of data from population based studies show that intake of magnesium is inversely related with the prevalence and incidence of metabolic syndrome. In addition, data from controlled randomized clinical trials provide evidence that oral magnesium supplementation restores serum magnesium levels decreasing inflammation and improving insulin sensitivity, high blood pressure, lipid profile, and serum glucose levels.

* Correspondence to: Fernando Guerrero-Romero MD, PhD, FACP, Siqueiros 225 esq./Castañeda, 34000 Durango, Dgo., Mex. Phone: (+52 618) 812-0997; Fax (+52 618) 813-2014; E-mail guerrero_romero@hotmail.com

Nonetheless, to determine whether low dietary intake of magnesium is associated with an increased risk for the metabolic syndrome and, its potential usefulness in the prevention strategies of cardiovascular disease and diabetes requires confirmation, and further research.

We review the clinical evidence that show the association between dietary intake of magnesium and the metabolic syndrome; furthermore, we present results from a randomized double-bind clinical trial showing the efficacy of oral magnesium supplementation in the reduction of inflammation.

Introduction

Magnesium is an essential cofactor of high-energy enzymatic pathways involved in the energetic metabolism, synthesis of protein, and modulation of glucose transport across cell membranes [1-3]. Furthermore, an interaction between magnesium and other ions occurs at the cellular level, regulating calcium, sodium, and potassium transmembrane movement [4, 5].

Magnesium deficiency is a common and frequently multifactorial entity [6], regularly induced by a diet and drinking water low in magnesium and/or increased magnesium loss [7, 8]. Hypomagnesemia has been associated with developing of type 2 diabetes [9], high blood pressure, [10] atherogenic alterations [11, 12], and micro-, and macro-vascular diabetic complications [13-15]. Furthermore, hypomagnesemia also has been strongly associated with metabolic syndrome [16].

The metabolic syndrome a co-occurrence of disturbed glucose metabolism, overweight and abdominal fat distribution, dyslipidemia, and high blood pressure has been associated with the subsequent development of cardiovascular disease and type 2 diabetes [17]. The *metabolic syndrome* was defined by the presence of at least three of the following risk factors: Fasting plasma glucose >100 mg/dL, abdominal obesity (waist circumference >102 cm in men and >88 in women), triglycerides ≥150 mg/dL, low HDL-cholesterol (<40 mg/dL in men and <50 mg/dL in women), and systolic and diastolic blood pressures ≥130 and 85 mmHg [19, 18]. The pathogenesis of the *syndrome* has multiple origins, but obesity and sedentary lifestyle coupled with diet and still largely unknown genetic factors clearly interact to produce the *syndrome* [20].

In addition, cross-sectional analyses of data from population based studies show an inverse correlation between both serum magnesium and dietary intake with the metabolic syndrome [16, 21].

On the other hand, Pickup et al [22] showed that elevated acute-phase/stress reactants (the innate immune system's response to environmental stress) and their major cytokine mediator are associated with the occurrence of metabolic syndrome, and may thus provide a unifying pathophysiological mechanism for this condition. Abnormalities of the innate immune system showed to be contributors to the hypertriglyceridemia, low HDL-cholesterol, hypertension, glucose intolerance, insulin resistance, and accelerated atherosclerosis [22].

On this regard, a growing body of evidence showing that coronary heart disease has an inflammatory component [23, 24] and that elevated plasma C-reactive protein (CRP) concentration predicts cardiovascular disease [25-27] is rapidly accumulating. In addition, data from observational studies show a strong relationship between hypomagnesemia and elevated serum concentrations of pro-inflammatory cytokines, CRP [28, 29], and pro-inflammatory neuropeptide levels [30] that may contribute to cardiovascular disease. Furthermore, recently, King et.al. [31] demonstrated that subjects with dietary intake of magnesium at levels below the recommended daily allowance are more likely to have elevation of CRP levels [31], defined as CRP serum concentration in the range of 3.0-10.0 mg/l [32].

We review the clinical evidence showing the association between dietary intake of magnesium and the metabolic syndrome; furthermore, we present results from a randomized double-bind clinical trial showing the efficacy of oral magnesium supplementation in the reduction of inflammation.

Dietary Intake of Magnesium

Magnesium is a widely occurring element, and its primary paths of entry into the organism are through water and food [33]. Magnesium absorption is inversely proportional to intake and occurs principally from the ileum and colon [6].

In addition to modern food processing, that cause magnesium lost in food, several other factors are involved in the reduction of magnesium within the ecosystem as whole; among these, acid rain causes exchanges between magnesium and aluminium in the soil that coupled with intensive farming have reduced magnesium within the food chain [6].

The U.S. Recommended Dietary Allowances (RDA) of magnesium for adult women is 320 mg/day and for adult men 420 mg/day [34, 35]. However, the RDA for magnesium in adults of various countries varies widely; as an example, in the Japanese women and men are 240 and 310 mg/day, in the English women and men 270 and 300 mg/day, in Australians women and men 270 and 320 mg/day, in Russian women and men 400 mg/day [36]. Although, small amounts of magnesium are required in the diet to ensure the capacity for energy expenditure and to maintain optimal physiological functions, surveys show that the dietary intake of magnesium is inadequate in the U.S. and other populations [37-40]. On this regard, about 23% of U.S. adults aged 25–74 years had a serum magnesium concentration lower than 1.9 mg/dL, a concentration that is consistent with hypomagnesemia [41], supporting the finding that dietary magnesium intake continues to be inadequate among large numbers of people in the US [40]; on the other hand, data on magnesium intake and serum magnesium concentrations in the vast majority of people living in developed and undeveloped countries is unknown. The findings of magnesium intake below recommendations should encourage the intake of foods with high magnesium content such as whole grains, nuts, shellfish, fish, green leafy vegetables, beans, dried fruit, cereals, and legumes [33, 42-44].

Despite the growing interest in the relations between dietary patterns and disease is necessary to keep in mind some limitations of the methodology for assessing micronutrients in diet: First, the main approach in the analysis of the link between dietary factors and the risk of chronic illnesses has been focused on individual nutrients or food items [45], which could be a limitation because the analysis of individual nutrients do not take into account the interactions of mixing different foods that could affect absorption of some micronutrients [46]; Second, measurement of the dietary data requires an appropriate instrument for capturing and analyzing the components of the foods of interest that minimize the bias in measuring magnesium intake; Third, because the tool used to evaluate the pattern of habitual food consumption generally are questionnaires listing food items to the choice of respondents, dietary changes during the period of study are not considered and the possibility of bias recall is high. Nonetheless, because the most frequent source of magnesium deficiency is an inadequate diet, results of follow-up studies evaluating the role of dietary magnesium intake on the risk of developing type 2 diabetes consistently show that deficient magnesium intake is associated with its development [9, 47-51].

Magnesium Intake and Systemic Low-Grade Inflammatory Syndrome

In response to stress and environmental insult, there is a significant change in the concentration of certain plasma proteins, the called acute-phase proteins [22, 52]. These proteins, synthesized in the liver by the stimulus of cytokines, have a major action that contributes to host defense and adaptation to insult [53]. The acute-phase reaction, a response of the innate immune system, is seen in many chronic inflammatory diseases. Among the main proinflammatory cytokines, Interleukine-1 (IL-1) and IL-6, and Tumor Necrosis Factor-alpha (TNF-α) act on the liver to stimuli the production of acute-phase proteins but also decrease the production of HDL-cholesterol [54-56]. On the other hand, among the main acute-phase proteins, the CRP, fibrinogen, serum amyloid, and others, are atherosclerotic risk factors contributing to hypertension, dyslipidemia, and insulin resistance [57, 58]. Thus, the mechanisms involved in the acute-phase response can be major contributors to the pathophysiology of many features of metabolic syndrome, type 2 diabetes, and cardiovascular disease [22, 59].

The antecedent of an association between magnesium and immune function derives from findings showing the early appearance of clinical signs of inflammation in magnesium deficient rats, the activation of immune cells during experimental magnesium deficiency, and the elevation of acute-phase proteins in the magnesium deficiency status [60-65].

The sequence of early events that produces the acute-phase response linked to magnesium deficiency is currently unknown; however, new data are emerging [61, 63, 66, 67]. It appears that abnormal calcium handling induced by extracellular magnesium deficiency may be the origin of an exacerbated inflammatory response [62], and that the activated or primed state of immune cells is an early event occurring in magnesium deficiency [62]. In addition, there is increasing evidence showing that these mechanisms could be mediated by an increase of substance P during magnesium deficiency.

Previously, we have reported data from a case-control study showing that hypomagnesemia is a trigger of both low-grade chronic inflammatory and metabolic syndrome [68], results agree with experimental data that suggest that hypomagnesemia elevates circulating pro-inflammatory neuropeptide levels [66], and clinical data showing that low serum magnesium levels and deficient dietary magnesium intake are strongly related to low-grade systemic inflammation [21, 31].

In this regard Barbagallo et.al. [69] have hypothesized that magnesium could be the missing link in the pathophysiology of insulin resistance, type 2 diabetes and cardiovascular disease. Based in the interaction hypomagnesemia → inflammation and hypomagnesemia → insulin resistance, we propose that magnesium deficiency may be the link between low-grade chronic inflammation and metabolic syndrome (Figure 1).

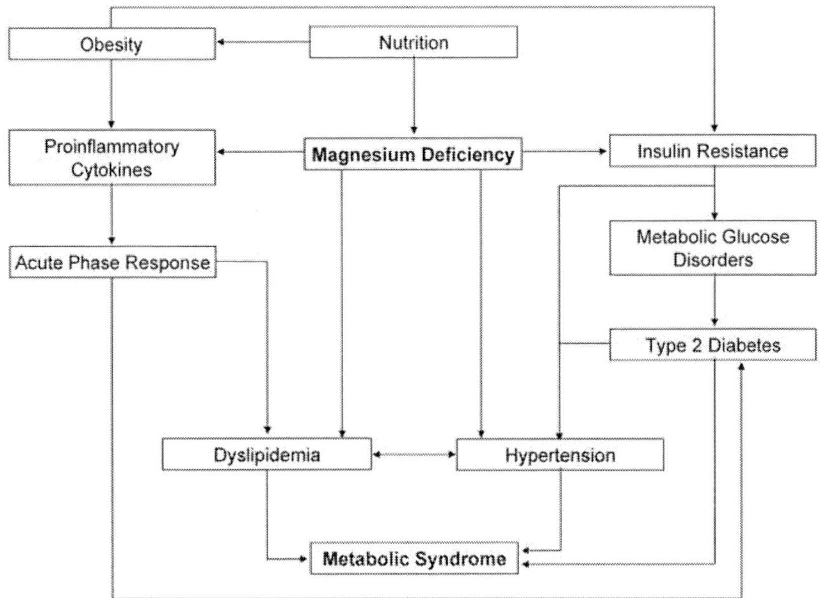

Figure 1. Relationship between magnesium deficiency with insulin resistance and the acute phase response in the pathophysiology of metabolic syndrome. Epidemiological, experimental, and clinical data supports the association between magnesium deficiency and both the triggering of acute phase response and insulin resistance that are in the base of the pathophysiology of metabolic syndrome.

Because available data regards the interaction between hypomagnesemia and inflammation have been obtained from cross-sectional analysis, recently we conducted a randomized double-bind clinical trial for evaluating the efficacy and security of oral magnesium supplementation in the reduction of inflammatory and pro-inflammatory markers. For this purpose, besides the institutional approval of protocol and after obtaining the subject informed consent, apparently healthy subjects were eligible to participate if they had both hypomagnesemia and elevated CRP and TNF-α levels.

Based on previous results on healthy subjects from our community, hypomagnesemia was defined by serum magnesium concentration equal or lower than 0.74 mmol/L [16, 29], and elevated CRP and TNF-α levels by serum concentration equal or greater than 3 mg/L, and ≥3.5 pg/mL, respectively [28, 68].

Chronic diarrhea, alcohol intake (equal or more than 30 g per day), smoking, diabetes, high blood pressure, malignancy, surgical stress, chronic diseases, diuretic therapy, and reduced renal function were exclusion criteria. In addition, subjects who received magnesium supplementation before randomization were not included.

The primary trial end point was the change in CRP and TNF-α levels. Sample size was determined based on a statistical power of 80%, alpha value 0.05, and allowing non-improve in the serum insulin level of 40 and 80% for the subjects who received magnesium supplementation and placebo, respectively. The required sample size to detect a treatment effect was of 26 subjects in each group [70]. To compensate potential withdrawn, finally 31 and 30 subjects were randomly allocated to daily receive either magnesium chloride ($MgCl_2$) 2.5 g (that represents approximately 300 mg/day of magnesium) or placebo during 12-weeks. Magnesium chloride solution (50 gr of $MgCl_2$ by 1000 ml of solution) was the magnesium supplement used. In fasting conditions, subjects in the $MgCl_2$ group drank 50 ml of the 5% solution; thus they received 2.5 g of $MgCl_2$ daily.

Adherence to magnesium supplementation was assessed every month by personal interview and measurement of residual solution of $MgCl_2$. All the participants and personnel assessing outcomes were blinded to group assignment.

There were not dropped out nor serious adverse events or side effects due to $MgCl_2$ or placebo. All the randomized subjects satisfactorily completed the follow-up. Adherence to treatment was achieved for 28 (90.3%) subjects in the $MgCl_2$ group and 29 (96.7%) subjects in the placebo group.

At baseline there were not differences by age, anthropometric, or laboratory characteristics between the magnesium-supplemented and control subjects (Table 1).

Subjects who received $MgCl_2$ significantly increased their serum magnesium concentrations compared with subjects in the placebo group (0.81 ± 0.09 versus 0.74 ± 0.11 mmol/L, $p<0.0001$). In addition, at end of follow-up, magnesium-supplemented subjects significantly reduced their CRP and TNF-α levels (Figure 2).

Our data show that restore of hypomagnesemia decrease inflammatory and pro-inflammatory markers in apparently healthy subjects with decreased serum magnesium levels. We can hypothesize that magnesium deficiency could be the trigger of the acute-phase response that and the release of CRP and TNF-α that may contribute to the development of metabolic syndrome.

Table 1. Baseline characteristics of subjects randomly allocated to receive either 12-weeks of 50 ml of magnesium chloride ($MgCl_2$) solution (50 g of $MgCl_2$ by 1000 ml of solution, equivalent to 300 mg of magnesium) or placebo

	$MgCl_2$ n = 31	Placebo n = 30	p value
Age, years	39.2 ± 7.3	40.1 ± 6.1	0.34
Body Mass Index, Kg/m^2	30.5 ± 4.7	31.1 ± 4.1	0.23
Fasting glucose, mg/dL	110.1 ± 17.2	107.6 ± 13.3	0.13
C-reactive protein, mg/L	10.2 ± 4.7	10.1 ± 3.9	0.21
TNF-alpha, pg/mL	7.9 ± 2.7	7.7 ± 3.1	0.09
Serum magnesium, mmol/L	0.72 ± 0.16	0.74 ± 0.15	0.08

Although this is the first report based on randomized clinical trial showing the efficacy and security of oral magnesium supplementation as an alternative treatment for the low-grade chronic inflammatory syndrome, its clinical implications in the prevention of metabolic syndrome remained to be established.

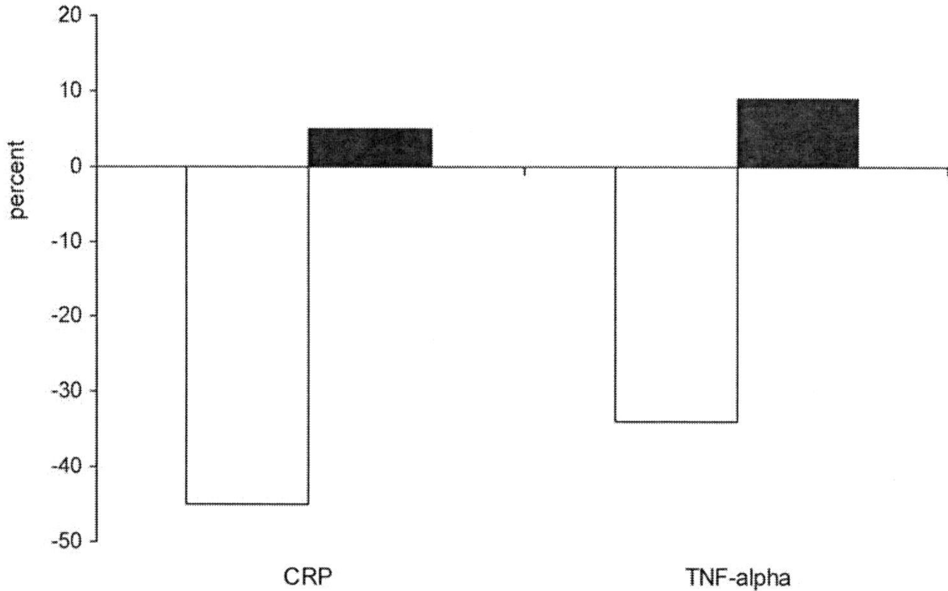

Figure 2. Variation of serum C Reactive protein (CRP) and Tumor Necrosis Factor Alpha (TNF-alpha) in the subjects who daily received 50 ml of magnesium chloride solution (50 g of MgCl2 by 1000 ml of solution, equivalent to 300 mg of magnesium) (white bar) or placebo (black bar). At 12-weeks of treatment, subjects receiving MgCl2 significantly reduced both CRP and TNF-alpha levels. Bars represent the percent variation between baseline and end conditions.

Magnesium Intake and Metabolic Syndrome

Whether low intake of magnesium is certainly associated with an increased risk of developing metabolic syndrome is important to determine in light of the syndrome's increasing prevalence in the U.S. population and the suboptimal intake of magnesium [40, 71].

Major determinants of the metabolic syndrome are obesity and insulin resistance [72, 73]. Because in the genesis of obesity, overeating and lack of physical activity are its main contributors, and obesity leads to alterations of the normal physiological balance of adipokines, insulin resistance, endothelial dysfunction, and a atherogenic state [74], components and style of diet play an important role in the development of metabolic syndrome; in addition, previously has been reported that hypomagnesemia and the low intakes of magnesium contribute to insulin resistance [47, 75, 76]. Thus, there is a rationale base supporting the hypothesis that inadequate diet with low dietary magnesium intake may play a role in the pathogenesis of metabolic syndrome.

Recently, Ford et.al. [71] using data from the Third National Health and Nutrition Examination Survey (1988 to 1994) test the hypothesis that dietary intake of magnesium is associated with the prevalence of metabolic syndrome. Their results showed an inverse association between dietary magnesium intake and the prevalence of metabolic syndrome in agree with findings from the Women's Health Study, and the Coronary Artery Risk Development in Young Adults Study [21, 77]. These based populations studies consistently indicate a protective role for the individuals in the highest magnesium intake. Data from the Third National Health and Nutrition Examination Survey (1988 to 1994) and Women's Health Study, were analyzed in a cross-sectional way; they showed an Odds Ratio, that computes the association between dietary magnesium and metabolic syndrome for the participants women, for the highest quintile of magnesium intake of 0.73 (95% CI, 0.60 – 0.88) and 0.55 (95% CI 0.2- 1.03), respectively [21, 71]. On the other hand, the Coronary Artery Risk Development in Young Adults Study [77], a 15 years follow-up study, prospectively analyzed the relationship between dietary magnesium and metabolic syndrome among young American people who were free from metabolic syndrome at baseline. They found that magnesium intake was associated inversely, in a dose-response manner, with the risk of incident metabolic syndrome; the Hazard Ratio for the subjects in the highest quartile of magnesium intake was 0.69 (95% CI 0.52 – 0.91).

Although results from these studies consistently shown an inverse relationship between dietary magnesium intake and metabolic syndrome, the interaction of nutrients other than magnesium and dietary fiber, that also are in the main sources of dietary magnesium were not controlled. Undoubtedly, further research is warranted to provide new data in this field.

However, taking into account that experimental and clinical evidence suggest that the amount of magnesium intake in the western diet is insufficient to meet individual needs and that magnesium deficiency may be related to the risk of high blood pressure, hyperglycemia, hypertriglyceridemia, low HDL-cholesterol, insulin resistance, and inflammation [78, 79, 80] there is strong biological plausibility for the direct impact of magnesium intake on metabolic and cardiovascular risk factors [81].

With regards of the association between magnesium dietary intake and the components of metabolic syndrome, data from the three large population based studies analyzing magnesium intake and metabolic syndrome [21, 71, 77] are inconsistent. On one hand, Ford et.al. [71] did not find association of none of the five components of metabolic syndrome with magnesium intake after adjustment for demographic variables and potential confounders. On the other hand, also after adjusted analysis, Song et.al. [21] reported that the prevalence of each of the components of the metabolic syndrome was lower in the women in the highest quintile of magnesium intake compared with women in the lowest quintile, and He et.al. [77] found that magnesium intake was inversely associated to components of metabolic syndrome, particularly between magnesium intake and fasting glucose, waist circumference, and HDL-cholesterol.

Although data are no entirely consistent, accumulating evidence from experimental, observational, clinical, and epidemiological studies suggests that magnesium deficiency is strongly related to individuals components of metabolic syndrome [82-86], suggesting that diets rich in magnesium could be beneficial for cardiometabolic health. Improves of insulin sensitivity and down-regulation of markers of inflammation [76, 79] may be the mechanisms by which a higher dietary magnesium intake reduce the risk of developing metabolic syndrome.

Conclusion

There is a growing body of evidence showing that magnesium intake is inversely associated with metabolic syndrome and its components. Deterioration of insulin sensitivity and the triggering of low inflammatory chronic syndrome seems to be the link between magnesium deficiency and metabolic syndrome. Results from long-term randomized clinical trials are needed to evaluate the safety and efficacy of diets rich in magnesium for reducing the incidence of metabolic syndrome.

References

[1] Guerrero-Romero F, Rodríguez-Morán M. Complementary therapies for diabetes: The case for chromium, magnesium, and antioxidants. *Arch. Med. Res.* 2005; 36: 250-57.

[2] Paolisso G, Barbagallo M. Hypertension, diabetes mellitus, and insulin resistance: the role of intracellular magnesium. *Am. J. Hypertens* 1997; 10: 346-355.

[3] Paolisso G, Scheen A, D'Onofrio F, Lefèbvre P. Magnesium and glucose homeostasis. *Diabetologia* 1990; 33: 511-514.

[4] Zofkova I, Kancheva RL. The relationship between magmnesium and calciotrophic hormones. *Magnes. Res.* 1995; 8: 77-84.

[5] Bara M, Guiet-Bara A, Durlach J. Regulation of sodium and potassium pathways by magnesium in cell membranes. *Magnes. Res.* 1993; 6: 167-177.

[6] Fawcett WJ, Haxby EJ, Male DA. Magnesium: physiology and pharmacology. *Br. J. Anaesth* 1999; 83: 302-320.

[7] Ryan MF. The role of magnesium in biochemistry: an overview. *Ann. Clin. Biochem.* 1991; 28: 19-26.

[8] Lefebvre PJ, Paolisso G, Scheen AJ. Magnesium and glucose metabolism. *Therapie* 1994; 49: 1-7.

[9] Kao WHL, Folsom AR, Nieto JF, Mo J-P, Watson RL, Brancati FL. Serum and dietary magnesium and the risk for type 2 diabetes mellitus. *Arch. Intern. Med.* 1999; 159: 2151-2159.

[10] Kisters K, Spieker C, Tepel M, Zidek W. New data about the effect of oral physiological magnesium supplementation on several cardiovascular risk factors (lipids and blood pressure). *Magnes. Res.* 1993; 6: 355-360.

[11] Guerrero-Romero F, Rodríguez-Morán M. Hypomagnesemia is linked to low serum HDL-cholesterol irrespective of serum glucose values. *J. Diabetes Complicat.* 2000; 14: 272-276.

[12] White JR Jr, Campbell RK Magnesium and diabetes: a review. *Ann. Pharmacother.* 1993; 27: 775-780.

[13] Grifò G, Lo Presti R, Montana M, Canino B, Caimi G. Plasma, erythrocyte and platelet magnesium in essential hypertension, diabetes mellitus without and with macrovascular complications and atherosclerotic vascular disease. *Recenti Prog. Med.* 1995; 86: 431-436.

[14] Rodríguez-Morán M, Guerrero-Romero F. Low serum magnesium levels and foot ulcers in subjects with type 2 diabetes. *Arch. Med. Res.* 2001; 32: 300-303.

[15] Grafton G, Bunce CM, Sheppard MC, Brown G, Baxter MA. Effect of Mg^{2+} on Na(+)-dependent inositol transport. Role for Mg^{2+} in etiology of diabetic complications. *Diabetes* 1992; 41: 35-39.

[16] Guerrero-Romero F, Rodríguez-Morán M. Low serum Magnesium levels and Metabolic Syndrome. *Acta Diabetológica* 2002; 39: 209-213.

[17] Liese AD, Mayer-Davis EJ, Haffner SM. Development of the multiple metabolic syndrome: an epidemiologic perspective. *Epidemiol. Rev.* 1998; 20: 157-172.

[18] Alberti KG, Zimmet PZ. Definition, diagnosis and classification of diabetes mellitus and its complications, I: diagnosis and classification of diabetes mellitus provisional report of a WHO consultation. *Diabet Med.* 1998; 15: 539-553.

[19] Executive Summary of The Third Report of The National Cholesterol Education Program (NCEP) Expert Panel on Detection, Evaluation, And Treatment of High Blood Cholesterol in Adults (Adult Treatment Panel III). *JAMA* 2001; 285: 2486-2497.

[20] Lakka H-M, Laaksonen DE, Lakka TA, Niskanen LK, Kumpusalo E, Tuomilehto J, Salonen JT. The Metabolic Syndrome and Total and Cardiovascular Disease Mortality in Middle-aged Men. *J*AMA 2002; 288: 2709-2716.

[21] Song Y, Ridker PM, Manson JE, Cook NR, Buring JE, Liu S. Magnesium intake, C-reactive protein, and the prevalence of metabolic syndrome in middle-aged and older U.S. women. *Diabetes Care* 2005; 28: 1438-1444.

[22] Pickup JC, Crook MA. Is type II diabetes mellitus a disease of the innate immune system?. *Diabetologia.* 1998; 41: 1241-1248.

[23] de Maat MP, Pietersma A, Kofflard M, Sluiter W, Kluft C. Association of plasma fibrinogen levels with coronary artery disease, smoking and inflammatory markers. *Atherosclerosis* 1996; 121: 185-191.

[24] Munro JM, Cotran RS. The pathogenesis of atherosclerosis: atherogenesis and inflammation. *Lab. Invest.* 1988; 58: 249-261.

[25] Thompson SG, Kienast J, Pyke SD, Haverkate F, van de Loo JC. Hemostatic factors and the risk of myocardial infarction or sudden death in patients with angina pectoris: European Concerted Action on Thrombosis and Disabilities Angina Pectoris Study Group. *N. Engl. J. Med.* 1995; 332: 635–641.

[26] Tracy RP, Lemaitre RN, Psaty BM, Ives DG, Evans RW, Cushman M, Meilahn EN, Kuller LH. Relationship of C-reactive protein to risk of cardiovascular disease in the elderly: results from the Cardiovascular Health Study and the Rural Health Promotion Project. *Arterioscler. Thromb. Vasc. Biol.* 1997; 17: 1121–1127.

[27] Kuller LH, Tracy RP, Shaten J, Meilahn EN. Relation of C-reactive protein and coronary heart disease in the MRFIT nested case-control study: Multiple Risk Factor Intervention Trial. *Am. J. Epidemiol.* 1996; 144:537-547.

[28] Rodríguez-Morán M, Guerrero-Romero F. Elevated concentrations of TNF-alpha are related to low serum magnesium levels in obese subjects. *Magnes. Res*. 2004; 17: 189-196.

[29] Guerrero-Romero F, Rodríguez-Morán M. Relationship between serum magnesium levels and C-reactive protein concentration, in non-diabetic, non-hypertensive obese subjects. *Int. J. Obes. Relat. Metab. Disord.* 2002; 26: 469-474.

[30] Kramer JH, Mak IT, Phillips TM, Weglicki WB. Dietary magnesium intake influences circulating pro-inflammatory neuropeptide levels and loss of myocardial tolerance to postischemic stress. *Exp. Biol. Med. (Maywood)* 2003; 228: 665-673.

[31] King DE, Mainous AG 3rd, Geesey ME, Woolson RF. Dietary magnesium and C-reactive protein levels. *J. Am. Coll. Nutr*. 2005; 24:166-171.

[32] Hutchinson W., Koenig W., Frölich M., Sund M., Lowe G., Pepys M.B. Immunoradiometric assay of circulating C-Reactive protein: Age related values in the adult general population. *Clin. Chem*. 2000; 46: 934-938.

[33] Tukiendorf A. Magnesium intake and hepatic cancer. In: Nishizawa Y, Morii H, Durlach J, Editors. *New perspectives in magnesium research: nutrition and health.* London, UK: Springer; 2006: 155-169.

[34] Lowenstein FW, Stanton MF Serum magnesium levels in the United States, 1971–1974. *J. Am. Coll. Nutr.* 1986; 5: 399-414.

[35] Institute of Medicine. Dietary reference intakes for calcium, phosphorus, magnesium, vitamin D, and fluoride. Washington, DC: National Academy Press 1997.

[36] Kimura M. Overview of magnesium nutrition. In: Nishizawa Y, Morii H, Durlach J, Editors. *New perspectives in magnesium research: nutrition and health.* London, UK: Springer; 2006:69-93.

[37] Pennington JA, Schoen S A. Total diet study: estimated dietary intakes of nutritional elements, 1982–1991. *Int. J. Vitam Nutr. Res.* 1996; 66: 350-362.

[38] Galan P, Preziosi P, Durlach V, Valeix P, Ribas L, Bouzid D, Favier A,.Hercberg S. Dietary magnesium intake in a French adult population. *Magnes. Res*. 1997; 10: 321-328.

[39] Ford ES. Race, education, and dietary cations: findings from the Third National Health and Nutrition Examination Survey. *Ethn. Dis*. 1998; 8:10-20.

[40] Ford ES, Mokdad AH. Dietary magnesium intake in a National Sample of U.S. adults. *J. Nutr.* 2003; 133: 2879-2882.

[41] Whang R,.Sims G. Magnesium and potassium supplementation in the prevention of diabetic vascular disease. *Med. Hypotheses* 2000; 55: 263-265.

[42] Liu S, Manson JE, Stampfer MJ, Hu FB, Giovannucci E, Colditz GA, Hennekens CH, Willett WC: A prospective study of whole-grain intake and risk of type 2 diabetes mellitus in US women. *Am. J. Public Health* 2000; 90: 1409–1415.

[43] van Dam RM, Hu FB, Rosenberg L, Krishnan S, Palmer JR. Dietary Calcium and Magnesium, Major Food Sources, and Risk of Type 2 Diabetes in U.S. Black Women. *Diabetes Care* 2006; 29: 2238-2243.

[44] Guerrero-Romero F, Rodríguez-Morán M. Magnesium intake and the incidence of type 2 diabetes. In: Nishizawa Y, Morii H, Durlach J, Editors. *New perspectives in magnesium research: nutrition and health.* London, UK: Springer; 2006: 143-154.

[45] Virtanen SM, Aro A. Dietary factors in the aetiology of diabetes. *Ann. Med.* 1994; 26: 469-478.

[46] Montonen J, Knekt P, Härkänen T, Järvinen R, Heliövaara M, Aromaa A, Reunanen A. Dietary patterns and the incidence of type 2 diabetes. *Am. J. Epidemiol.* 2005; 161: 219-227.

[47] Song Y, Manson JE, Buring JE, et al. Dietary Magnesium Intake in Relation to Plasma Insulin Levels and Risk of Type 2 Diabetes in Women. *Diabetes Care* 2004 27: 59-65.

[48] Salmeron J, Ascherio A, Rimm EB, et al. Dietary fiber, glycemic load, and risk of NIDDM in men. *Diabetes Care* 1997; 20: 545-50.

[49] Salmeron J, Manson JE, Stampfer MJ, et al. Dietary fiber, glycemic load, and risk of non-insulin-dependent diabetes mellitus in women. *JAMA* 1997; 277: 472-77.

[50] Lopez-Ridaura R, Willett WC, Rimm EB, et al. Magnesium Intake and Risk of Type 2 Diabetes in Men and Women. *Diabetes Care* 2004; 27: 134-40.

[51] Meyer KA, Kushi LH, Jacobs Jr DR, et al. Carbohydrates, dietary fiber, and incident type 2 diabetes in older women. *Am. J. Clin. Nutr.* 2000; 71: 921-930.

[52] Baumann H, Gauldie J. The acute phase response. *Immunol. Today* 1994;15: 74-80.

[53] Kushner I, Rzewnicki DL. The acute phase response: general aspects. *Baillieres Clin. Rheumatol.* 1994; 8: 513-530.

[54] Conraads VM, Bosmans JM, Schuerwegh AJ, De Clerck LS, Bridts CH, Wuyts FL, Stevens WJ, Vrints CJ. Association of lipoproteins with cytokines and cytokine receptors in heart failure patients. Differences between ischaemic versus idiopathic cardiomyopathy. *Eur. Heart J.* 2003; 24: 2221-2226.

[55] Bolton CH, Downs LG, Victory JG, Dwight JF, Tomson CR, Mackness MI, Pinkney JH. Endothelial dysfunction in chronic renal failure: roles of lipoprotein oxidation and pro-inflammatory cytokines. *Nephrol. Dial Transplant.* 2001; 16: 1189-1197.

[56] Barter PJ, Nicholls S, Rye K-A, Anantharamaiah GM , Navab M, Fogelman AM. Antiinflammatory Properties of HDL. *Circ. Res.* 2004; 95: 764-772.

[57] Inayat-ur-Rahman, Malik SA, Khan WA. Relation of serum sialic acid with serum lipids in cardiac patients. *Pak. J. Pharm. Sci.* 2005; 18: 71-73.

[58] Malik Sh, Wong ND, Franklin S, Pio J, Fairchild C, Chen R. Cardiovascular Disease in U.S. Patients With Metabolic Syndrome, Diabetes, and Elevated C-Reactive Protein. *Diabetes Care* 2005; 28: 690 - 693.

[59] Ridker PM, Buring JE, Cook NR, Rifai N. C-Reactive Protein, the Metabolic Syndrome, and Risk of Incident Cardiovascular Events: An 8-Year Follow-Up of 14 719 Initially Healthy American Women. *Circulation* 2003; 107: 391-397.

[60] Laires MJ, Monteiro C. Exercise and magnesium. In: Nishizawa Y, Morii H, Durlach J, Editors. *New perspectives in magnesium research: nutrition and health.* London, UK: Springer; 2006: 173-185.

[61] Malpuech-Brugère C, Nowacki W, Rock E, Gueux E, Mazur A, Rayssiguier Y. Enhanced tumor necrosis factor-alpha production following endotoxin challenge in

rats is an early event during magnesium deficiency. *Biochim. Biophys. Acta* 1999; 1453: 35-40.

[62] Malpuech-Brugère C, Rock E, Astier C, Nowacki W, Mazur A, Rayssiguier Y. Exacerbated immune stress response during experimental magnesium deficiency results from abnormal cell calcium homeostasis. *Life Sci.* 1998; 63: 1815-1822.

[63] Malpuech-Brugère C, Nowacki W, Daveau M, Gueux E, Linard C, Rock E, Lebreton J, Mazur A, Rayssiguier Y. Inflammatory response following acute magnesium deficiency in the rat. *Biochim. Biophys. Acta* 2000; 1501: 91-98.

[64] Weglicki WB, Phillips TM, Freedman AM, Cassidy MM, Dickens BF. Magnesium-deficiency elevates circulating levels of inflammatory cytokines and endothelin. *Mol. Cell Biochem.* 1992; 110: 169-173.

[65] Weglicki WB, Phillips TM. Pathobiology of magnesium deficiency: a cytokine/neurogenic inflammation hypothesis. *Am. J. Physiol.* 1992; 263 (3 Pt 2): R734-737.

[66] Dong A, Caughey WS, Du Clos TW. Effects of calcium, magnesium, and phosphorylcholine on secondary structures of human C-reactive protein and serum amyloid P component. *J. Biol. Chem.* 1994; 269: 6424-8430.

[67] Dobrinich R, Spagnuolo PJ. Binding of C-reactive protein to human neutrophils. Inhibition of respiratory burst activity. *Arthritis Rheum.* 1991; 34: 1031-1038.

[68] Guerrero-Romero F, Rodríguez-Moran M. Hypomagnesemia, oxidative stress, inflammation, and metabolic syndrome. *Diabet Metab. Res. Rev.* 2006; 22: 471-476.

[69] Barbagallo M, Dominguez LJ, Galioto A, Ferlisi A, Cani C, Malfa L, Pineo A, Busardo A, Paoliso G. Role of magnesium in insulin action, diabetes, and cardio-metabolic syndrome *X. Mol. Aspects Med.* 2003; 24: 39-52.

[70] Mejía-Aranguré JM, Fajardo-Gutierrez A, Gómez-delgado A, et al. El tamaño de la muestra. Un enfoque práctico en la investigación clínica pediátrica. *Bol. Med. Hos. Infant Mex.* 1995; 52: 381-391.

[71] Ford ES, Li C, McGuire LC, Mokdad AH, Liu S. Intake of dietary magnesium and the prevalence of the metabolic syndrome among U.S. adults. *Obesity* 2007; 15: 1139-1146.

[72] Isomaa B. A major health hazard: the metabolic syndrome. *Life Sci.* 2003; 73: 2395-2411.

[73] Hanley AJ, Wagenknecht LE, D'Agostino RB Jr, Zinman B, Haffner SM. Identification of subjects with insulin resistance and beta-cell dysfunction using alternative definitions of the metabolic syndrome. *Diabetes* 2003; 52: 2740-2747.

[74] Ritchie SA, Connell JM. The link between abdominal obesity, metabolic syndrome and cardiovascular disease. *Nutr. Metab. Cardiovasc. Dis.* 2007; 17: 319-326.

[75] McCarty MF. Magnesium may mediate the favorable impact of whole grains on insulin sensitivity by actino as a mild calcium antagonist. *Med. Hypotheses* 2005; 64: 619-627.

[76] Rumawas ME, McKeown NM, Rogers G, Meigs JB, Wilson PWF, Jacques PF. Magnesium intake is related to improved insulin homeostasis in the Framingham Offspring Cohort. *J. Am. Coll. Nutr.* 2006; 25: 486-492.

[77] He K, Liu K, Daviglus ML, Morris SJ, Loria CM, Van Horn L, Jacobs DR Jr, Savage PJ. Magnesium intake and incidence of metabolic syndrome among young adults. *Circulation* 2006; 113: 1675-82.

[78] He K, Song Y, Belin RJ, Chen Y. Magnesium intake and the metabolic syndrome: epidemiologic evidence to date. *J. Cardiometab. Syndr.* 2006; 1: 351-355.

[79] Rayssiguier Y, Gueux E, Nowacki W, Rock E, Mazur A. High fructuose consumption combined with low dietary magnesium intake may increase the incidence of the metabolic syndrome by reducing inflammation. *Magnes. Res.* 2006; 19: 237-243.

[80] Song Y, Li TY, van Dam RM, Manson JE, Hu FB. Magnesium intake and plasma concentrations of markers of systemic inflammation and endothelial dysfunction in women. *Am. J. Clin. Nutr.* 2007; 85: 1068-1074.

[81] Bo S, Pisu E. Role of dietary magnesium in cardiovascular disease prevention, insulin sensitivity and diabetes. *Curr. Opin. Lipidol.* 2008; 19: 50-56.

[82] Mizushima S, Cappuccio FP, Nichols R, Elliott P. Dietary magnesium intake and blood pressure: a qualitative overview of the observational studies *J. Hum. Hypertens* 1998; 12: 447-453.

[83] Singh RB, Rastogi SS, Mani UV, Seth J, Devi L. Does dietary magnesium modulate blood lipids? *Biol. Trace Elem. Res.* 1991; 30: 59-64.

[84] De Leeuw I, Vansant G, Van Gaal L. Magnesium and obesity: influence of gender, glucose tolerance, and body fat distribution on circulating magnesium concentrations. *Magnes. Res.* 1992; 5: 183-187.

[85] Rodriguez-Hernandez H, Gonzalez JL, Rodriguez-Moran M, Guerrero-Romero F. Hypomagnesemia, insulin resistance, and non-alcoholic steatohepatitis in obese subjects. *Arch. Med. Res.* 2005; 36: 362-366.

[86] Jee SH, Miller ER III, Guallar E, Singh VK, Appel LJ, Klag MJ. The effect of magnesium supplementation on blood pressure: a meta-analysis of randomized clinical trials. *Am. J. Hypertens* 2002; 15: 691-696.

Reviewed by

Kuninobu Yokota MD, PhD
Associate Professor
Department of Internal Medicine
Jikei University School of Medicine
Tokyo, Japan
yokota@jikei.ac.jp

In: Dietary Magnezium: New Research
Editor: Andrew W. Yardley

ISBN 978-1-60692-109-8

Chapter V

Relation of Vitamin D, Calcium, and Magnesium to the Risk of Type 2 Diabetes Mellitus

***Sara Chacko*[1] *and Simin Liu*[2]**
[1]Department of Epidemiology, University of California, Los Angeles
[2]Departments of Epidemiology and Medicine, University of California, Los Angeles

Abstract

An increasing body of evidence suggests that low vitamin D status may impair both insulin secretion and action, ultimately increasing the risk of type 2 diabetes mellitus (DM). Experimentally, vitamin D repletion improves insulin sensitivity and insulin secretion in animal studies of rats. Cross-sectional studies in humans suggest an inverse association between circulating vitamin D levels and impaired glucose tolerance, insulin resistance, and risk of type 2 diabetes. Prospective data, albeit limited, also indicate an inverse association between intake of dietary and supplemental vitamin D and type 2 diabetes risk. Calcium and magnesium may exert both independent and interactive effects on the risk of type 2 diabetes through metabolically related pathways. Genetic variants of these pathways, including the vitamin D receptor (VDR) pathway and calcium and magnesium homeostasis related pathways, also appear to play a role in affecting the risk of type 2 diabetes in humans.

I. Introduction

Several lines of evidence support the hypothesis that low vitamin D status is associated with impaired β-cell function, insulin resistance, impaired glucose tolerance, and type 2 diabetes. Experimental studies have identified vitamin D receptors (VDR) on the pancreatic β-cells that may promote transcription of genes (human insulin gene) necessary for insulin secretion[1]. Low bioavailability of vitamin D can therefore negatively impact insulin production and potentially lead to impaired glucose tolerance and type 2 diabetes, although the exact mechanism of this action and the extent of influence on β-cell function and insulin resistance are not fully understood.

The vitamin D endocrine system is complex, involving multiple pathways and interactions, and it is possible that the effects of vitamin D on insulin and glucose metabolism are mediated by metabolically related minerals. Vitamin D is principally responsible for calcium and phosphorus homeostasis and may play a role in magnesium absorption. Accumulating evidence suggests that calcium and magnesium may exert independent and interactive effects on insulin secretion, insulin resistance, and type 2 diabetes, although the extent of influence and interaction with vitamin D is uncertain.

This chapter will review and summarize the physiology and metabolism of vitamin D in the body and consider potential interactions with calcium, magnesium, and other minerals. Animal and epidemiologic evidence linking low vitamin D status to insulin secretion, insulin resistance, and type 2 diabetes will also be assessed. We will also explore potential biological mechanisms and future research directions with a special emphasis on genetic polymorphisms of the vitamin D receptors (VDR) and magnesium and calcium homeostasis related pathways.

II. A Brief Overview of the Vitamin D Endocrine System

A. Overview

Vitamin D consists of a group of fat-soluble steroid prohormones that are essential for healthy body functioning. There are two main forms of vitamin D, cholecalciferol (vitamin D_3), and ergocalciferol (vitamin D_2). Vitamin D_3 can be obtained in small amounts from fatty fish such as salmon, mackerel, tuna, and cod. In addition, some dairy and cereal products are fortified with vitamin D_3 in the U.S. Yet, the major source of vitamin D in the body is still synthesized in the skin after direct exposure to sunlight or ultraviolet light whereby 7-dehydrocholestrol in the plasma membrane of the epidermal cells is converted to cholecalciferol. The amount of cholecalciferol the skin produces depends on the duration of exposure, time of day, season, latitude of the location, sunscreen use and skin pigmentation [2]. Vitamin D_2 is produced by ultraviolet irradiation of plant sterols and is added to some foods. After consumption of vitamin D containing food or endogenous production in the body, vitamin D is further metabolized by the liver and the kidney into the hormonally active form of the vitamin, 1,25-dihydroxyvitamin D ($25(OH)_2D$). (Hereinafter, vitamin D refers to both cholecalciferol [vitamin D_3] and ergocalciferol [vitamin D_2] unless otherwise specified). The first step in vitamin D metabolism is transport to the liver where it is hydroxylated into 25-hydroxyvitamin D (25(OH)D) and released into the blood stream. If there are adequate stores of 25(OH)D circulating in the bloodstream, it is then converted into the vitamin D hormone 1,25-dihydroxyvitamin D ($1,25\ (OH)_2D$), or calcitriol, in the kidney. The production of $1,25\ (OH)_2D$ in the kidney is homeostatically regulated through a negative feedback loop controlled by parathyroid hormone (PTH). When serum calcium (Ca^{2+}) levels drop, PTH is secreted from the parathyroid gland and directly stimulates 1,25 $(OH)_2D$ production in the kidney to increase Ca^{2+} absorption and ensure the maintenance of calcium homeostasis. Conversely, 1,25 $(OH)_2D$ synthesis is suppressed in states of hypercalcemia due to low secretion of PTH (Figure 1)[3].

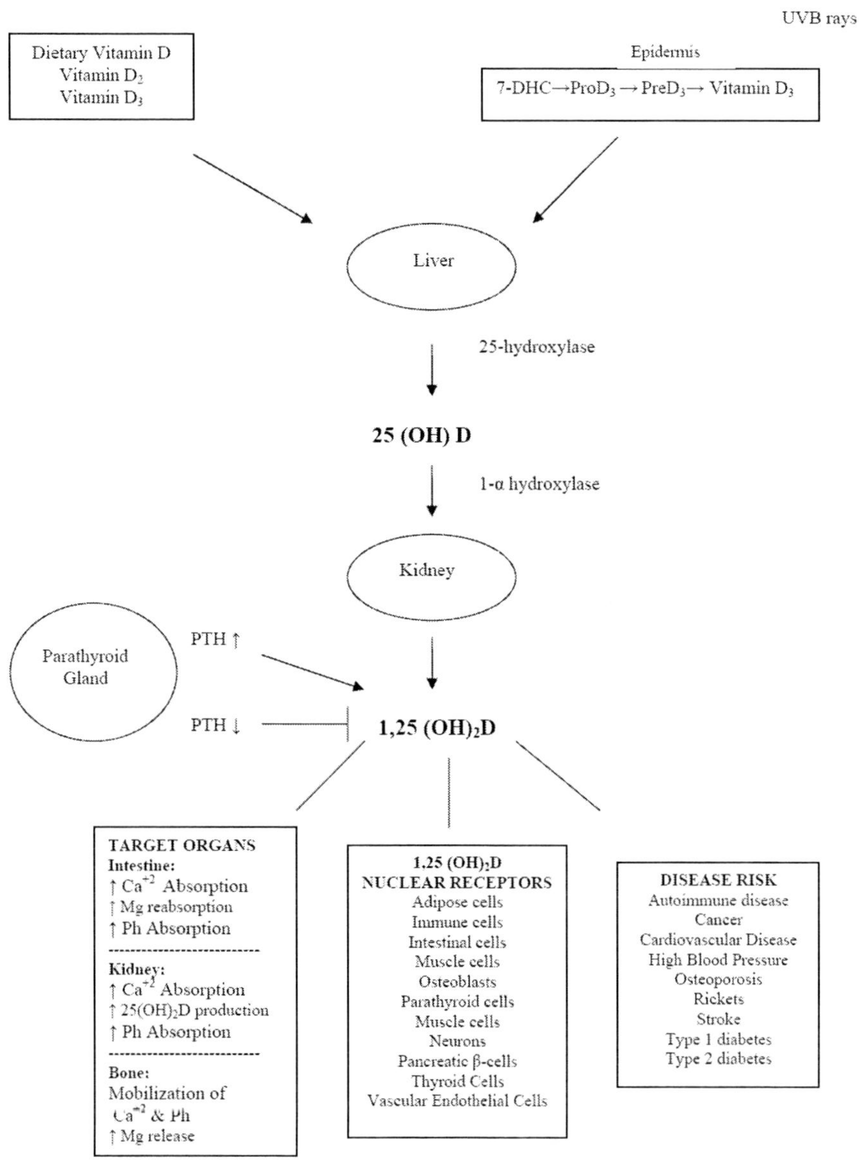

Figure 1. Vitamin D Endocrine System.

1,25 $(OH)_2D$ is a potent steroid hormone with strong regulatory effects on calcium homeostasis, and it is considered the active metabolite of vitamin D in the body. 1,25 $(OH)_2D$ binds to vitamin D receptors (VDR) which can be found in more than thirty cell types throughout the body, including intestinal cells, muscle cells, osteoblasts, parathyroid cells, epidermal cells, vascular endothelial cells, neurons, immune cells, and pancreatic β-cells [4]. VDR acts as a transcription factor to regulate the rate of gene transcription in many cell types throughout the body, exerting effects on calcium homeostasis, cell proliferation and differentiation, immune function, and various endocrine functions including insulin resistance [5].

B. Interaction with Calcium and Phosphorous

The major physiologic functions of vitamin D in the body include the regulation of calcium and phosphorous homeostasis in the blood and the promotion of bone mineralization and growth. Target organs of the system include the intestine, bone, and kidney[6]. Homeostatic control of extracellular calcium (Ca^{2+}) is essential for numerous cellular and tissue functions, and a feedback system involving vitamin D controls the balance of intra- and extracellular calcium[7]. Levels of extracellular Ca^{2+} must be maintained within the range of 7 mgCa/100 ml to 12 mg/100 ml for optimal physiological functioning[8]. When Ca^{2+} concentrations fall below the optimal level, 1,25 $(OH)_2D$ acts to increase Ca^{2+} through increasing the absorption of calcium from the gastrointestinal tract and reabsorption of calcium into the kidney. 1,25 $(OH)_2D$ binds to nuclear receptors in the intestinal cells which stimulate the synthesis of messenger RNA molecules that code for calcium binding protein (CaBP), a protein responsible for transporting calcium into the bloodstream. Synthesis of CaBP is dependent on the presence of 1,25 $(OH)_2D$ in the blood. Therefore, if circulating serum vitamin D falls below the optimal level (80 nmol/L; 32 ng/dL)[9-12], dietary calcium absorption is impaired and stores of calcium from the bones must be mobilized to maintain normal functioning of the neuromuscular system.

Phosphorous is an essential mineral required by the body for bone and teeth mineralization, ATP production, utilization of macronutrients for growth, and cell and tissue repair[13]. Excessive serum phosphate can inhibit the production of 1,25 $(OH)_2D$ in the kidneys, reduce extracellular Ca^{2+} concentrations, and increase the production of parathyroid hormone (PTH)[14], which may lead to secondary hyperparathyroidism, a condition associated with osteoporosis and bone degradation. 1,25 $(OH)_2D$ acts to maintains normal phosphorous levels in the blood through a mechanism similar to the control of extracellular Ca^{2+}. 1,25 $(OH)_2D$ increases absorption of dietary phosphorus in the gut, reabsorption in the kidney, and mobilization of phosphate from the bone through stimulation of osteoclastic activity[5].

C. Interaction with Calciotropic Hormones

Calcium homeostasis is principally mediated by the actions of the calciotropic hormones including 1,25 $(OH)_2D$, PTH, and calcitonin. 1,25 $(OH)_2D$ interacts with PTH and calcitonin to exert direct and indirect effects on hundreds of physiological processes. PTH, released in response to low extracellular levels of calcium (Ca^{2+}), is an important endocrine regulator of calcium homeostasis and stimulates the production of 1,25 $(OH)_2D$ in the kidney. A negative feedback loop exists between calcium, PTH, and 1,25 $(OH)_2D$ that ensures that extracellular calcium levels (Ca^{2+}) are maintained within the narrow limits required for cellular function. PTH works to maintain Ca^{2+} levels through several mechanisms including the stimulation of the production of 1,25 $(OH)_2D$ in the kidney and subsequent absorption of calcium in the small intestine, the mobilization of calcium from the bone, and suppression of calcium loss in urine [15]. Calcitonin, a calciotropic hormone produced primarily in the C cells of the thyroid gland, is also involved in the endocrine control of calcium. Calcitonin exerts effects on the bone and kidney to decrease elevated extracellular Ca^{2+} levels in the blood and maintain calcium balance in the body [16].

Calcium homeostasis is essential for numerous physiological functions including proper functioning of the neuromuscular system, secretion of hormones and enzymes, blood clotting, and the mineralization of bone and teeth. Given the close metabolic interconnections of the hormones involved in the homeostatic control of calcium, it is imperative to consider the joint and interactive effects when discussing the physiological effects of vitamin D.

D. Interaction with Magnesium

Vitamin D may also play an important role in magnesium absorption[17], although the extent of influence is not completely understood. Magnesium, an essential intracellular cation that acts as a co-factor in hundreds of enzymatic reactions in the body, has been shown to interact with calciotropic hormones and is highly involved in calcium homeostasis [18]. Just as PTH is secreted in response to low extracellular concentrations of Ca^{2+}, PTH is released in response to low extracellular concentrations of Mg [19]. PTH stimulates Mg reabsorption in the Loop of Henle and the distal tubule [20, 21], releases Mg from the bone [18], and increases intestinal absorption[22, 23]. In addition, PTH leads to increased production of 1,25 $(OH)_2D$ in the kidney which may mediate this process further enhancing Mg absorption in the intestine (Figure 2) [24, 25].

III. Vitamin D Status

Serum levels of 25(OH)D are currently the best marker of vitamin D bioavailability in humans and are used to measure vitamin D status [26]. There is currently no clear consensus among researchers as to what constitutes a deficiency in vitamin D. One proposed categorization includes deficiency (0-25 nmol/l; 0-10ng/ml), insufficiency (<25-50.0 nmol/l; <10-20ng/ml), hypovitaminosis D (<50-100 nmol/l; <20-40 ng/ml), adequacy (70-100 to 250 nmol/l; 28-40 to 100 ng/ml), and toxicity (>250 nmol/l; >100 ng/ml) [27]. Recent work in the field suggests that higher levels of vitamin D may have beneficial effects on a number of adverse health outcomes. It has been suggested that the optimal physiologic level of serum vitamin D for calcium absorption, PTH concentration, and a number of other health outcomes including bone health, lower-extremity function, dental health, and colorectal cancer prevention falls between 75 nmol/L (30 ng/mL) to 100 nmol/L (40 ng/dL)[9-12, 28, 29].

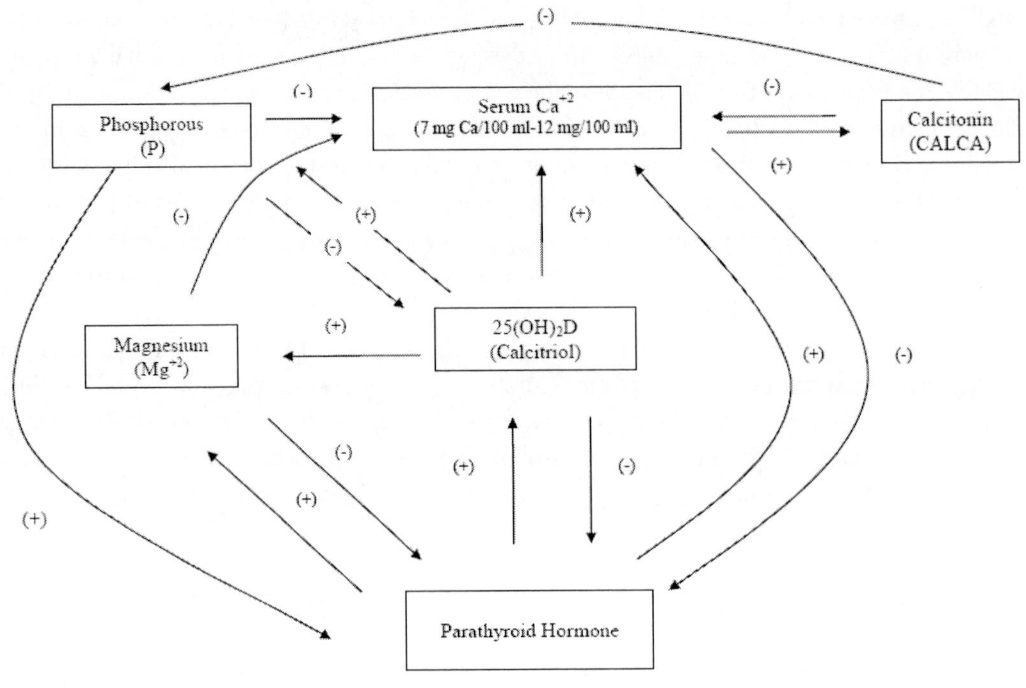

Figure 2. The Interaction between Vitamin D, Calcium, Phosporous, Magnesium and Capciotropic Hormones.

Low vitamin D status is an increasingly recognized problem worldwide, and recently it has been identified as an "epidemic" in the United States. [11]. A number of factors, including limited sun exposure, dark skin pigmentation, lack of dietary vitamin D, and obesity have been identified as risk factors for low vitamin D status. High risk groups for low vitamin D status include the elderly, especially those living in nursing homes [30]; the obese [31, 32]; and dark skinned individuals who do not produce adequate amounts of cholecalciferol from sunlight exposure due to high skin pigmentation [2, 33, 34]. However, increasing evidence suggests low vitamin D status is also common among apparently healthy populations, especially in the winter time. One cross-sectional study assessing serum vitamin D levels in Boston found a 36% prevalence of vitamin D insufficiency among healthy young adults aged 18-29 (n=69) at the end of winter [35].

A. Vitamin D Status and the Elderly

Low vitamin D status among the elderly is a well-documented problem and may lead to decreased bone and muscle strength and the increased incidence of bone fractures due to impaired calcium absorption [30]. Several serological studies have found a high prevalence of vitamin D deficiency among older populations [36, 37]. This may be partially explained by a decrease in the concentration of important vitamin D precursors, including 7-

dehydrocholesterol and previtamin D_3, in the skin of older individuals. A reduction in these vitamin D precursors can potentially result in the decreased production of vitamin D_3. McLaughlin et al.[38] found a strong negative association ($r = -0.89$) between age and levels of 7-dehydrocholesterol in the skin independent of the total mass of the epidermis. Furthermore, the production of previtamin D_3 in the epidermis and dermis was more than two times greater among 8-year-olds (442 ng/cm^2 preD-3) than among 82-year-olds (183 ng/cm^2 preD-3) after exposure to ultraviolet radiation. These findings suggest that aging affects the ability of skin to produce the necessary precursors for vitamin D synthesis, making elderly individuals more susceptible to low vitamin D status. The elderly may also increase their risk of vitamin D deficiency by staying indoors longer or consuming a diet poor in vitamin D[2].

B. Vitamin D Status and Obesity

Overweight and obese individuals are also at high-risk for low vitamin D status. Although this association is not completely understood, one possible explanation is that overweight individuals have inadequate exposure to UV radiation in sunlight due to clothing choices or limited mobility[39]. Alternatively, it is possible that increased production of 1,25 $(OH)_2D$ in obese individuals exerts negative feedback on hepatic synthesis of 25(OH)D[40].

It has also been suggested that vitamin D may accumulate in excess adipose tissue in obese individuals resulting in reduced bioavailability of the vitamin in the bloodstream, and several recent reports indicate that total adiposity may be an important predictor of low vitamin D status. In a study of the cutaneous synthesis of vitamin D_3 in response to UV-B irradiation (n=13 controls, BMI: 22.2 ± 0.04; n=13 obese participants, BMI: 38 ± 1.7), basal concentrations of 7-dehydrocholesterol and vitamin D_3 were not significantly different between obese and control participants. However, 24 hours after exposure to whole body irradiation (wavelength 260-330 nm), the increase in circulating vitamin D_3 concentrations was significantly less in obese participants than in controls (Difference between basal and post-irradiation vitamin D_3 concentrations: Controls: 38.3 ± 5.5 nmol/L vs obese participants: 17.4 ± 3.6 nmol/L; $p=0.0029$)[41]. These findings support the hypothesis that vitamin D synthesized by the skin is not readily available in the bloodstream in obese individuals, perhaps due to excessive storage in body fat. In addition, total body fat percentage measured with dual-energy x-ray absorptiometry (DXA) was negatively associated with circulating levels of 25(OH)D ($r= -0.13$, $p=.013$) in a cross-sectional study of healthy women (n=410, aged 20-80 years old, BMI ranging from 17-30 kg/m^2) after controlling for race, age, season, and dietary vitamin D intake [42]. More recently, DXA total body fat percentage was negatively associated with 25(OH)D levels in a sample of men and women (n=453) aged 65 years and older ($r= -0.261$, $p< 0.001$). The association was attenuated with the use of anthropometric measures (i.e BMI, waist circumference, waist-to-hip ratio) indicating that fat mass, not total body weight, is the most important factor driving the inverse relation between obesity and circulating 25(OH)D concentrations [43].

However, it is also possible that obesity is the consequence of low vitamin D status. Excess parathyroid hormone (PTH), released in response to low circulating 25(OH)D concentrations, stimulates the production of 1,25 $(OH)_2D$ in the kidney to increase extracellular calcium (Ca^{2+}) concentrations and maintain calcium homeostasis. However, excess 1,25 $(OH)_2D$ also stimulates the influx of extracellular Ca^{2+} into the adipocytes, and thus may enhance lipogenesis and weight gain [44, 45]. Several studies have reported an inverse relation between calcium levels and obesity [46-49].

Irrespective of the underlying biological mechanism, cross-sectional studies of obese individuals consistently show decreased serum vitamin D levels in overweight and obese individuals [31, 32, 39, 43, 50-53]. A small cross-sectional study (n=13 obese white participants; n=13 nonobese white participants) showed that serum 25(OH)D levels were significantly lower in obese white subjects than non obese subjects (Mean 25(OH)D levels in obese 11 ± 1 ng/ml vs. Nonobese: 16 ± 2 ng/ml; $p< 0.05$) [32]. Among morbidly obese females (n=60) tested for vitamin D deficiency, 62% were found to be below the "normal" range (defined as 16-74 ng/ml). In addition, serum vitamin D levels were negatively correlated to BMI ($r=-0.49$; $p<0.001$) [31]. Among middle-aged Caucasian subjects from the 1958 British birth cohort (n=1,798), serum 25(OH)D levels decreased with increasing BMI (25(OH)D <75 nmol/l among 80% of obese participants vs 68% of nonobese subjects; p for trend < 0.001)[54]. Results from the Third National Health and Nutrition Examination Survey (NHANES III, 1988-1994) were consistent with these findings. After controlling for multiple risk factors, the odds of abdominal obesity increased linearly across decreasing quintiles of serum concentrations of 25(OH)D [25(OH)D ≥96.4 nmol/l: OR= 0.30 (0.21,0.42); 78.2-96.3 nmol/l: OR=0.55 (0.41, 0.72); 63.5-78.1 nmol/L: OR=0.65 (0.52,0.81); 48.5-63.4 nmol/l: OR=0.78 (0.61,0.98); p for trend < .0001) [53]. Furthermore, among 10,066 women aged ≥45 years in the Women's Health Study, means of waist circumference and BMI increased significantly across decreasing quintiles of total vitamin D intake [Waist circumference: Highest quintile of vitamin D intake (511-2369 IU/day): 39.7 inches; Lowest quintile (6.0-159 IU/day): 43.5 inches, p for trend = 0.0004; BMI: Highest quintile: 14.4 kg/m^2; Lowest quintile: 20.2 kg/m^2, p for trend < 0.0001][55].

C. Vitamin D Status and Ethnicity

Ethnic, cultural, and geographic factors such as skin color, dress, diet, and latitude influence vitamin D status, and substantial variation in vitamin D status is observed across ethnic groups and countries. Ethnic groups with dark skin pigmentation, especially African Americans, are at increased risk for low vitamin D status due to high levels of melanin in the skin. Research suggests that melanin in the skin competes with 7-dehydrocholesterol (7-DHC) for UVB rays, thereby limiting the synthesis of vitamin D-3 in individuals with dark skin [56]. Observational studies assessing vitamin D status in humans show that African-Americans have lower circulating levels of 25(OH)D and are more likely to be vitamin D deficient that other ethnic groups [33, 50, 56-58]. Mean levels of 25(OH)D were found to be lower in African Americans than in Caucasians in a clinical intervention study (n=26) assessing the vitamin D endocrine system [6±1 vs 20±2 ng/ml, $p<0.001$][57]. Likewise, in a cross-sectional study of 379 obese African American and Caucasian adults, 43% of African Americans had 25(OH)D levels ≤ 37.5 nmol/L as compared with 11.7% of the Caucasians.

[50]. Furthermore, results from NHANES III (1988-1994) suggest that almost 50% of African American women of reproductive age in the United States have 25(OH)D levels $\leq$ 37.5 nmol/L, indicating high levels of vitamin D deficiency [33].

Low vitamin D status is also common in many Asian countries and the Middle East [59]. In a cross-sectional survey of adolescent girls in Beijing (n=1,277),[60] more than 40% of girls had 25(OH)D concentrations of <12.5 nmol/L. The latitude of Beijing and the lack of sunlight in the winter may partially explain this high prevalence of low vitamin D status. Similarly, low serum concentrations of vitamin D were reported in a young adult population of Japanese women[61], with 42.1% of the population having serum 25(OH)D concentrations < 30 nmol/L. Low vitamin D status is prevalent among Indian populations as well. In a study of postmenopausal women living in south India (n=164) [62], varying degrees of low vitamin D status were reported in approximately 82% of the women. Likewise, in a population of pregnant women in northern India (n=207) [63], 43% of the population had serum 25(OH)D concentrations <10 ng/ml, and 67% had concentrations <15 ng/ml. Middle Eastern populations such as the Lebanese[64], Turkish[65, 66], Jordanians[67], Iranians[68], and Saudi Arabians[69] also exhibit low vitamin D status. Prevailing patterns of dress among Muslims may explain the high prevalence of low vitamin D status in India and the Middle East where many women wear the traditional veil covering most of the body. Cross-sectional studies [64, 65, 67] suggest a higher prevalence of low vitamin D status among veiled females when compared with non-veiled females and males, indicating that culture and dress may be an important predictor of vitamin D status.

D. Health Effects of Low Vitamin D Status

Severe vitamin D deficiency was first defined as a serious health problem in Europe and North America during the late 19th and early 20th century when infants began developing rickets, a disease characterized by weakening of the bones and muscles, due to lack of sunlight exposure[3]. This disorder is now rare in the United States, although it can be found in developing countries and among some high-risk groups. Milder forms of low vitamin D status, however, are now endemic across all areas of the world and are related to an increasing number of illnesses and disorders, including cardiovascular disease, hypertension, inflammatory and autoimmune diseases, and type 2 diabetes [4].

Vitamin D is essential for the absorption of calcium and phosphorous in the body, and inadequate levels of vitamin D can result in impaired intestinal absorption of calcium and phosphorous leading to decreased bone mineral density, bone fragility, and bone loss [70]. This increases the risk of bone fractures and falls, especially in the elderly [30]. In addition, low levels of calcium in the blood can lead to secondary hyperparathyroidism, the overproduction of parathyroid hormone in the body, further worsening deleterious effects on the bone.

Given that vitamin D may play a role in the intestinal absorption of magnesium, it is possible that low vitamin D status may also lead to number of health effects mediated by the effects of low intracellular Mg concentrations [$(Mg^{2+})_i$]. Previous reports indicate that $(Mg^{2+})_i$ levels are frequently low in diabetic and hypertensive patients[71-74], and it is possible that

$(Mg^{2+})_i$ plays an important role in insulin-mediated glucose uptake and vascular tone. In addition, dietary magnesium intake is associated with a number of health conditions including cardiovascular disease[75], stroke[76], hypertension[77], and type 2 diabetes[74, 78], suggesting that magnesium exerts a range of health effects that could potentially be associated with low vitamin D status and impaired Mg absorption.

In recent years, research attention has shifted toward the investigation of the role of vitamin D in the pathogenesis of chronic diseases, including type 2 diabetes. An accumulating body of research suggests that the role of vitamin D in the human body extends far beyond calcium absorption and bone mineralization, although the interactions with calcium, magnesium, and other minerals remain an essential part of inquiry in this area. The identification of VDR in numerous tissues throughout the body has generated much research interest in a wide range of potential health effects of vitamin D. Increasing evidence indicates that vitamin D influences the immune system and response to infections, the development of inflammatory and autoimmune diseases, and chronic diseases such as cancer, cardiovascular disease, and diabetes mellitus. It has even been suggested that fluctuating vitamin D levels are responsible for the seasonality of epidemic flu [79]. The evidence for these relationships has been reviewed extensively elsewhere [4, 11, 70]. Hereinafter, we will focus our discussion on the role of vitamin D in the development of type 2 diabetes, the animal and epidemiologic evidence examining this association, and potential biological mechanisms including possible interactions with calcium, magnesium, and other minerals.

IV. Vitamin D and Type 2 Diabetes

A. Animal Evidence

The discovery of VDR in the pancreatic β-cells in chicks over 25 years ago provided evidence that vitamin D may affect insulin secretion [80, 81]. This finding, combined with the identification of vitamin D-dependent calcium-binding protein (CaBP) in the pancreas of several other animals [82-84] prompted a host of depletion and repletion studies of vitamin D in animals that consistently demonstrate the importance of vitamin D in the pancreatic secretion of insulin.

Vitamin D repletion significantly improved insulin secretion in an *in vitro* study of isolated perfused pancreases from vitamin D-deficient rats [85]. Over a 30 minute period of glucose and arginine perfusion, insulin secretion was reduced by 48% in those pancreases not replenished with vitamin D. Kadowaki and Norman [86] reported similar effects in a series of *in vitro* experiments in isolated perfused rat pancreases controlling for the effects of caloric intake and serum calcium levels. In the first experiment, vitamin D deficient (-D) and vitamin D sufficient (+D) rats were pair-fed, receiving identical quantities of food, to assure equal caloric intake. After treatment with arginine-glucose, the +D rats exhibited significantly higher insulin secretion than the –D rats, suggesting that vitamin D status, not caloric intake, was responsible for the insulin response. The second experiment investigated the effects of varying calcium levels on the insulin response. Results indicated that serum calcium levels did not influence arginine-glucose-induced insulin secretion in rats [86].

In vivo studies have reported comparable findings regarding the effects of vitamin D on insulin secretion. Vitamin D deficient rats injected with 1,25 $(OH)_2D$ exhibited over an 100% increase in peripheral blood levels of insulin (17 microunits/ml increase) as compared with the control group[87]. Similarly, among live +D rats and -D rats, glucose-mediated insulin secretion and glucose tolerance declined significantly in the -D rats as compared with the +D rats after a glucose load. Additionally, repletion with vitamin D recovered insulin function and improved glucose tolerance in the –D rats [88]. Findings from an intervention study of the effects of vitamin D-deficiency on insulin secretion and glucose tolerance in rabbits were consistent. Rabbits on a vitamin D-deficient diet exhibited a significant reduction in insulin secretion and glucose tolerance after only 2 months on the diet. Furthermore, repletion with an injection of vitamin D restored normal insulin function [89].

It has been suggested that reductions in insulin secretion observed in –D rats can be explained, at least partially, by the difference in caloric intake between the –D and +D rats. In a study assessing the effects of decreased food intake and vitamin D-deficiency on impaired glucose secretion in rats, Chertow et al. [90] observed an association between vitamin D-deficiency and inhibition of insulin release, but only in the rats were not pair-fed. When +D and –D rats were pair fed, there was no significant difference in insulin secretion. This study suggests that total caloric intake, not vitamin D deficiency, is responsible for impaired insulin secretion. However, subsequent studies explored this possibility with similar methods and concluded that the effect of caloric intake on insulin secretion was secondary to the effect of vitamin D status [86]. Overall, the totality of the evidence supports the role of vitamin D in pancreatic insulin secretion.

Little is known about the direct effects of vitamin D on insulin resistance in animals, and scant animal research has investigated this topic. In several *in vitro* studies of rat adipocytes, pre-treatment with 100 nM 1,25 $(OH)_2D$ suppressed insulin-induced glucose uptake via activation of the PKCβ pathway[91, 92]. These findings suggest that excess calcitriol in insulin-responsive cells can lead to hyperglycemia and insulin resistance. Elevated levels of 1,25 $(OH)_2D$ are generally the result of low circulating 25(OH)D levels and impaired calcium absorption, and excess 1,25 $(OH)_2D$ has been shown to stimulate the influx of intracellular free calcium $[Ca^{2+}]$ into adipocytes, leading to weight gain, insulin resistance, and the development of type 2 diabetes in humans[44].

B. Evidence from Studies in Humans

In addition to animal studies, numerous clinical and epidemiologic studies have investigated the association of serum and dietary vitamin D with insulin secretion, impaired glucose tolerance, insulin resistance and type 2 diabetes in humans.

Cross-Sectional Evidence

A number of cross-sectional studies have reported inverse associations between vitamin D and risk factors for type 2 diabetes, including decreased insulin secretion, glucose intolerance, insulin resistance, as well as established type 2 diabetes (Table 1).

Table 1. Cross-sectional studies of Vitamin D and Type 2 Diabetes

Reference	Study Population	Outcome	Outcome Measurement	Results
Scragg et al. 1995	5,677 men and women aged 40-64 yrs: New Zealand	IGT Type 2 Diabetes	Fasting & 2-hr plasma glucose/ Serum insulin level T2D	Inverse association btw 25(OH)D and T2D/IGT [Mean (SD) of cases vs controls: 69(31) vs 76(34) nmol/l; p=.001]
Baynes et al. 1997	142 elderly Dutchmen aged 70-88: Seven Countries Study	IGT Type 2 Diabetes	Fasting and 2-hr plasma glucose	Inverse association btw 25(OH)D and insulin secretion & glucose [Insulin concentration AUC: r= -0.23, p<0.05; Glucose AUC: r=-0.23, p<0.01]
Isaia et al. 2001	799 postmenopausal white women: Italy	Type 2 Diabetes	Self-report of T2D	Inverse association btw 25(OH)D and T2D (Mean (SD) of cases vs controls (11(9.8) vs 9(11.3) ng/ml, p<0.01)
Chiu et al. 2004	126 healthy glucose-tolerant subjects (Mean age 26): California	IGT β-cell function Insulin Sensitivity	Fasting & 2-hr plasma glucose / 1st and 2nd phase insulin response (Hyperglycemic clamp)	Inverse association btw 25(OH)D and fasting glucose [OGTT: β_{120min}= -0.52]; Positive association btw 25(OH)D and insulin sensitivity (r=0.46, p<.0001)
Scragg et al. 2004	6,228 adults aged ≥20yrs: NHANES III	IGT Type 2 Diabetes	T2D: Fasting and 2 hr plasma glucose	Inverse association btw 25(OH)D & IR: Whites [$\beta_{LOG\ HOMA\ IR}$ (SE) = -0.009 (0.004); p=0.058]; Mex Amer [$\beta_{LOG\ HOMA\ IR}$ (SE) = -0.016 (0.005); =.0024]
Ford et al. 2005	8,421 adults aged ≥20yrs: NHANES III	Metabolic Syndrome	NCEP criteria	Inverse association btw 25(OH)D and hyperglycemia [Highest quartile of 25(OH)D: OR=.44 (0.29, 0.68)]
Need et al. 2005	753 postmenopausal white women	IGT	Fasting plasma glucose	Inverse association btw 25(OH)D and fasting glucose (r=-0.15, p<0.01)
Hyponnen and Power 2006	7,189 Caucasians aged 45 years: British birth Cohort	IGT	HbA1C (%)	Inverse association btw 25(OH)D and A1C [25(OH)D ≥75 nmol/l: HbA1C = 5.12%; 25(OH)D <25 nmol/l: HbA1C = 5.37%; p for trend <0.0001)
Hahn et al. 2006	120 female patients with polycystic ovarian syndrome (Mean age: 28): Germany	IGT Insulin Sensitivity	Fasting & 2-hr plasma glucose and insulin	Inverse association btw 25(OH)D and insulin resistance (r=-0.19, p=0.03) and hyperinsulinemia (r=-0.19, p=0.04)

IGT= Impaired glucose tolerance; OGTT= Oral glucose tolerance test; IR= Insulin resistance.

Table 2. Prospective cohort studies of Vitamin D and Type 2 Diabetes

Reference	Study Population	Outcome	Outcome Measurement	Results
Liu et al. 2005	10,066 female health professionals ≥45 years: Women's Health Study	Type 2 Diabetes	Self-report	Inverse association btw total and dietary vitamin D and metabolic syndrome [Highest total quartile: OR=0.89 (0.72-1.09); Highest dietary quartile: OR=0.85 (0.70-1.02)] ; No association after controlling for dietary Ca
Pittas et al. 2006	83,779 female nurses aged 30-55 years: Nurses Health Study	Type 2 Diabetes	Self-report	Inverse association btw total vitamin D and risk of T2DM [Highest total quartile: OR=0.77 (0.63-0.94); Highest dietary quartile: OR=0.81 (0.64-1.01)]; No association after controlling for Mg and Ca

Table 3. Clinical Intervention studies of Vitamin D and Type 2 Diabetes

Reference	Study Population	Treatment	Follow-up	Outcome	Results
Gedik et al. 1986	4 severe vitamin D-deficient females 10 healthy controls	2,000 IU vitamin D3/d	6 months	Insulin Secretion	Improved insulin secretion after treatment [Insulin AUC (mu/min) Pre-treat: 9.09 ± .07 Post-treat:13.6 ±0.5; P<0.05]
Orwoll et al. 1994	35 established type 2 diabetics	1 ug/d calcitriol for 4 days	1 month	IGT Insulin Secretion	No improvement in insulin secretion or glucose among established diabetics; Improvement in diabetics [Change in insulin AUC: <3 yrs: 337 ±301 pmol/L vs. >6yrs: 0.7±93 pmol/L]
Boucher et al. 1995	44 "at risk" (IGT) cases and 15 "low" controls	Single bolus injection of 100,000 IU vitamin D3	12 weeks	IGT Type 2 Diabetes	Improved insulin secretion in IGT group [Specific insulin (mIU/l): Pre-treat: 36.8±24.4; Post-treat: 96.2±82.4; p<0.01] Abnormal glucose tolerance unchanged
Fliser et al. 1997	18 healthy males (mean age 26±3yrs)	1.5 ug/d calcitriol	7 days	Fasting plasma glucose	No significant change in mean glucose or insulin
Borissova et al. 2003	10 postmenopausal females with T2DM 17 matched controls	1332 IU vitamin D	1 month	Insulin Secretion IGT	Baseline FPIS: 34.7±12.9 mU/l vs. Post-treat FPIS: 46.6±16.1 mU/l; p<0.05
Pittas 2007	314 adults aged 65 years and over	Combined vitamin D and Ca (700IU vitamin D3 & 500mg Ca)	3 years	IGT Insulin resistance	Increases in FPG & IR smaller in treated than placebo group [Increases: Treatment FPG: 0.02 ± 0.09 nmol/L vs. Placebo FPG: 0.34 ± 0.11 nmol/L; Treatment IR: 0.05± 0.19; Placebo: 0.91 ± 0.31, p=0.031).

IGT= Impaired glucose tolerance; IR= Insulin resistance; Insulin AUC= Insulin area under the curve; FPG= Fasting plasma glucose.

With regard to insulin secretion and glucose metabolism, 25(OH)D concentrations were inversely associated with insulin secretion and OGTT glucose concentrations (Insulin concentration AUC: $r= -0.23$, $p<0.05$; Glucose AUC: $r=-0.23$, $p<0.01$) among elderly Dutchmen (n=142) aged 70-88 years[93]. Similarly, Need et al[94] reported an inverse association between serum 25(OH)D levels and fasting glucose ($r=-0.150$, $p<0.001$) among postmenopausal white women (n=753; aged 34-94 years). Among 8,421 men and nonpregnant women ≥20 years who had fasted ≥8 hours (NHANES III, 1988-1994), a test for a linear trend indicated increasing risk for hyperglycemia across decreasing quintiles of vitamin D intake [25(OH)D ≥ 96.4 nmol/l: OR of hyperglycemia = 0.44 (0.29,0.68); 25(OH)D: 48.5-63.4 nmol/l: OR of hyperglycemia = 0.92 (0.69, 1.23) $p<.001$][53]. In this same population, Vitamin D status was inversely associated with fasting and 2-hr glucose in non-Hispanic whites [25(OH)D: ≥ 80.0 nmol/l: Fasting glucose OR= 0.25 (0.11,0.60); 2-hr glucose OR=0.25 (0.11, 0.60)] and Mexican Americans [25(OH)D: ≥ 80.0 nmol/l: Fasting glucose OR= 0.17 (0.08, 0.37); 2-hr glucose OR= 0.45(0.15, 1.38)], but not in non-Hispanic blacks[58]. The lack of inverse association among non-Hispanic blacks may possibly be explained by the small numbers of African Americans within the highest quartile of serum vitamin D, although it has been suggested that African Americans metabolize vitamin D and other related hormones differently that other ethnic groups[57].

Long term measures of glucose metabolism (i.e. HbA1C) were also associated with vitamin D status. In the 1958 British birth cohort (n=7,189), as 25(OH)D levels decreased, HbA1C levels increased [25(OH)D ≥75 nmol/l: HbA1C = 5.12%; 25(OH)D <25 nmol/l: HbA1C = 5.37%; p for trend <0.0001)[54]. The effect was strongest for 25(OH)D concentrations ≤65 nmol/L, suggesting an interaction between 25(OH)D and glucose levels. In addition, adjustment for BMI and waist circumference weakened the negative association between 25(OH)D and HbA1C [Unadjusted percentage change in A1C per 10-unit increase in 25(OH)D: -0.49 (-0.58, -0.40); vs Adjusted for BMI and A1C: -0.16 (-0.22, -0.10), indicating that BMI may mediate the relation between 25(OH)D concentration and glucose metabolism.

Inverse associations between 25(OH)D concentrations and insulin resistance have also been reported. Among healthy, glucose-tolerant subjects living in California (n=126), 25(OH)D concentrations were positively associated with insulin sensitivity ($r=0.4600$, $p<.0001$), first-phase insulin response ($r=-0.2513$, $p=.0045$), and second-phase insulin response ($r=-0.3487$, $p=0.0001$) measured with the hyperglycemic clamp. No association was reported between 25(OH)D concentration and β-cell function. However, the significant inverse association between 25(OH)D levels and fasting glucose concentrations [Regression coefficients: $\beta_{fasting}= -0.114$; $\beta_{30min}= -0.092$; $\beta_{60min}= -0.698$; $\beta_{90min}= -0.605$; $\beta_{120min}= -0.52$] indicates that low 25(OH)D levels do exert effects on β-cell function. If β-cell function was optimal, then glucose concentrations would be expected to remain normal even with low circulating 25(OH)D. Among the NHANES III population[58], insulin resistance was inversely associated with vitamin D levels among non-Hispanic whites [$\beta_{LOG\ HOMA\ IR}$ (SE) = -0.009 (0.004); p=0.058] and Mexican Americans [$\beta_{LOG\ HOMA\ IR}$ (SE) = -0.016 (0.005); p=0.0024]. Consistent with these findings, 25(OH)D was inversely associated with insulin resistance among German women with polycystic ovarian syndrome (PCOS)[52].

In addition to risk factors for type 2 diabetes, cross-sectional studies suggest an association between low 25(OH)D concentrations and prevalent type 2 diabetes. Scragg et al[95] assessed serum 25(OH)D levels among workforce members aged 40-64 years in New Zealand (n=5,677). After adjustment for potential confounders, serum 25(OH)D levels were significantly lower in both newly diagnosed diabetics and impaired glucose tolerant cases when compared with controls matched on sex, age, ethnicity, and date of interview [Mean (SD): 69 (31) vs 76 (34) nmol/l; p=0.0016). Adjusted odds ratios associated with serum 25(OH)D levels showed a decreased risk of type 2 diabetes among the middle [OR=.57 (0.32, 1.02), p=0.059] and highest [OR=.36, (0.19,0.71), p=0.003) tertiles of 25(OH)D concentrations when compared with the lowest. Similarly, among 799 postmenopausal Italian women (n=66 diabetics)[96], mean levels of serum 25(OH)D were significantly lower in diabetic patients than in controls (Means of 25(OH)D ± SD: 11 ± 9.8 vs. 9 ± 11.3 ng/ml, p<0.008) and the prevalence of vitamin D-deficiency was higher among this group (Diabetics: 39% vs. Controls: 25%).

Prospective Cohort Evidence

Several prospective cohort studies have investigated the long-term effects of vitamin D on insulin secretion, glucose metabolism, insulin resistance, and incident type 2 diabetes (Table 2). Liu et al[55] reported an inverse association between total and dietary vitamin D and the metabolic syndrome over an average of 8.8 years of follow-up in the Women's Health Study (n=10,066) [Highest total vitamin D quartile: OR=0.89 (0.72,1.09); Highest dietary vitamin D quartile: OR=0.85 (0.70,1.02)]. After controlling for calcium however, the association between total and dietary vitamin D and metabolic syndrome disappeared, suggesting calcium as a potential mediator of this relation. Similarly, total and dietary vitamin D intake were inversely associated with risk of type 2 diabetes over a 20-year follow up period in the Nurses Health Study[97] (n=83,779) [Highest total quartile: OR=0.77 (0.63, 0.94); Highest dietary quartile: OR=0.81 (0.64, 1.01)], but the linear trend was not significant after controlling for both dietary calcium and magnesium intake, indicating that the effects of vitamin D may be mediated by these metabolically related micronutrients.

Clinical Intervention Trials

Although the majority of research exploring the role of vitamin D in the pathophysiology of diabetes thus far has been cross-sectional in nature, several clinical trials have explored the effects of vitamin D supplementation on type 2 diabetes with varied results (Table 3).

Insulin secretion, but not glucose levels, improved significantly after vitamin D treatment in several small clinical trials[98-100]. After 6 months of treatment with 2,000 IU vitamin D3 daily (n=4 female patients with severe vitamin D deficiency; n=10 healthy volunteers), insulin secretion in the vitamin D-deficient group improved significantly [Insulin AUC (mu/min) Pre-treat: 9.09 ± .07 vs. Post-treat:13.6 ±0.5; P<0.05], surpassing baseline levels in the healthy group. Insulinogenic indices followed a similar pattern and rose significantly after treatment in the vitamin D-deficient group [Pre-treatment: 1.71±0.4 vs. Post-treatment: 2.48±0.3]. Plasma glucose levels remained unchanged after treatment[98]. Consistent findings were reported in a trial of East London Asians [n=44 subjects "at risk" for diabetes (spot blood glucose level > 6.0 mmol/l < 2 hr post cibum, or > 4.6 mmol/l > 2 hr post cibum on two separate occasions), n=15 age and sex-matched "low risk" controls]. Eight to twelve weeks after a single bolus injection of 100,000 IU of vitamin D, insulin secretion, but not glucose levels improved significantly [Specific insulin (mIU/l): Pre-treatment: 36.8±24.4; Post-treatment: 96.2±82.4; $p<0.01$][99]. Similarly, first phase insulin secretion (FPIS) improved significantly in diabetics (n=10 postmenopausal females with type 2 diabetes, n=17 age- and BMI-matched controls) after treatment with 1332 IU vitamin D daily for 1 month [Baseline FPIS: 34.7±12.9 mU/l vs. Post-treatment FPIS: 46.6±16.1 mU/l; $p<0.05$]. In addition, there was a strong correlation between the change in FPIS and the change in 25(OH)D levels ($r=0.7234$, $p=0.018$), indicating a role of vitamin D in insulin secretion[100].

With regard to insulin resistance, two trials[100, 101] have reported positive effects of vitamin D supplementation. In the largest double-blinded, randomized controlled trial to date (n=314 Caucasian adults aged 65 years and over)[101], participants were randomly assigned to a combined calcium-vitamin D supplement (700 IU vitamin D3, 500 mg CA) or placebo for 3 years. Among impaired glucose tolerant participants, increases in fasting plasma glucose and insulin resistance (measured by HOMA-IR) over the study period were significantly smaller than those increases in the placebo group [Increases: Treatment Fasting Plasma Glucose (FPG): 0.02 ± 0.09 nmol/L vs. Placebo FPG: 0.34 ± 0.11 nmol/L; Treatment IR: 0.05± 0.19; Placebo: 0.91 ± 0.31, $p=0.031$). In a smaller trial of type 2 diabetics[100], HOMA-IR decreased after one month of treatment with vitamin D [Post-treatment: 7.82±2.31 mU/l.mmol/l vs. Pretreatment: 6.15 mU/l.mmol/l; $p>0.8$], although the change was not significant.

However, several clinical trials have observed no effect on insulin secretion, glucose homeostasis, and insulin resistance[102, 103]. In a randomized, placebo-controlled, crossover trial of 1,25 dihydroxyvitamin D3 treatment (1 μg/day for 4 days) in established diabetics (n=35, aged 40-70 years)[102], no effect on fasting insulin or glucose concentrations was reported. However, those subjects with a shorter duration of diabetes showed greater improvements in insulin secretion after administration of vitamin D [Change in insulin area under the curve for diabetics <3 yrs duration: 337 ±301 pmol/L vs. 3-6 yrs: 3.6± 122 pmol/l vs. >6 yrs: 0.7±93 pmol/l], suggesting that vitamin D does not influence insulin secretion in established diabetics, but may exert effects earlier in the development of the disease. Similarly, in a randomized, placebo-controlled study of 1,25 $(OH)_2D_3$ treatment (1.5 *u*g/ day for seven days) in healthy white males (n=18)[103], there were no significant changes in mean glucose, insulin, or insulin sensitivity after treatment [Pre-treatment mean glucose disposal rate: 7.0±1.4 $mgkg^{-1}min^{-1}$; Post-treatment: 7.2±1.4 $mgkg^{-1}min^{-1}$). However, mean PTH levels decreased [Pre-treatment: 2.6± 0.9 $pmol/l^{-1}$ vs. Post-treatment: 1.7±0.9] and urinary excretion increased [Pre-treatment: 4.3±1.5 vs. Post-treatment: 6.0±2.2 pmol/l] after treatment, indicating biological actions of 1,25 $(OH)_2D_3$.

Taken together, these studies suggest that vitamin D supplementation may have beneficial effects on type 2 diabetes. Diverse study populations, vitamin D supplements, doses, and follow-up periods make comparisons difficult; however, the majority of the evidence seems to support the advantageous role of vitamin D supplementation in improving markers of type 2 diabetes, especially when given in larger doses for longer durations of time.

V. Potential Biological Mechanisms

A. Insulin Secretion

Independent Effects of Vitamin D

Vitamin D is necessary for normal pancreatic secretion of insulin, and animal models consistently show an improved insulin response to glucose stimulation after treatment with vitamin D_3[85-87]. Reports from studies in humans described earlier in this review support this model[54, 58, 95, 98-100, 102, 104]. The presence of specific vitamin D receptors on the pancreatic β-cells and evidence of involvement in gene transcription provides a plausible biological explanation for this association.

Joint Effects of Vitamin D and Calcium

Several lines of evidence suggest that calcium may be a potential mediator of the relation between vitamin D and insulin secretion. In an *in vitro* study of rat pancreatic islets, Kikuchi et al examined the role of intracellular calcium ($[Ca^{2+}]_i$)stores on insulin release. Control islets were those with normal $[Ca^{2+}]_i$ levels, and a second set of islets was loaded with $[Ca^{2+}]_i$. Glucose-stimulated first-phase insulin release was 3.5 times greater in the islets loaded with $[Ca^{2+}]_i$. These findings suggest that calcium may play a role in first phase insulin release in rats [105]. Similarly, in a study assessing the respective role of vitamin D and calcium on insulin response, calcium repletion alone normalized glucose tolerance and insulin secretion in vitamin D-depleted rats [106].

Insulin secretion is dependent on the balance between extracellular and intracellular calcium levels[107], and evidence that intracellular Ca^{2+} ($[Ca^{2+}]_i$) levels in various cell types rise with the administration of vitamin D provides additional support for the mediating role of calcium in insulin secretion[108-110]. It is possible that vitamin D stimulates the entry of extracellular (Ca^{2+}) into the β-cells through voltage dependent Ca^{2+} channels and leads to the activation of second messenger systems involving protein kinase A and cAMP [111]. A vitamin D induced influx of $[Ca^{2+}]_i$ into the β-cells may potentially affect the balance between intra- and extracellular calcium levels and affect insulin secretion through a nongenomic pathway. However, the role of vitamin D and calcium in insulin secretion is still disputed due to animal models demonstrating the independent role of vitamin D[86, 88, 89] combined with evidence from clinical intervention studies in humans demonstrating improved insulin secretion after treatment with vitamin D[98-100]. Based on the totality of the evidence, it is likely that vitamin D and calcium exert both independent and interactive effects on insulin secretion. However, further research assessing the independent effects of each on insulin secretion is essential to further our understanding of the role of vitamin D in the development of type 2 diabetes.

Joint Effects of Vitamin D and Magnesium

Vitamin D plays a role in the absorption of magnesium, and it is well-established that magnesium is a key regulator of insulin and glucose metabolism[71, 78]. Clinical and prospective studies in humans[112, 113] suggest that dietary magnesium may improve insulin secretion and glucose response. However, the direct effects of magnesium on insulin secretion are not completely understood. Magnesium is required for insulin secretion from the pancreatic β-cells, and a deficiency in magnesium has been shown to lead to impaired insulin secretion and disturbances in glucose homeostasis in animal models[114, 115]. *In vitro* studies[116, 117] suggest that the balance of extra- and intracellular Mg^{2+} in the pancreatic β-cells may regulate the secretion of insulin. Given that intracellular Mg^{2+} is dependent upon the influx of extracellular Mg^{2+} through the voltage dependent Ca^{2+} channels, it is possible that extracellular Mg^{2+} competitively inhibits this pathway and in turn, inhibits the secretion of insulin which is dependent on this pathway[117]. Another possible mechanism through which the balance of intra- and extracellular Mg^{2+} may affect insulin secretion is the hypothesis that extracellular Mg^{2+} plays a role in ATP-sensitive potassium channels involved in insulin secretion[116]. However, the role of magnesium in the pancreatic secretion of insulin is still unclear, and it is possible that the effects of magnesium on glucose metabolism are mediated via effects on insulin sensitivity[71, 78, 118, 119].

B. Insulin Resistance

Independent Effects of Vitamin D

Vitamin D receptors (VDR) identified on numerous cell types throughout the body, including insulin responsive tissues such as muscle cells[120], suggest that vitamin D may affect insulin responsiveness and glucose uptake. Vitamin D may regulate insulin receptor gene expression at the genomic level by increasing the total insulin receptor number through an increase in the levels of mRNA of the insulin receptor gene. An increase in insulin receptors may potentially increase the binding of insulin, stimulating the cascade of intracellular events leading to the translocation of GLUT-4 transporter to the plasma membrane and greater influx of glucose into cell[121, 122]. This effect has been demonstrated in human promonocytic cells, generally considered to be a good *in vitro* model to study insulin receptors, and it is possible that this same biological process occurs in other insulin responsive cells, such as muscle and adipose tissue.

Joint Effects of Vitamin D and Calcium

Vitamin D may also indirectly affect insulin resistance by influencing intracellular free calcium ($[Ca^{2+}]_i$) levels in insulin responsive target tissues. 1,25 $(OH)_2D$ stimulates the influx of calcium into insulin responsive cells such as adipocytes[46] and can lead to elevated $[Ca^{2+}]_i$ levels. An optimal range of $[Ca^{2+}]_i$ is required for insulin-stimulated glucose transport in skeletal muscle and adipose tissue[123, 124], and high levels of $[Ca^{2+}]_i$ in adipocytes can contribute to insulin resistance [125, 126]. It is possible that elevated levels of $[Ca^{2+}]_i$ inhibit the dephosphorylation of the glucose transporter, Glut4, and decrease insulin-stimulated glucose tranport[127]. Increased $[Ca^{2+}]_i$ may also affect insulin sensitivity via protein kinase C activation and inactivation of the insulin receptor[128]. Inverse associations between vitamin D status and insulin resistance observed in several cross-sectional studies[52, 53, 58, 104] support the role of vitamin D in insulin resistance. However, the inverse association was not independent of calcium intake in the Women's Health Study[55], suggesting a possible mediating role of calcium. Results from intervention trials are limited and report inconsistent findings[100, 103]. Based on this evidence, it seems reasonable to conclude that vitamin D and insulin resistance are inversely associated, although the exact causal mechanism, and whether the association is driven by low vitamin D status or a related mineral such as calcium, remains to be determined.

Joint Effects of Vitamin D and Magnesium

Intracellular Mg^{2+} concentrations are known to be an important mediator of insulin action and glucose homeostasis, and depletion of intracellular Mg^{2+} is a well-recognized characteristic of type 2 diabetes [73, 118, 119]. Insulin has been shown to regulate influx of Mg^{2+} into the intracellular space [129], and Mg^{2+} also influences the action of insulin. Decreased intracellular Mg^{2+} concentrations are associated with an impairment in insulin action and glucose uptake in insulin sensitive tissues such as skeletal muscle tissue[130], heart muscles[131], and adipocytes[132]. Animal models[133] suggest that a defect in the tyrosine kinase activity of insulin receptors may be responsible for the decrease in insulin sensitivity associated with decreased intracellular Mg^{2+} concentrations, a plausible explanation given the critical role of intracellular Mg^{2+} in the Mg-ATP complex and phosphorylation reactions, including phosphorylation of the insulin receptor [134]. Although the connection between vitamin D and magnesium is not fully characterized, vitamin D may possibly influence the balance of intra- and extra-cellular Mg^{2+} in insulin-responsive tissues through its effects on the absorption of Mg in the small intestine, thereby exerting effects on insulin resistance via alterations in Mg^{2+} concentrations.

VI. Genetic Variants

A. Vitamin D Receptor (VDR) Polymorphisms

Biological actions of vitamin D are mediated by the vitamin D receptor (VDR), a ligand-activated member of the steroid/thyroid hormone-receptor superfamily[3]. Vitamin D influences gene transcription through a series of steps involving high affinity and highly selective bonds to the VDR. 1,25 $(OH)_2$ D binds to retinoid X receptor (RXR), forming a heterodimer which binds to specific DNA sequence elements in the promoter regions of hormone responsive genes called Vitamin D Response Elements (VDRE)[6]. The VDR gene is located on chromosome 12cen-q12 and contains 14 exons[135]. Genetic variations in the VDR may potentially lead to deleterious effects on gene expression, including the dysregulation of insulin and glucose levels in the body and the development of type 2 diabetes.

Genetic polymorphisms, or common genetic variants that appear in more than 1% of the population, have been identified on the VDR gene in humans[3]. Examples of polymorphisms identified in the VDR gene include *Tru*9I, *Fok*I, *Taq*I, *Bsm*I, *Eco*RV, and *Apa*I[136]. The effects of VDR polymorphisms on type 1 diabetes have been studied extensively in varied populations, and published findings have been conflicting[137-141]. The b allele of the *Bsm*I polymorphism was associated with susceptibility to Type 1 diabetes in a population of South Indians (53/84; p=0.016) [139]. *Bsm*I and *Apa*I were linked to Type

1 diabetes in a Taiwanese population [*BsmI*: BB OR=6.74 (4.54, 8.94); *Apa*I: AA OR=2.46 (1.68,3.24)][141]. No such associations were found in Finnish[138] and Chilean[140] populations. In a recent meta-analysis of the studies in this area, little evidence was found to suggest an association between VDR polymorphisms, including *Apa*I, *Bsm*I, *Fok*I, and *Taq*, and type 1 diabetes[142]. However, it is plausible that there are alternative VDR polymorphisms other than those well-studied that may play a role in type 1 diabetes.

The role of VDR polymorphisms in insulin secretion, glucose homeostasis, insulin resistance, and risk of type 2 diabetes has been explored in several studies, and findings have been inconsistent. In a study of healthy Bangladeshi Asians (n=171)[143], the *Apa*I, *Bsm*I, and *Taq*I polymorphisms were positively associated with insulin secretion but not insulin resistance [Insulin secretion Index (ISI): *Apa*I: AA genotype = 146.8 (112.8, 191.0); aa = 68.5 (48.9-95.8); *Bsm*I: BB = 120.5(89.0, 163.1); bb = 80.7 (64.6, 100.7); *Taq*I: TT = 87.5 (72.2, 106.0); tt = 173.3 (102.0, 294.4)]. In the Rancho Bernardo Study[144], a community-based study of nondiabetic Caucasians (n=1,545), the *Apa*I polymorphism was associated with the prevalence of glucose intolerance [AA genotype: 30.9%; aa: 39.9%, p for trend <0.05], and fasting plasma glucose was significantly higher in individuals with the aa genotype compared to those with the AA genotype (5.43 ± 0.56 mmol/L vs. 5.35 ± 0.57 mmol/L, $p<0.05$]. The *Bsm*I polymorphism was associated with insulin resistance, with higher insulin resistance reported among individuals with the bb genotype [HOMA IR: BB genotype: 2.8 ± 1.5 vs bb: 3.2 ± 2.2, $p<0.05$].

With regard to prevalent type 2 diabetes, several studies reported no association with VDR polymorphisms[144-146]. Specifically, *Bsm*I, *Tru9*I, and *Apa*I were not associated with prevalent type 2 diabetes in a population of French Caucasians (n=309 diabetic patients; 143 healthy controls)[145], and the *Fok*I, *Apa*I, *Bsm*I, and *Taq*I were not associated with type 2 diabetes in a homogenous Polish population (n=308 diabetic patients, 240 healthy controls)[146]. However, the B allele of the *Bsm*I polymorphism was associated with increased odds of having prevalent type 2 diabetes [BB genotype: OR=3.64 (1.53, 8.55), p=0.002] in a population of German patients at high risk for coronary artery disease (n=293)[147].

Further research is required to unravel the role of VDR polymorphisms in the development of type 2 diabetes. It is likely that conflicting findings in this area stem from inadequate power to detect associations, a common problem among genetic association studies, combined with tight linkage disequilibrium between several of the selected polymorphisms (i.e. ApaI, BsmI, TaqI, EcoRV). In addition, most of the VDR polymorphisms studied thus far are located in nonfunctional introns of the VDR gene.

Observed associations may reflect linkage disequilibrium with a functional variant elsewhere in the VDR gene that has not been considered[135]. Further exploration of these selected polymorphisms and other potential candidate genes in larger studies is essential to deepen our understanding of the molecular impact of genetic variants of the VDR in the development of Type 2 diabetes.

B. Magnesium and Calcium Homeostasis-Related Genetic Variants

Magnesium and calcium homeostasis in the body is tightly regulated, and imbalances in intra- and extracellular levels of these ions can disrupt a number of cellular and systemic processes that may play a role in the pathogenesis of disease, including type 2 diabetes. Recently, several genes encoding proteins responsible for Mg^{2+} cellular influx have been identified, including members of the transient receptor potential (TRP) family of cation channels[148-150]. TRPM6, an Mg^{2+} and Ca^{2+} channel permeable channel localized in the kidney tubules and intestinal epithelia, has been shown to play a critical role in intestinal and renal Mg^{2+} absorption[151]. Mutations in TRPM6 lead to hypomagnesemia with secondary hypocalcemia, an autosomal recessive disorder characterized by impaired intestinal Mg^{2+} absorption, decreased PTH, and decreased serum Ca^{2+} levels[148, 149]. TRPM7, a closely related intracellular ligand-gated ion channel, may interact with TRPM6 to form channel complexes regulating the influx of Mg^{2+} into the cell[150, 152]. These findings suggest that TRPM6 and TRPM7 play a crucial role in intracellular Mg levels, a key factor in insulin and glucose metabolism[71, 78]. Similarly, TRP channels play an important role in Ca^{2+} signaling and may exert effects on a range of Ca^{2+} dependent functions including the balance of intra- and extracellular calcium, known to affect insulin secretion[107] and insulin resistance[124, 125]. Given the close interconnection between TRP channels and mineral absorption and homeostasis, defects in these ion channels are critically important to examine in future research into the pathogenesis of type 2 diabetes. It is possible that genetic variation in these channels may help to explain variations in risk of type 2 diabetes in the general population.

Conclusion

The link between low vitamin D status and type 2 diabetes is of critical public health importance due to the severity of the diabetes epidemic and the urgent need for prevention efforts. An extensive body of literature suggests the potential important role of low vitamin D status in the development of type 2 diabetes. However, the vitamin D endocrine system is an elaborate system, involving a complex interplay of interactions between calcium, phosphorus, magnesium, and other minerals and hormones. Disentangling the independent and interactive effects of these factors is of critical importance, and further research is essential in this area. To date, the majority of the human research in this area has been cross-sectional in design, hindering the ability to make causal inferences. Future research should therefore focus on assessing the effects of vitamin D supplementation in prospective studies of large and diverse populations with careful assessment of vitamin D status as well as in randomized controlled settings in diverse populations. In addition, mechanistic and interaction studies assessing the role of metabolically related minerals are needed to understand the interrelations among vitamin D and insulin secretion, insulin resistance, and type 2 diabetes. Consideration of gene-environment interactions, including genetic variants of the vitamin D receptor and other pathways involved in mineral homeostasis should also be investigated further. Research of this nature is essential to further our understanding of the pathophysiology of type 2 diabetes and the potential use of vitamin D and other minerals in primary prevention and treatment.

References

[1] Boucher, B.J., Inadequate vitamin D status: does it contribute to the disorders comprising syndrome 'X'? *Br. J. Nutr.*, 1998. 79(4): p. 315-27.

[2] Holick, M.F., McCollum Award Lecture, 1994: vitamin D--new horizons for the 21st century. *Am. J. Clin. Nutr.,* 1994. 60(4): p. 619-30.

[3] Feldman, D., F.H. Glorieux, and J.W. Pike, eds. *Vitamin D.* 1997, Academic Press: San Diego.

[4] Zittermann, A., Vitamin D in preventive medicine: are we ignoring the evidence? *Br. J. Nutr.*, 2003. 89(5): p. 552-72.

[5] Dusso, A.S., A.J. Brown, and E. Slatopolsky, Vitamin D. *Am. J. Physiol. Renal. Physiol.*, 2005. 289(1): p. F8-28.

[6] Holick, M.F., Vitamin D: *Physiology, Molecular Biology, and Clinical Applications.* 1999, Totowa: Humana Press Inc. 458.

[7] Hurwitz, S., Homeostatic control of plasma calcium concentration. *Crit. Rev. Biochem. Mol. Biol.,* 1996. 31(1): p. 41-100.

[8] Norman, A.W., The vitamin D endocrine system. *Physiologist,* 1985. 28(4): p. 219-32.

[9] Vieth, R., Why the optimal requirement for Vitamin D3 is probably much higher than what is officially recommended for adults. *J. Steroid. Biochem. Mol. Biol.*, 2004. 89-90(1-5): p. 575-9.

[10] Vieth, R., et al., The urgent need to recommend an intake of vitamin D that is effective. *Am. J. Clin. Nutr.*, 2007. 85(3): p. 649-50.

[11] Holick, M.F., The vitamin D epidemic and its health consequences. *J. Nutr.,* 2005. 135(11): p. 2739S-48S.

[12] Hollis, B.W., Circulating 25-hydroxyvitamin D levels indicative of vitamin D sufficiency: implications for establishing a new effective dietary intake recommendation for vitamin D. *J. Nutr.*, 2005. 135(2): p. 317-22.

[13] Takeda, E., et al., Inorganic phosphate homeostasis and the role of dietary phosphorus. *J. Cell Mol. Med.*, 2004. 8(2): p. 191-200.

[14] Amato, D., et al., Acute effects of soft drink intake on calcium and phosphate metabolism in immature and adult rats. *Rev. Invest Clin.*, 1998. 50(3): p. 185-9.

[15] Poole, K.E. and J. Reeve, Parathyroid hormone - a bone anabolic and catabolic agent. *Curr. Opin. Pharmacol.,* 2005. 5(6): p. 612-7.

[16] Huang, C.L., et al., Molecular physiology and pharmacology of calcitonin. *Cell Mol. Biol.* (Noisy-le-grand), 2006. 52(3): p. 33-43.

[17] Moon, J., The role of vitamin D in toxic metal absorption: a review. *J. Am. Coll Nutr.*, 1994. 13(6): p. 559-64.

[18] Zofkova, I. and R.L. Kancheva, The relationship between magnesium and calciotropic hormones. *Magnes Res.,* 1995. 8(1): p. 77-84.

[19] Loughead, J.L., et al., A role for magnesium in neonatal parathyroid gland function? *J. Am. Coll Nutr.*, 1991. 10(2): p. 123-6.

[20] Bailly, C., N. Roinel, and C. Amiel, Stimulation by glucagon and PTH of Ca and Mg reabsorption in the superficial distal tubule of the rat kidney. *Pflugers Arch.*, 1985. 403(1): p. 28-34.

[21] Morel, F., Sites of hormone action in the mammalian nephron. *Am. J. Physiol.*, 1981. 240(3): p. F159-64.

[22] Hulter, H.N. and J.C. Peterson, Renal and systemic magnesium metabolism during chronic continuous PTH infusion in normal subjects. *Metabolism*, 1984. 33(7): p. 662-6.

[23] Rude, R.K., Magnesium metabolism and deficiency. *Endocrinol. Metab. Clin. North Am.*, 1993. 22(2): p. 377-95.

[24] Miller, E.R., et al., Mineral Balance Studies with the Baby Pig: Effects of Dietary Vitamin D2 Level Upon Calcium, Phosphorus and Magnesium Balance. *J. Nutr.*, 1965. 85: p. 255-9.

[25] Karbach, U. and K. Ewe, Calcium and magnesium transport and influence of 1,25-dihydroxyvitamin D3. In vivo perfusion study at the colon of the rat. *Digestion*, 1987. 37(1): p. 35-42.

[26] Hollis, B.W., Assessment of vitamin D nutritional and hormonal status: what to measure and how to do it. *Calcif Tissue Int.*, 1996. 58(1): p. 4-5.

[27] Zittermann, A., Vitamin D and disease prevention with special reference to cardiovascular disease. *Prog. Biophys. Mol. Biol.*, 2006. 92(1): p. 39-48.

[28] Bischoff-Ferrari, H.A., et al., Estimation of optimal serum concentrations of 25-hydroxyvitamin D for multiple health outcomes. *Am. J. Clin. Nutr.*, 2006. 84(1): p. 18-28.

[29] Heaney, R.P., The Vitamin D requirement in health and disease. *J. Steroid Biochem. Mol. Biol.,* 2005. 97(1-2): p. 13-9.

[30] Lips, P., Vitamin D deficiency and secondary hyperparathyroidism in the elderly: consequences for bone loss and fractures and therapeutic implications. *Endocr. Rev.*, 2001. 22(4): p. 477-501.

[31] Buffington, C., et al., Vitamin D Deficiency in the Morbidly Obese. *Obes. Surg.*, 1993. 3(4): p. 421-424.

[32] Liel, Y., et al., Low circulating vitamin D in obesity. *Calcif Tissue Int.*, 1988. 43(4): p. 199-201.

[33] Nesby-O'Dell, S., et al., Hypovitaminosis D prevalence and determinants among African American and white women of reproductive age: third National Health and Nutrition Examination Survey, 1988-1994. *Am. J. Clin. Nutr.*, 2002. 76(1): p. 187-92.

[34] Willis, C.M., et al., A prospective analysis of plasma 25-hydroxyvitamin D concentrations in white and black prepubertal females in the southeastern United States. *Am. J. Clin. Nutr.,* 2007. 85(1): p. 124-30.

[35] Tangpricha, V., et al., Vitamin D insufficiency among free-living healthy young adults. *Am. J. Med.,* 2002. 112(8): p. 659-62.

[36] Gloth, F.M., 3rd, et al., Vitamin D deficiency in homebound elderly persons. *Jama*, 1995. 274(21): p. 1683-6.

[37] LeBoff, M.S., et al., Occult vitamin D deficiency in postmenopausal US women with acute hip fracture. *Jama*, 1999. 281(16): p. 1505-11.

[38] MacLaughlin, J. and M.F. Holick, Aging decreases the capacity of human skin to produce vitamin D3. *J. Clin. Invest*, 1985. 76(4): p. 1536-8.

[39] Compston, J.E., et al., Vitamin D status and bone histomorphometry in gross obesity. *Am. J. Clin. Nutr.*, 1981. 34(11): p. 2359-63.

[40] Bell, N.H., S. Shaw, and R.T. Turner, Evidence that 1,25-dihydroxyvitamin D3 inhibits the hepatic production of 25-hydroxyvitamin D in man. *J. Clin. Invest.,* 1984. 74(4): p. 1540-4.

[41] Wortsman, J., et al., Decreased bioavailability of vitamin D in obesity. *Am. J. Clin. Nutr.*, 2000. 72(3): p. 690-3.

[42] Arunabh, S., et al., Body fat content and 25-hydroxyvitamin D levels in healthy women. *J. Clin. Endocrinol. Metab.*, 2003. 88(1): p. 157-61.

[43] Snijder, M.B., et al., Adiposity in relation to vitamin D status and parathyroid hormone levels: a population-based study in older men and women. *J. Clin. Endocrinol. Metab.*, 2005. 90(7): p. 4119-23.

[44] Zemel, M.B., Regulation of adiposity and obesity risk by dietary calcium: mechanisms and implications. *J. Am. Coll. Nutr.*, 2002. 21(2): p. 146S-151S.

[45] McCarty, M.F. and C.A. Thomas, PTH excess may promote weight gain by impeding catecholamine-induced lipolysis-implications for the impact of calcium, vitamin D, and alcohol on body weight. *Med. Hypotheses.*, 2003. 61(5-6): p. 535-42.

[46] Zemel, M.B., et al., Regulation of adiposity by dietary calcium. *Faseb J.,* 2000. 14(9): p. 1132-8.

[47] Heaney, R.P., Normalizing calcium intake: projected population effects for body weight. *J. Nutr.*, 2003. 133(1): p. 268S-270S.

[48] Davies, K.M., et al., Calcium intake and body weight. *J. Clin. Endocrinol. Metab.*, 2000. 85(12): p. 4635-8.

[49] Drapeau, V., et al., Modifications in food-group consumption are related to long-term body-weight changes. *Am. J. Clin. Nutr.*, 2004. 80(1): p. 29-37.

[50] Yanoff, L.B., et al., The prevalence of hypovitaminosis D and secondary hyperparathyroidism in obese Black Americans. *Clin. Endocrinol.* (Oxf), 2006. 64(5): p. 523-9.

[51] Parikh, S.J., et al., The relationship between obesity and serum 1,25-dihydroxy vitamin D concentrations in healthy adults. *J. Clin. Endocrinol. Metab.*, 2004. 89(3): p. 1196-9.

[52] Hahn, S., et al., Low Serum 25-Hydroxyvitamin D Concentrations are Associated with Insulin Resistance and Obesity in Women with Polycystic Ovary Syndrome. *Exp. Clin. Endocrinol. Diabetes,* 2006. 114(10): p. 577-83.

[53] Ford, E.S., et al., Concentrations of serum vitamin D and the metabolic syndrome among U.S. adults. *Diabetes Care*, 2005. 28(5): p. 1228-30.

[54] Hypponen, E. and C. Power, Vitamin D status and glucose homeostasis in the 1958 British birth cohort: the role of obesity. *Diabetes Care*, 2006. 29(10): p. 2244-6.

[55] Liu, S., et al., Dietary calcium, vitamin D, and the prevalence of metabolic syndrome in middle-aged and older U.S. women. *Diabetes Care*, 2005. 28(12): p. 2926-32.

[56] Clemens, T.L., et al., Increased skin pigment reduces the capacity of skin to synthesise vitamin D3. *Lancet*, 1982. 1(8263): p. 74-6.

[57] Bell, N.H., et al., Evidence for alteration of the vitamin D-endocrine system in blacks. *J. Clin. Invest.*, 1985. 76(2): p. 470-3.

[58] Scragg, R., M. Sowers, and C. Bell, Serum 25-hydroxyvitamin D, diabetes, and ethnicity in the Third National Health and Nutrition Examination Survey. *Diabetes Care*, 2004. 27(12): p. 2813-8.

[59] Lips, P., Vitamin D status and nutrition in Europe and Asia. *J. Steroid. Biochem. Mol. Biol.,* 2007. 103(3-5): p. 620-5.

[60] Fraser, D.R., Vitamin D-deficiency in Asia. *J. Steroid. Biochem. Mol. Biol.*, 2004. 89-90(1-5): p. 491-5.

[61] Nakamura, K., et al., Low serum concentrations of 25-hydroxyvitamin D in young adult Japanese women: a cross sectional study. *Nutrition,* 2001. 17(11-12): p. 921-5.

[62] Harinarayan, C.V., Prevalence of vitamin D insufficiency in postmenopausal south Indian women. *Osteoporos Int.*, 2005. 16(4): p. 397-402.

[63] Sachan, A., et al., High prevalence of vitamin D deficiency among pregnant women and their newborns in northern India. *Am. J. Clin. Nutr.,* 2005. 81(5): p. 1060-4.

[64] Gannage-Yared, M.H., et al., Hypovitaminosis D in a sunny country: relation to lifestyle and bone markers. *J. Bone Miner Res.*, 2000. 15(9): p. 1856-62.

[65] Alagol, F., et al., Sunlight exposure and vitamin D deficiency in Turkish women. *J. Endocrinol. Invest*, 2000. 23(3): p. 173-7.

[66] Atli, T., et al., The prevalence of Vitamin D deficiency and effects of ultraviolet light on Vitamin D levels in elderly Turkish population. *Arch. Gerontol. Geriatr.*, 2005. 40(1): p. 53-60.

[67] Mishal, A.A., Effects of different dress styles on vitamin D levels in healthy young Jordanian women. *Osteoporos Int.,* 2001. 12(11): p. 931-5.

[68] Hashemipour, S., et al., *Vitamin D deficiency and causative factors in the population of Tehran.* BMC Public Health, 2004. 4: p. 38.

[69] Sedrani, S.H., A.W. Elidrissy, and K.M. El Arabi, Sunlight and vitamin D status in normal Saudi subjects. *Am. J. Clin. Nutr.,* 1983. 38(1): p. 129-32.

[70] Lips, P., Vitamin D physiology. *Prog. Biophys. Mol. Biol.*, 2006. 92(1): p. 4-8.

[71] Paolisso, G. and M. Barbagallo, Hypertension, diabetes mellitus, and insulin resistance: the role of intracellular magnesium. *Am. J. Hypertens.,* 1997. 10(3): p. 346-55.

[72] Resnick, L.M., Cellular ions in hypertension, insulin resistance, obesity, and diabetes: a unifying theme. *J. Am. Soc. Nephrol.,* 1992. 3(4 Suppl): p. S78-85.

[73] Resnick, L.M., et al., Intracellular and extracellular magnesium depletion in type 2 (non-insulin-dependent) diabetes mellitus. *Diabetologia,* 1993. 36(8): p. 767-70.

[74] Ma, J., et al., Associations of serum and dietary magnesium with cardiovascular disease, hypertension, diabetes, insulin, and carotid arterial wall thickness: the ARIC study. Atherosclerosis Risk in Communities Study. *J. Clin. Epidemiol.,* 1995. 48(7): p. 927-40.

[75] Arsenian, M.A., Magnesium and cardiovascular disease. *Prog. Cardiovasc. Dis.,* 1993. 35(4): p. 271-310.

[76] Ascherio, A., et al., Intake of potassium, magnesium, calcium, and fiber and risk of stroke among US men. *Circulation,* 1998. 98(12): p. 1198-204.

[77] Mizushima, S., et al., Dietary magnesium intake and blood pressure: a qualitative overview of the observational studies. *J. Hum. Hypertens.*, 1998. 12(7): p. 447-53.

[78] Barbagallo, M. and L.J. Dominguez, Magnesium metabolism in type 2 diabetes mellitus, metabolic syndrome and insulin resistance. *Arch. Biochem. Biophys.*, 2007. 458(1): p. 40-7.

[79] Cannell, J.J., et al., Epidemic influenza and vitamin D. *Epidemiol. Infect.*, 2006. 134(6): p. 1129-40.

[80] Pike, J.W., L.L. Gooze, and M.R. Haussler, Biochemical evidence for 1,25-dihydroxyvitamin D receptor macromolecules in parathyroid, pancreatic, pituitary, and placental tissues. *Life Sci.*, 1980. 26(5): p. 407-14.

[81] Christakos, S. and A.W. Norman, Studies on the mode of action of calciferol. XXIX. Biochemical characterization of 1,25-dihydroxyvitamin D3 receptors in chick pancreas and kidney cytosol. *Endocrinology*, 1981. 108(1): p. 140-9.

[82] Arnold, B.M., et al., Radioimmunoassay studies of intestinal calcium-binding protein in the pig. II. The distribution of intestinal CaBP in pig tissues. *Can. J. Physiol. Pharmacol.*, 1975. 53(6): p. 1135-40.

[83] Christakos, S., et al., Studies on the mode of action of calciferol. XIII. Development of a radioimmunoassay for vitamin D-dependent chick intestinal calcium-binding protein and tissue distribution. *Endocrinology*, 1979. 104(5): p. 1495-503.

[84] Morrissey, R.L., et al., Calcium-binding protein: its cellular localization in jejunum, kidney and pancreas. *Proc. Soc. Exp. Biol. Med.*, 1975. 149(1): p. 56-60.

[85] Norman, A.W., et al., Vitamin D deficiency inhibits pancreatic secretion of insulin. *Science*, 1980. 209(4458): p. 823-5.

[86] Kadowaki, S. and A.W. Norman, Dietary vitamin D is essential for normal insulin secretion from the perfused rat pancreas. *J. Clin. Invest.*, 1984. 73(3): p. 759-66.

[87] Clark, S.A., W.E. Stumpf, and M. Sar, Effect of 1,25 dihydroxyvitamin D3 on insulin secretion. *Diabetes*, 1981. 30(5): p. 382-6.

[88] Cade, C. and A.W. Norman, Vitamin D3 improves impaired glucose tolerance and insulin secretion in the vitamin D-deficient rat in vivo. *Endocrinology*, 1986. 119(1): p. 84-90.

[89] Nyomba, B.L., R. Bouillon, and P. De Moor, Influence of vitamin D status on insulin secretion and glucose tolerance in the rabbit. *Endocrinology*, 1984. 115(1): p. 191-7.

[90] Chertow, B.S., et al., Cellular mechanisms of insulin release: the effects of vitamin D deficiency and repletion on rat insulin secretion. *Endocrinology*, 1983. 113(4): p. 1511-8.

[91] Huang, Y., et al., Effect of 1 alpha,25-dihydroxy vitamin D3 and vitamin E on insulin-induced glucose uptake in rat adipocytes Dominant negative protein kinase Cbeta improves 1alpha, 25-dihydroxy vitamin D3-induced insulin resistance. *Diabetes Res. Clin. Pract.*, 2002. 55(3): p. 175-83.

[92] Natsume, Y., et al., Dominant negative protein kinase Cbeta improves 1alpha, 25-dihydroxy vitamin D3-induced insulin resistance. *Endocr. Res.*, 2003. 29(4): p. 457-64.

[93] Baynes, K.C., et al., Vitamin D, glucose tolerance and insulinaemia in elderly men. *Diabetologia*, 1997. 40(3): p. 344-7.

[94] Need, A.G., et al., Relationship between fasting serum glucose, age, body mass index and serum 25 hydroxyvitamin D in postmenopausal women. *Clin. Endocrinol.* (Oxf), 2005. 62(6): p. 738-41.

[95] Scragg, R., et al., Serum 25-hydroxyvitamin D3 levels decreased in impaired glucose tolerance and diabetes mellitus. *Diabetes Res. Clin. Pract.*, 1995. 27(3): p. 181-8.

[96] Isaia, G., R. Giorgino, and S. Adami, High prevalence of hypovitaminosis D in female type 2 diabetic population. *Diabetes Care,* 2001. 24(8): p. 1496.

[97] Pittas, A.G., et al., Vitamin D and calcium intake in relation to type 2 diabetes in women. *Diabetes Care*, 2006. 29(3): p. 650-6.

[98] Gedik, O. and S. Akalin, Effects of vitamin D deficiency and repletion on insulin and glucagon secretion in man. *Diabetologia,* 1986. 29(3): p. 142-5.

[99] Boucher, B.J., et al., Glucose intolerance and impairment of insulin secretion in relation to vitamin D deficiency in east London Asians. *Diabetologia*, 1995. 38(10): p. 1239-45.

[100] Borissova, A.M., et al., The effect of vitamin D3 on insulin secretion and peripheral insulin sensitivity in type 2 diabetic patients. *Int. J. Clin. Pract.*, 2003. 57(4): p. 258-61.

[101] Pittas, A.G., et al., The Effects of Calcium and Vitamin D Supplementation on Blood Glucose and Markers of Inflammation in Non-diabetic Adults. *Diabetes Care*, 2007.

[102] Orwoll, E., M. Riddle, and M. Prince, Effects of vitamin D on insulin and glucagon secretion in non-insulin-dependent diabetes mellitus. *Am. J. Clin. N*utr., 1994. 59(5): p. 1083-7.

[103] Fliser, D., et al., No effect of calcitriol on insulin-mediated glucose uptake in healthy subjects. *Eur. J. Clin. Invest.,* 1997. 27(7): p. 629-33.

[104] Chiu, K.C., et al., Hypovitaminosis D is associated with insulin resistance and beta cell dysfunction. *Am. J. Clin. Nutr.,* 2004. 79(5): p. 820-5.

[105] Kikuchi, M., et al., Biphasic insulin release in rat islets of Langerhans and the role of Intracellular Ca++ stores. *Endocrinology*, 1979. 105(4): p. 1013-9.

[106] Beaulieu, C., et al., Calcium is essential in normalizing intolerance to glucose that accompanies vitamin D depletion in vivo. *Diabetes,* 1993. 42(1): p. 35-43.

[107] Milner, R.D. and C.N. Hales, The role of calcium and magnesium in insulin secretion from rabbit pancreas studied in vitro. *Diabetologia,* 1967. 3(1): p. 47-9.

[108] Farach-Carson, M.C., I. Sergeev, and A.W. Norman, Nongenomic actions of 1,25-dihydroxyvitamin D3 in rat osteosarcoma cells: structure-function studies using ligand analogs. *Endocrinology*, 1991. 129(4): p. 1876-84.

[109] Tornquist, K. and A.H. Tashjian, Jr., Dual actions of 1,25-dihydroxycholecalciferol on intracellular Ca2+ in GH4C1 cells: evidence for effects on voltage-operated Ca2+ channels and Na+/Ca2+ exchange. *Endocrinolog*y, 1989. 124(6): p. 2765-76.

[110] Civitelli, R., et al., Nongenomic activation of the calcium message system by vitamin D metabolites in osteoblast-like cells. *Endocrinology*, 1990. 127(5): p. 2253-62.

[111] de Boland, A.R. and A.W. Norman, Influx of extracellular calcium mediates 1,25-dihydroxyvitamin D3-dependent transcaltachia (the rapid stimulation of duodenal Ca2+ transport). *Endocrinology,* 1990. 127(5): p. 2475-80.

[112] Paolisso, G., et al., Dietary magnesium supplements improve B-cell response to glucose and arginine in elderly non-insulin dependent diabetic subjects Impaired insulin-induced erythrocyte magnesium accumulation is correlated to impaired insulin-mediated glucose disposal in type 2 (non-insulin-dependent) diabetic patients. *Acta Endocrinol.* (Copenh), 1989. 121(1): p. 16-20.

[113] Song, Y., et al., Dietary magnesium intake in relation to plasma insulin levels and risk of type 2 diabetes in women. *Diabetes Care*, 2004. 27(1): p. 59-65.

[114] Gueux, E. and Y. Rayssiguier, The effect of magnesium deficiency on glucose stimulated insulin secretion in rats. *Horm. Metab. Res.*, 1983. 15(12): p. 594-7.

[115] Matsunobu, S., et al., Insulin secretion and glucose uptake in hypomagnesemic sheep fed a low magnesium, high potassium diet. *J. Nutr. Biochem.*, 1990. 1(3): p. 167-71.

[116] Ishizuka, J., et al., In vitro relationship between magnesium and insulin secretion. *Magnes. Res.,* 1994. 7(1): p. 17-22.

[117] Murakami, M., et al., Role of extracellular magnesium in insulin secretion from rat insulinoma cells. *Proc. Soc. Exp. Biol. Med.,* 1992. 200(4): p. 490-4.

[118] Yajnik, C.S., et al., Fasting plasma magnesium concentrations and glucose disposal in diabetes. *Br. Med.* J. (Clin Res Ed), 1984. 288(6423): p. 1032-4.

[119] Takaya, J., H. Higashino, and Y. Kobayashi, Intracellular magnesium and insulin resistance. *Magnes. Res.*, 2004. 17(2): p. 126-36.

[120] Simpson, R.U., G.A. Thomas, and A.J. Arnold, Identification of 1,25-dihydroxyvitamin D3 receptors and activities in muscle. *J. Biol. Chem.*, 1985. 260(15): p. 8882-91.

[121] Leal, M.A., et al., The effect of 1,25-dihydroxyvitamin D3 on insulin binding, insulin receptor mRNA levels, and isotype RNA pattern in U-937 human promonocytic cells. *Exp. Cell Res.*, 1995. 217(2): p. 189-94.

[122] Maestro, B., et al., Stimulation by 1,25-dihydroxyvitamin D3 of insulin receptor expression and insulin responsiveness for glucose transport in U-937 human promonocytic cells. *Endocr. J.,* 2000. 47(4): p. 383-91.

[123] Zemel, M.B., Insulin resistance vs. hyperinsulinemia in hypertension: insulin regulation of Ca2+ transport and Ca(2+)-regulation of insulin sensitivity. *J. Nutr.*, 1995. 125(6 Suppl): p. 1738S-1743S.

[124] Draznin, B., et al., The existence of an optimal range of cytosolic free calcium for insulin-stimulated glucose transport in rat adipocytes. *J. Biol. Chem.,* 1987. 262(30): p. 14385-8.

[125] Draznin, B., et al., Possible role of cytosolic free calcium concentrations in mediating insulin resistance of obesity and hyperinsulinemia. *J. Clin. Invest.*, 1988. 82(6): p. 1848-52.

[126] Segal, S., et al., Postprandial changes in cytosolic free calcium and glucose uptake in adipocytes in obesity and non-insulin-dependent diabetes mellitus. *Horm. Res.,* 1990. 34(1): p. 39-44.

[127] Begum, N., et al., GLUT-4 phosphorylation and its intrinsic activity. Mechanism of Ca(2+)-induced inhibition of insulin-stimulated glucose transport. *J. Biol. Chem.,* 1993. 268(5): p. 3352-6.

[128] Zemel, M.B., Nutritional and endocrine modulation of intracellular calcium: implications in obesity, insulin resistance and hypertension. *Mol. Cell Biochem.*, 1998. 188(1-2): p. 129-36.

[129] Hwang, D.L., C.F. Yen, and J.L. Nadler, Insulin increases intracellular magnesium transport in human platelets. *J. Clin. Endocrinol. Metab.*, 1993. 76(3): p. 549-53.

[130] Naitoh, T., et al., Intracellular Ca2+ and Mg2+ regulation for insulin-stimulated glucose uptake into mouse diaphragm muscles. *Jpn. J. Pharmacol.,* 1991. 56(2): p. 241-4.

[131] Paxton, R. and L. Ye, Regulation of heart insulin receptor tyrosine kinase activity by magnesium and spermine. *Mol. Cell Biochem.*, 2005. 277(1-2): p. 7-17.

[132] Nadler, J. and S. Scott, Evidence that pioglitazone increases intracellular free magnesium concentration in freshly isolated rat adipocytes. *Biochem. Biophys. Res. Commun.*, 1994. 202(1): p. 416-21.

[133] Suarez, A., et al., Impaired tyrosine-kinase activity of muscle insulin receptors from hypomagnesaemic rats. *Diabetologia*, 1995. 38(11): p. 1262-70.

[134] Barbagallo, M., et al., Altered ionic effects of insulin in hypertension: role of basal ion levels in determining cellular responsiveness. *J. Clin. Endocrinol. Me*tab., 1997. 82(6): p. 1761-5.

[135] Zmuda, J.M., J.A. Cauley, and R.E. Ferrell, Molecular epidemiology of vitamin D receptor gene variants. *Epidemiol. Rev*., 2000. 22(2): p. 203-17.

[136] Reis, A.F., O.M. Hauache, and G. Velho, Vitamin D endocrine system and the genetic susceptibility to diabetes, obesity and vascular disease. *A review of evidence. Diabetes Metab*., 2005. 31(4 Pt 1): p. 318-25.

[137] Skrabic, V., et al., Vitamin D receptor polymorphism and susceptibility to type 1 diabetes in the Dalmatian population. *Diabetes Res. Clin. Pract*., 2003. 59(1): p. 31-5.

[138] Turpeinen, H., et al., Vitamin D receptor polymorphisms: no association with type 1 diabetes in the Finnish population. *Eur. J. Endocrinol*., 2003. 149(6): p. 591-6.

[139] McDermott, M.F., et al., Allelic variation in the vitamin D receptor influences susceptibility to IDDM in Indian Asians. *Diabetologia,* 1997. 40(8): p. 971-5.

[140] Angel, B., et al., Vitamin D receptor polymorphism and susceptibility to type 1 diabetes in Chilean subjects: a case-parent study. *Eur. J. Epidemiol.,* 2004. 19(12): p. 1085-7.

[141] Chang, T.J., et al., Vitamin D receptor gene polymorphisms influence susceptibility to type 1 diabetes mellitus in the Taiwanese population. *Clin. Endocrinol.* (Oxf), 2000. 52(5): p. 575-80.

[142] Guo, S.W., et al., Meta-analysis of vitamin D receptor polymorphisms and type 1 diabetes: a HuGE review of genetic association studies. *Am. J. Epidemiol.,* 2006. 164(8): p. 711-24.

[143] Hitman, G.A., et al., Vitamin D receptor gene polymorphisms influence insulin secretion in Bangladeshi Asians. *Diabetes,* 1998. 47(4): p. 688-90.

[144] Oh, J.Y. and E. Barrett-Connor, Association between vitamin D receptor polymorphism and type 2 diabetes or metabolic syndrome in community-dwelling older adults: the Rancho Bernardo Study. *Metabolism,* 2002. 51(3): p. 356-9.

[145] Ye, W.Z., et al., Vitamin D receptor gene polymorphisms are associated with obesity in type 2 diabetic subjects with early age of onset. *Eur. J. Endocrinol.,* 2001. 145(2): p. 181-6.

[146] Malecki, M.T., et al., Vitamin D receptor gene polymorphisms and association with type 2 diabetes mellitus in a Polish population. *Exp. Clin. Endocrinol. Diabetes*, 2003. 111(8): p. 505-9.

[147] Ortlepp, J.R., et al., The vitamin D receptor gene variant is associated with the prevalence of type 2 diabetes mellitus and coronary artery disease. *Diabet. Med.,* 2001. 18(10): p. 842-5.

[148] Schlingmann, K.P., et al., Hypomagnesemia with secondary hypocalcemia is caused by mutations in TRPM6, a new member of the TRPM gene family. *Nat. Genet.,* 2002. 31(2): p. 166-70.

[149] Walder, R.Y., et al., Mutation of TRPM6 causes familial hypomagnesemia with secondary hypocalcemia. *Nat. Genet.,* 2002. 31(2): p. 171-4.

[150] Nadler, M.J., et al., LTRPC7 is a Mg.ATP-regulated divalent cation channel required for cell viability. From worm to man: three subfamilies of TRP channels. *Nature,* 2001. 411(6837): p. 590-5.

[151] Voets, T., et al., TRPM6 forms the Mg2+ influx channel involved in intestinal and renal Mg2+ absorption. TRP channels in disease TRPM7: channeling the future of cellular magnesium homeostasis? *J. Biol. Chem.,* 2004. 279(1): p. 19-25.

[152] Chubanov, V., et al., Disruption of TRPM6/TRPM7 complex formation by a mutation in the TRPM6 gene causes hypomagnesemia with secondary hypocalcemia. *Proc. Natl. Acad. Sci. USA,* 2004. 101(9): p. 2894-9.

In: Dietary Magnezium: New Research
Editor: Andrew W. Yardley

ISBN 978-1-60692-109-8

Chapter VI

Enhancement of Magnesium Content in Plants by Exploiting Ionomics and Transcriptomics

Christian Hermans* and Nathalie Verbruggen
Laboratory of Plant Physiology and Molecular Genetics,
Université Libre de Bruxelles, Campus Plaine CP242, Bd du Triomphe,
1050 Brussels, Belgium

Abstract

Plant and crop nutrition drives all terrestrial food-webs. Nutrient composition of crops can be manipulated through agronomy and genetics to optimize the delivery of essential minerals to humans and livestock. Our aim is to dissect and exploit the physiological and genetic bases for magnesium homeostasis in plants. Understanding how plants regulate Mg uptake from the rhizophere, as well as transport and cycling could have significant implications for plant nutrition and human health. With the knowledge of genes governing Mg homeostasis, it will be possible to reduce the need for fertilisers and to develop crops that grow efficiently on nutrient-poor soils. Furthermore, biofortification strategies through conventional breeding and transgenic approaches could lead to Mg-rich edible parts of crops, which would offer humans improved sources of this essential cation and overcome mineral malnutrition.

1. Magnesium in Plant Physiology

Plants require magnesium to harvest solar energy and to drive photochemistry. This is probably the most eminent physiological function of this metal *in planta*. Other roles such as the cation-mediated grana stacking of thylakoid membrane (Kaftan et *al*., 2002), the

* Corresponding author: chermans@ulb.ac.be

activation of enzymes in metabolic biochemistry (Cowan, 2002), including those in the Calvin cycle (Pakrasi et *al*., 2001), the nucleotidyl phosphate Mg-chelated forms in the cell energy budget (Igamberdiev and Kleczkowski, 2001), the involvement in nucleic acids folding and the chemical catalysis of RNA splicing (Pyle, 2002), and the involvement in antioxidative mechanisms (Camak and Kirby, 2008) have been the substance of numerous reviews. Our intent here is not to cover extensively that literature but to provide some interesting accounts of recent publications on Mg physiology in plants. In particular, focus will be (1) on the impact of Mg deficiency on sugar partitioning and biomass allocation and (2) on mechanisms regulating Mg homeostasis with possible applications in biofortification.

1.1. Incidence of Magnesium Deficiency in Forestry and Agriculture

Magnesium deficiency in plants is a widespread problem, affecting productivity and quality in agriculture (Bennett, 1997; Aitken et *al*., 1999; Graeft et *al*., 2001; Ding et *al*., 2006), in horticulture (Shaahan et *al*., 1999; Troyanos et *al*., 2000) and forestry (Mehne-Jakobs, 1995; Mitchell et *al*., 1999; Laing et *al*., 2000, Sun et *al*., 2001). Mg deficiency is distributed worldwide in forest regions, and is associated with the 'upper mid crown yellowing' of conifers in New Zealand (Mitchell et *al*., 1999) and the 'new type forest decline' or 'crown thinning' in Europe and the North-Eastern part of North America. Intensive monitoring of forest ecosystems across Europe also revealed that one third of the beech stands are subject to Mg limitation, based on foliar mineral analyses (BFH, 2000). In agriculture, the incidence of Mg deficiency symptoms is increasing, due to greater crop growth rates, which increases the demand on soil Mg, and intensive harvesting. Signs of Mg deficiency in most crop plants usually make their appearance first on old mature and recently expanded leaves, and systematically progress from them towards the youngest ones. Visible symptoms of Mg starvation are manifested as chloroses between leaf veins, which remain green (see Figure 1 for symptoms in sugar beet).

The energy-intensive manufacture and application of mineral fertilizers has been used for decades to increase crop yield and to attempt to biofortify crops in industrialized countries. However, the future of sustainable farming in these countries requires that mineral fertilizer applications are optimized to minimize environmental pollution and to preserve economic margins. In fast-developing countries such as China, the introduction of chemical fertilizers is a blessing for the agriculture but turns out to be a curse for the environment mainly due to leaching of mineral in groundwater basin and increased riverine transport (Liu et *al*., 2008). Because not all farmers understand the importance of balanced application of nutrients (Jiyun et *al*., 1999), a nutrient disequilibria in the agroecosystem mirrored by a lack of secondary essential elements (e.g. magnesium) has begun to have an impact on production worldwide. Irrational application is leading to a relative increase of K^+ and Ca^{2+} content in soil, compared to Mg^{2+}. Since high levels of these cations exert a competitive inhibition of Mg^{2+} uptake in plants (Marschner, 1995), induced Mg deficiency is becoming more and more frequent. Experiments in controlled conditions illustrate this occurrence. For example, increasing K^+ concentration in nutrient solution reduces Mg^{2+} inflow and concentration in plants and aggravates Mg deficiency symptoms (Troyanos et *al*., 2000; Ding et *al*., 2006).

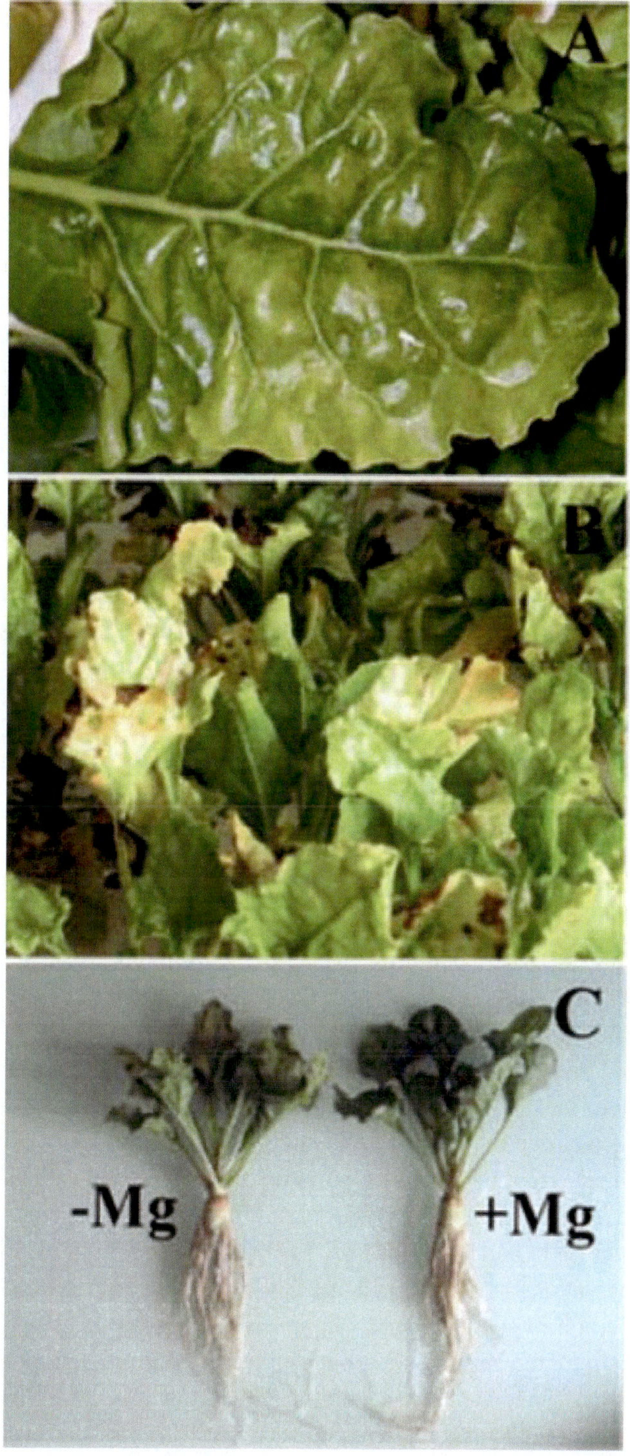

Figure 1. Magnesium deficiency symptoms observed in sugar beet. (A) Interveinal chlorosis in most recently developed leaf. (B) Chlorosis and necrotic necrotic lesion in plants at a severe stage of deficiency. (C) Comparison of Mg deficient (left) and control (right) plants, 22 d after omitting Mg from the nutrient solution.

1.2. Involvement of Magnesium in Assimilates Partitioning

Plants are photoautotrophic organisms, as they convert solar light as a useful biological energy source to fix atmospheric CO_2 and to build complex carbohydrates components. However, plants also contain sink organs (typically roots, fruits and immature leaves), which are heterotrophic and therefore require a carbon import from photosynthesizing organs. Sink and source organs are separated from each other in space but connected together through the phloem vasculature. Partitioning is the differential distribution of photosynthates within the whole plant. Phloem loading of sucrose (the carbon currency for long distance transport) in sieve elements of source leaves is considered as an essential step of carbon exportation and partitioning to sink organs (Figure 2B). These tissues are of economic importance because they are the crop final products (e.g. cereal grains, sugar beet taproots, potato tubers,…). Few reports exist concerning the effects of a Mg shortage on physiological processes but those that do exist, essentially describe an early impairment in sugar partitioning (in Arabidopsis: Hermans and Verbruggen, 2005; bean plants: Fisher and Bremer, 1993, Cakmak et *al.*, 1994 a,b; rice: Ding et *al.*, 2006; spinach: Fisher et *al.*, 1998; spruce: Mehne-Jakobs, 1995 and sugar beet Hermans et *al.*, 2004, 2005). Proper knowledge of the molecular mechanisms underpinning this metal role in sugar partitioning and biomass allocation is currently scarce. One dramatic effect of Mg starvation is sucrose and starch accumulation in source leaves, before any noticeable effect on photosynthetic activity. A later effect of Mg deficiency is a reduction of plant growth. On one hand, Mg deficiency is described not redirecting carbon resources to root growth and deeply impact on biomass allocation (Cakmak et *al.*, 1994 a,b; Ericsson and Kahr, 1995). On the other hand, some species like Arabidopsis (Hermans and Verbruggen, 2005, Hermans et *al.*, 2006), rice (Ding et *al.*, 2006) and sugar beet (Hermans et *al.*, 2004, 2005) do not present a decrease in root biomass or it comes relatively late after the outbreak of chlorotic symptoms in aerial parts.

Figure 2 illustrates the susceptibility of sucrose partitioning to low Mg availability in sugar beet. As a first step in the study of altered sucrose partitioning upon Mg deficiency, the ^{14}[C]-sucrose distribution in sugar beet was analyzed (Figure 2A). Mg-deficient and control plants were abraded and labelled apoplasmically with ^{14}[C]-sucrose according to Grusak et *al.* (1990) in order to track sucrose movement. Whole plants were autoradiographed. Fewer ^{14}[C]-sucrose molecules were exported from the young mature leaf to sink organs of Mg deficient plant compared to the radioactive pattern from old mature leaf (Figure 2A). There is a debate as to the cause of restricted growth of sink organs. It has been proposed that either (i) a decrease in sucrose export is responsible for the inhibition of growth of sink organs (in bean plants, Cakmak at *al.*, 1994 a,b) or that (ii) a decrease in the metabolic activity in sink organs causes inhibition of sucrose export (in spinach, Fisher et *al.*, 1998). (i) According to Cakmak et *al.* (1994a,b), the high susceptibility of sucrose partitioning to low Mg levels may be related to the carrier-mediated uptake of sucrose in the conducting complex of phloem (Figure 2B). Mg is possibly involved in sucrose phloem loading because it interacts with nucleotidyl tri-phosphates (Igamberdiev and Kleczkowski, 2003) fuelling the H^+-ATPases which creates the protonmotive force energizing the sucrose symporters. Likewise, pyrophosphatases, playing a role in the long-distance transport of sugars (Lerchl et *al.*, 1995), also require Mg for pyrophosphate hydrolysis.

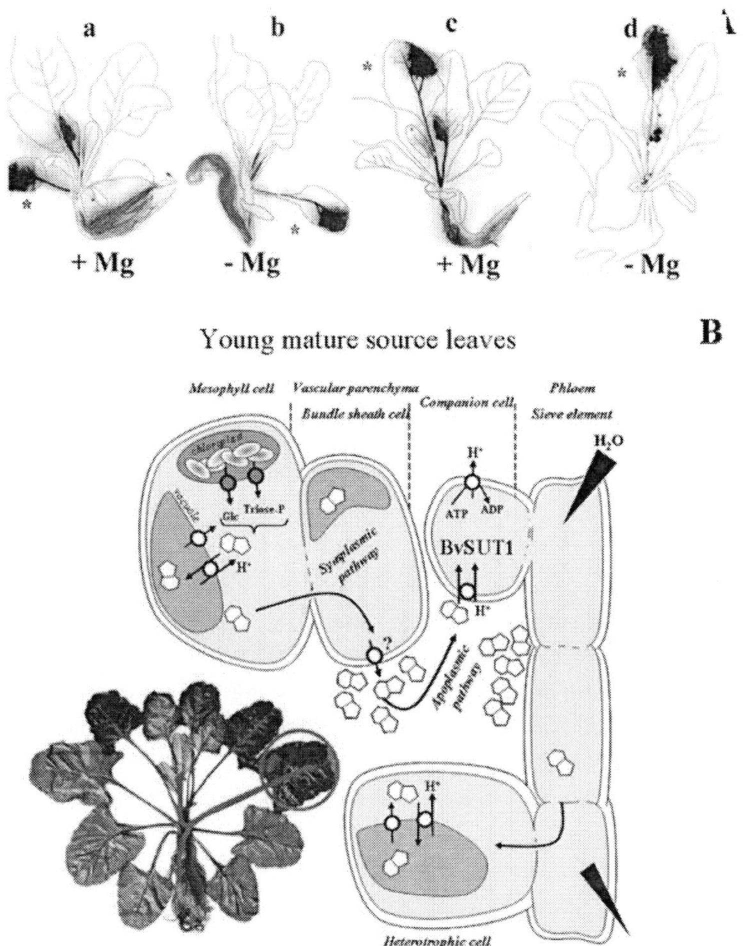

Figure 2. Model of sugar partitioning and biomass allocation upon Mg deficiency in sugar beet. (A) Autoradiographs of whole sugar beet plants labelled with 14C-sucrose. Transfer to Mg free solution was done with plants having 4 expanded leaves and labelling study was performed at d 11 after Mg withdrawal. Plants were labeled apoplasmically after deposition of 25µl droplets containing 14[C]sucrose (37kBq) on abraded zones of old mature leaves (a,b) or young mature leaves (c,d) which are indicated by asterisks. Plants were kept in light for 3.5 hours and thereafter immediately frozen and lyophilized before exposure to x-ray film. Quantification of labeled sucrose molecules between donor blade, petiole and sink organs (taproot, root and youngest immature leaves) is reported somewhere in Hermans et al. (2005). (B) Sucrose pathways for long distance transport between source leaves and sink organs upon Mg starvation. Sucrose is synthesized in mesophyll cell of source tissues and its production is balanced between export and storage in vacuole. From its point of synthesis, sucrose is loaded into the SECC (sieve element – companion cell) complex via an apoplasmic route (N.B. in sugar beet, the SECC complex is almost isolated from the surrounding cells, making it indispensable to include an apoplasmic step). The entry into the SECC complex is mediated by sucrose/H+ symporters (e.g. BvSUT1), which are localized in companion cells or sieve tube elements. The H+ potential difference is generated by H+-ATPase localized in the plasma-membrane of companion cells. Phloem loading of assimilates results in a difference in water potential that causes water uptake into SECC complex. Phloem unloading in sink may occur through plasmodesmata or via an apoplasmic path (not represented for clarity reason).

Figure 2. (Continued) The model here represents the partitioning of sucrose from young mature source leaves to sink immature leaves in an Mg deficient plant. Mg starvation increases the concentrations of sugars and starch (visible in black after staining with iodine) in leaves. A clear inverse relationship between leaf Mg concentrations and sugar content is demonstrated in sugar beet (Hermans et al., 2005). It is proposed that reduced sucrose export is due to impaired phloem loading, because this process requires Mg (as MgATP substrate for H+-pumps). In our model, the sucrose allocation to the root is proportionally less affected than that to the youngest leaves because sucrose export is relatively unaffected from the oldest leaves, which contain higher Mg content and which are preferentially feeding the roots. Since carbon allocation to the youngest leaves is likely more affected than carbon allocation to the root, an increase in root:shoot ratio is observed in that species.

All these arguments suggest that phloem loading in source leaves may be limited by low Mg availability. (ii) According to Fischer et *al.* (1998), a congestion of metabolites in source leaves from *Spinacia oleracea* arises from a limited consumption in sink leaves. In that work, phloem loading did, however, not appear to be the most susceptible process, as sucrose content in phloem sap of mature leaves was identical in Mg-deficient plants and in control plants. Limited use of assimilates in sink organs could result from growth inhibition by low Mg supply. As a result, sucrose would accumulate in source organs. This in turn points to a regulation of sucrose synthesis in the source depending on consumption in the sink tissues. Recent works support the hypothesis that Mg deficiency in Arabidopsis and sugar beet affects sucrose export from source leaves (starting with the youngest mature ones), rather than sink metabolism (Hermans et *al.*, 2004; Hermans and Verbruggen, 2005; Hermans et *al.*, 2006).

The present experiment also provides an explanation of the unrestricted root growth under low Mg status observed in certain species (Arabidopsis and sugar beet). In fact, the proximity between source and sink organs is a significant factor in the distribution of photosynthates between organs. Generally, the upper mature leaves are thought to provide photosynthates to the growing shoot tip and young immature leaves; whereas the lower oldest leaves predominantly supply the root system, and the intermediate leaves export in both directions. This model of distribution can significantly differ between species and during plant development though. Upon Mg deficiency, sucrose export to the root is proportionally less affected than that to the youngest leaves in sugar beet (Figure 2A). Those leaves, where the deficiency symptoms first manifest, have the highest starch and sucrose contents (Figure 2B) and the lowest Mg content among all plant organs (Hermans et *al.*, 2005), and they provide less carbon resources to growing shoot. Consequently, the overall aerial biomass is decreased compared to control plants. With the ongoing severity of the deficiency, intermediate and lower leaves also accumulate higher starch amount; and finally the root and taproot growth was restricted when treatment is prolonged.

2. Magnesium in Human Nutrition

2.1. Incidence of Magnesium Deficiency in Human Body

Main plant derived sources of magnesium are cereals, nuts and green vegetables, which contain chlorophyll (Buttriss, 2003). In most instances, elevated Mg content in edible plant tissue improves the nutritional quality for animal and human diet (Shaul, 2002). Mg deficiency in human body is recognized as a worldwide clinical problem and is related to muscle dysfunction, myocardial ischemia, migraines, attention deficit disorder, ... (Meij et *al.*, 2002). Mg starvation is one of the most under-recognized electrolyte disorders causing arrhythmia and sudden cardiac death (Klevay and Milne, 2002; Chiu et *al.*, 2005). Inadequate diet containing low Mg is primarily responsible of hypomagnesaemia. Human Mg concentration in the body depends on the balance between intestinal absorption and renal excretion (Schlingmann et *al.*, 2007). There are also indications of genetic inheritance in Mg requirement and hypomagnesaemia susceptibility, primarily due to defect in Mg intestinal absorption and renal-wastage. The involvement of TRPM6 and TRPM7, members of transient receptor potential (TRP) ion channels family, was demonstrated in the intestinal Mg absorption process and body Mg homeostasis (Schlingmann et *al.*, 2007; Chubanov et *al.*, 2007). Knowledge of these novel Mg transporters and platforms for future investigations for a better understanding of Mg deficiency disorders were recently reviewed by Quamme (2008). Hypomagnesaemia is also a serious disorder for ruminants, finding its roots in low Mg content of grass or forages, especially in the spring when lactation demands substantial Mg amount.

2.2. Research on Magnesium Homeostasis: Insights on Mechanisms in Regulating Magnesium Content in Edible Plants

Our pursued goal is the acquisition of new molecular knowledge of Mg homeostasis and of responses to external Mg supply in the model plant *Arabidopsis thaliana*. In particular, the research is based on the variation of Mg content in tissues, as well as the identification and the dissection of transcriptome changes associated to Mg availability (Figure 3). Comparative genomics through a model-to-crop pipeline (Arabidopsis-Brassica) could allow the development of crops that grow efficiently on nutrient-poor soils, and to reduce the need for fertilizers. Furthermore, Mg homeostasis research in plants could also lead to Mg-rich food, which would offer humans improved sources of that essential element. Biofortification is the process of increasing the bioavailable nutrients (such as vitamins and essential mineral elements) in edible portions of crops through fertilizer application, conventional breeding or transgenic strategies (Broadley and White, 2005; Zhu et *al.*, 2007; Mayer et *al.*, 2008). Through this process, we, scientists, can provide cultivators with crop varieties that through the higher nutritive provision can overcome mineral malnutrition.

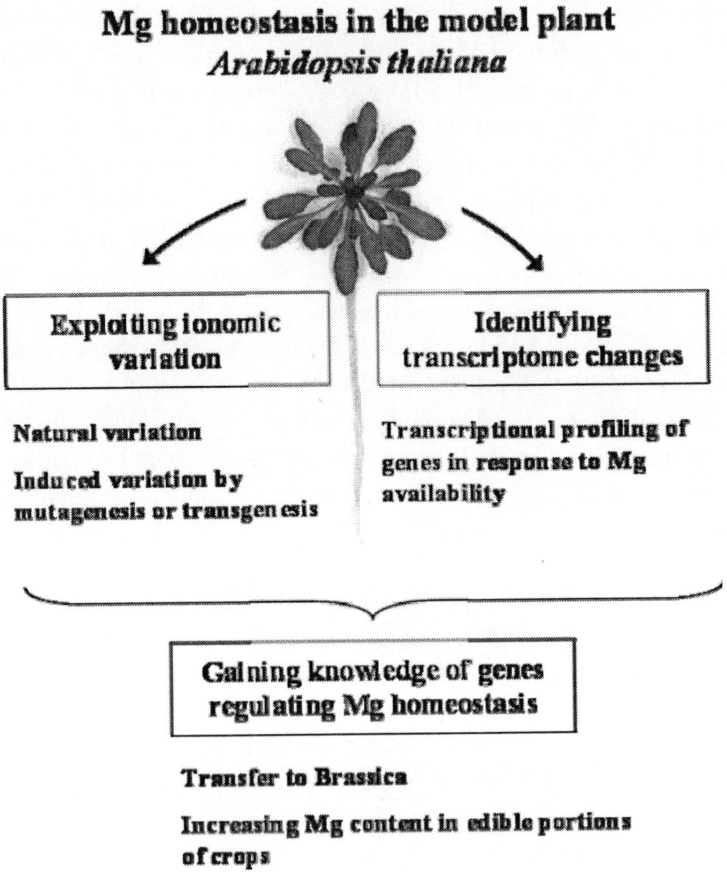

Mg homeostasis in the model plant *Arabidopsis thaliana*

Exploiting ionomic variation

Natural variation

Induced variation by mutagenesis or transgenesis

Identifying transcriptome changes

Transcriptional profiling of genes in response to Mg availability

Gaining knowledge of genes regulating Mg homeostasis

Transfer to Brassica

Increasing Mg content in edible portions of crops

Figure 3. Research strategies developed in order to dissect the mechanisms of magnesium homeostasis in the model plant *Arabidopsis thaliana*. (i) The exploitation of the variation in the ionome is realized through the study of the natural variation of the Mg content in accessions of Arabidopsis, the characterization of mutants impaired in their Mg content (Ionomics data base mutants and insertion mutants for permeases potentially involved in Mg transport). (ii) The identification of transcriptomic changes in response to Mg deficiency and restoration is realized through different profiling methods (e.g. cDNA-AFLP and microarrays). A transfer of the knowledge acquired in the model species *Arabidopsis thaliana* to closely related crops of the *Brassicaceae* family is foreseen.

Successful creation of genotypes with increased nutrient densities has already been accomplished for some minerals, such as a carrot with increased Ca content (Park et *al*., 2005) and with better body absorption *in fine* in mice and humans (Morris et *al*., 2008).

Transgenic approaches to biofortification have mainly focused on micronutrient (e.g. Fe and Zn), but rarely on Mg despite the recognition of its deficiency in human diet. This is probably due to the fact that tissue Mg concentration typically shows less, but nevertheless significant, variation among genotypes (reviewed in Broadley and White, 2005). Here, we propose to briefly depict some intervention strategies recently developed to increase Mg dietary value of plants.

2.2.1. Exploiting Magnesium Content Variation Induced by Mutagenesis or Genetic Engineering in Plants

Arabidopsis Mutants Which Contain Abnormal Levels of Mg

The ionome is defined as the mineral nutrient and trace element (both essential and non-essential) composition of an organism (Lahner et *al.*, 2003). The study of the plant ionome (so called ionomics) involves the quantitative measurement of the composition in elements and changes in this composition associated with physiological stimuli, developmental state and genetic modifications. The analytical technologies, bioinformatics aspects and workflow tools (PiiMS- Purdue Ionomics formation Management System) of ionomics were recently reviewed by Salt et *al.* (2008). In early development of their project, Lahner et *al.* (2003) isolated more than fifty mutants in a fast neutron mutagenized *Arabidopsis thaliana* population, with altered mineral profile in the shoot. The characterization of four mutants with abnormal Mg content compared to wild type plant was undertaken (Figure 4A).

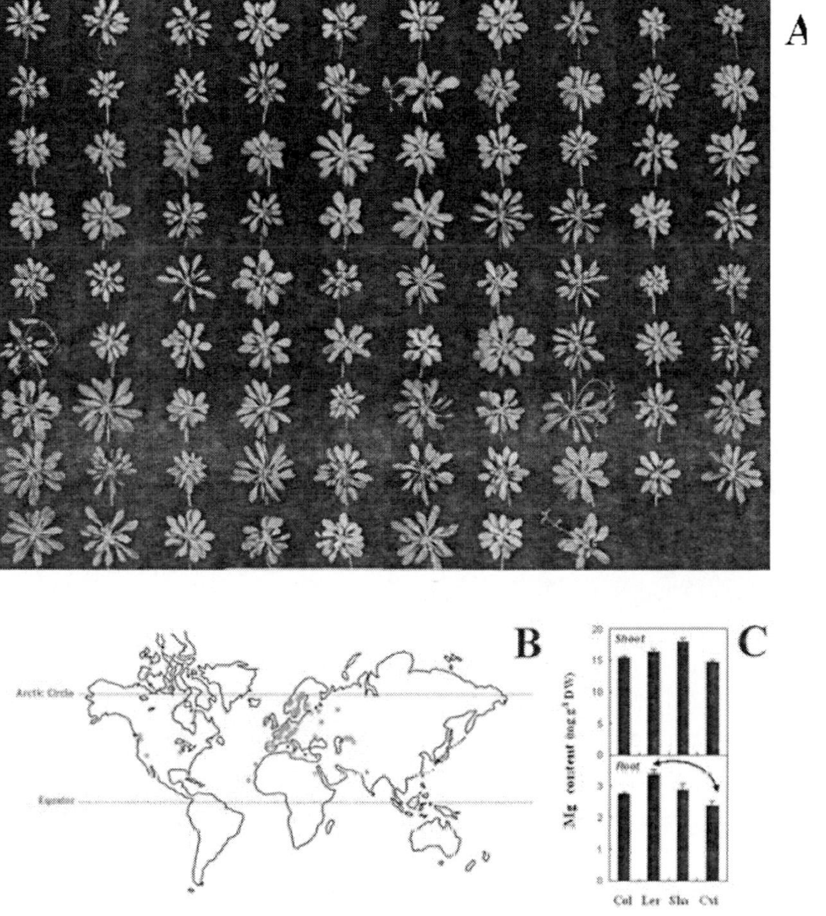

Figure 4. Studying the mutagenized induced variation of Mg content in Arabidopsis thaliana (A) Hydroponics culture of wild type and four of the Ionomics Project (Lahner et al., 2003) mutants. (B) Changes in the mineral profile of mutants compared to wild type. Mutant 79:48 presents lower Mg content than WT, while 117:20, 132:01 and 136:31 have higher Mg content.

A striking correlation between magnesium, arsenic and lithium incorporation was observed. This observation points to possible negative side effect of Mg biofortification in plants. Genetic analysis is under way to investigate co-segregation of higher content in Mg, As and Li. Positional cloning and microarray-based cloning procedures are both used to identify the mutations in genes responsible for Mg-profile changes and visual phenotypes.

Genetic Engineering of Mg Transporters

To date, the Mg transporters characterized *in planta* are the Mg^{2+}/H^{+} exchanger AtMHX (Shaul et *al.*, 1999) and the MRS2 homologues family (Schock et *al.*, 2000; Li et *al.*, 2001; Gardner et *al.*, 2003). An early attempt to modify the expression of Mg transporter in plant was realized by Deng et *al.* (2006).

These authors expressed the Arabidopsis transporter gene *AtMGT1/AtMRS2-1* under the control of the cauliflower mosaic virus CaMV 35S promoter (which is strong and constitutive) in *Nicotiana benthamiana*. *AtMGT1* overexpression favorably increased by 30% the Mg content in transgenic plants. This result is therefore encouraging for the development of further transgenic strategies for Mg nutritional enhancement of plants.

2.2.2. Exploiting Natural Magnesium Content Variation in Arabidopsis Populations

The natural variation in *Arabidopsis thaliana* ecotypes (Figure 5A) can be exploited to identify *loci* controlling Mg concentration in tissues. These ecotypes which grow on a wide range of soil conditions (Figure 5B) provide a rich source of genetic diversity to explore potentially adaptive differences in the ionome. Magnesium partitioning between organs throughout the life cycle of Arabidopsis presents contrasted patterns between a small numbers of ecotypes studied so far (Waters and Grusak, 2008). With a high marker density (over 250,000 single nucleotide polymorphisms, or one SNP every 500 base pairs in the Arbidopsis genome) and the existence of over 1,000 accessions, association mapping, also referred as linkage disequilibrium mapping (Kim et *al.*, 2006), is emerging as a powerful tool for identifying alleles or *loci* responsible for the natural variation of a given trait. The genetic basis of adaptively traits to the abiotic environment in *Arabidopsis thaliana*, such as flowering-time, has already begun to be investigated through the genome-wide association mapping strategy (Zhao et *al.*, 2007).

Likewise, a similar strategy is currently adopted in collaboration with D. Salt (Purdue University, IN) and M. Nordborg (University of Southern California, CA) groups, initially based on the analysis of numerous essential and non-essential ions in both roots and shoots of 96 accessions developed by Nordborg et *al.* (2005).

This collection includes stock center accessions and hierarchical sample from natural populations. The accessions are grown hydroponically (Figure 5A,C), in order to find those showing the most contrasted phenotypes (low and high Mg tissue concentration), and to search for genetic determinants of Mg content.

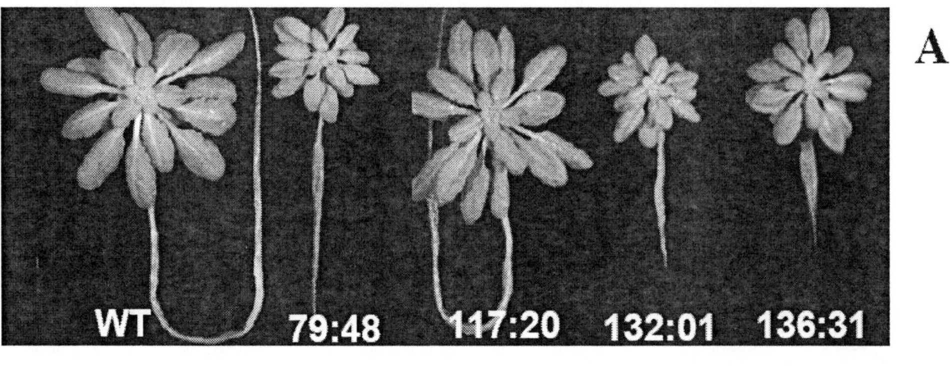

B

Line	Li	Na	Mg	P	K	Ca	Cr	Mn	Fe	Co	Ni	Cu	Zn	As	Se	Mo	Cd	Pb
79:48			-18						-21							37		
117:20	93		93		-24		68							104	60	20		
132:01	32		53		30	15								112		-40		
136:31	47		79		121		-36							195	22			

Figure 5. Studying the natural variation of Mg content in Arabidopsis thaliana accessions. (A) Accessions of the collection of Nordborg et al. (2005) grown hydroponically. (B) Geographic distribution of the Arabidopsis accessions of the Nordborg collection indicated by red spots. (C) Preliminary results of the Mg content analysis in root and shoot of four principal accessions Columbia (Col), Lansdberg (Ler), Shadara (Sha) and Cape Verde (Cvi).

2.2.3. Identifying Transcriptome Changes in Early and Late Signalling of Mg Deficiency

With the emergence of microarray technologies to monitor gene expression, plant physiologists have begun to investigate the rapid transcriptional changes associated with imbalance of mineral elements (Wang et *al.*, 2003; Misson et *al.*, 2005; Muller et *al.*, 2007). At present no transcriptomics data on Mg are available but we have undertaken a genome-wide analysis of the rapid (within hours) and late (within days) responses to Mg deprivation in *Arabidopsis thaliana* (Figure 6). This study was performed on the root and young mature leaves, which are the first target of Mg deficiency (Hermans and Verbruggen, 2005). Because genechips hybridizations are costly, a cDNA-AFLP approach covering on estimation 5% of the Arabidopsis transcriptome was chosen as a pilot experiment, in order to decide about the sampling time for further microarray studies. Subsequently, a microarray study was done with full genome chips. A functional analysis of the differentially expressed genes is currently under progress to uncover some of the relationships of specific downstream events (e.g. sugar accumulation and chlorophyll degradation in leaves) to the signaling pathways that control Mg deficiency responses in Arabidopis. A study of the expression of certain genes is performed upon macro element deficiencies in order to assess the specificity of the response to Mg deficiency. That would help in the development of novel molecular diagnostic markers of incipient Mg deprivation and of smart plant technology (Hammond et *al.*, 2003) to monitor plant Mg status. The whole data will enable to understand plant response to Mg deprivation and allow developing new tools for Mg biofortification purpose.

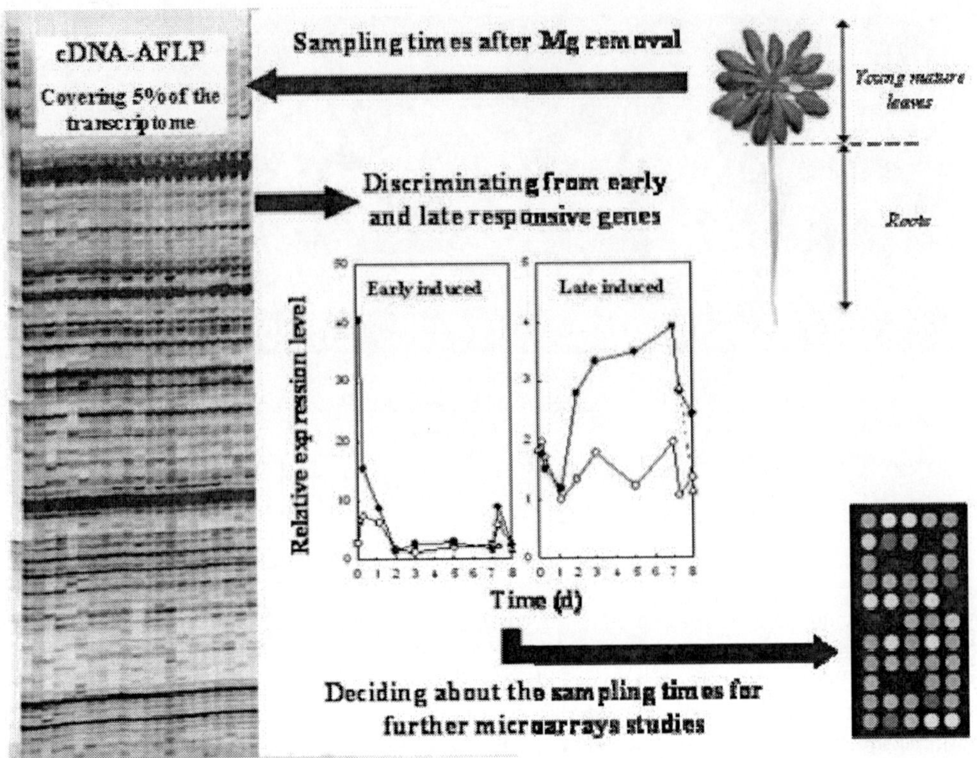

Figure 6. Transcriptomic study of Mg deficiency in Arabidopsis thaliana. Example of cDNA-AFLP gel and transcript derived fragment differentially (≥ 2 fold) regulated by Mg starvation treatment. Open symbols: control fully supplied samples, closed symbols: Mg deficient samples. Sampling times used for microarrays studies are decided base on that pilot experiment.

2.2.4. Transferring the Benefits from Arabidopsis Research to Brassica

Cultivated Brassica species are the group of crops most closely related to *Arabidopsis thaliana*. Comparative genomics through a model-to-crop pipeline will allow genes controlling tissue Mg content, including those identified in the strategies that we previously described, to be studied in crop systems with relative ease. Ongoing genome sequencing of *Brassica oleracea* will hasten this effort in the near future. We will be able to test the hypothesis that shoot Mg content is controlled by conserved *loci* in the closely-related model and *Brassica oleracea* (Broadley et *al*., 2008). The ultimate goal would be to improve mineral composition of Brassica. Genetic and environmental factors impacting plant Mg concentrations will be quantified to determine the robustness of transgenic biofortification strategies.

In conclusion, a proper understanding of Mg homeostasis in plant at a basic research level is the key to the development of strategies to conserve natural resources, increase crop yield but also to boost the nutritional value of crops, which would be of benefit to human health. Improving Mg content in plants is not a trivial task. Nevertheless, Mg supplements from plant origin could reduce the incidence and severity of hypomagnesaemia diseases in humans.

Acknowledgments

The authors thank the Belgian Science Policy for financial support (project PAIVI/33, return grant of C.H) and the Fonds National de la Recherche Scientifique FRNS-FRS.

References

Aitken RL, Dickson T, Hailes KJ and Moody PW (1999) Response of field-grown maize to applied magnesium in acidic soil in north-eastern Australia. *Australian Journal of Agricultural Research* 50: 191-198.

BFH, Federal Research Centre for Forestry and Forest Products (2000). Forest condition in Europe, 2000 executive report. ISSN 1020-587x.

Bennett WF (1997) Nutrients deficiencies and toxicities in crop plants. APS Press, The American Phythopathological Society.

Broadley MR, Hammond JP, King GJ, Astley D, Bowen HC, Meacham MC, Mead A, Pink DAC, Teakle GR, Hayden RM, Spracklen WP and White PJ (2008) Shoot calcium and magnesium concentrations differ between subtaxa, are highly heritable, and associate with potentially pleiotropic loci in *Brassica oleracea*. *Plant Physiology* 146:1707-1720.

Buttriss J (2003) Introduction: Plant foods and health pg15. *In* Plants: diet and health, Goldberg G (ed), Blackwell Publishing, The British Nutrition Foundation.

Cakmak I, Hengeler C and Marschner H (1994a) Partitioning of shoot and root dry matter and carbohydrates in bean plants suffering from phosphorus, potassium and magnesium deficiency. *Journal of Experimental Botany* 45: 1245-1250.

Cakmak I, Hengeler C and Marschner H (1994b). Changes in phloem export of sucrose in leaves in response to phosphorus, potassium and magnesium deficiency in bean plants. *Journal of Experimental Botany* 45: 1251-1257.

Cakmak I and Kirkby EA (2008) Role of magnesium in carbon partitioning and alleviating photooxidative damage. *Physiologia Plantarum* In press ISSN 0031-9317.

Chiu HF, Chen CC, Tsai SS, Wu TN and Yang CY (2005) Relationship between magnesium levels in drinking water and sudden infant death syndrome. *Magnesium Research* 18: 12-8.

Chubanov V, Schlingmann KP, Wäring J, Heinzinger J, Kaske S, Waldegger S, Schnitzler MM and Gudermann T (2007) Hypomagnesemia with secondary hypocalcemia due to a missense mutation in the putative pore-forming region of TRPM6. *Journal of Biological Chemistry* 282: 7656-7667.

Cowan JA (2002) Structural and catalytic chemistry of magnesium-dependent enzymes. *Biometals* 15: 225-235.

Deng W, Luo K, Li D, Zheng X, Wei X, Smith W, Thammina C, Lu L, Li Y and Pei Y (2007) Overexpression of an Arabidopsis magnesium transport gene, *AtMGT1*, in *Nicotiana benthamiana* confers Al tolerance. *Journal of Experimental Botany* 57: 4235 – 4243.

Ding Y, Luo W and Xu G (2006) Characterisation of magnesium nutrition and interaction of magnesium and potassium in rice. *Annals of Applied Biology* 149: 111-123.

Fisher ES and Bremer E (1993) Influence of magnesium deficiency on rates of leaf expansion, starch and sucrose accumulation and net assimilation in *Phaseolus vulgaris*. *Physiologia Plantarum* 89: 271-276.

Fisher ES, Lohaus G, Heineke D and Heldt HW (1998) Magnesium deficiency results in accumulation of carbohydrates and amino acids in source and sink leaves of spinach. *Physiologia Plantarum* 102: 16-20.

Gardner RC (2003) Genes for magnesium transport. *Current Opinion in Plant Biology* 6: 263-267.

Graeft S, Steffens D and Schubert S (2001) Use of reflectance measurements for the early detection of N, P, Mg and Fe deficiencies in *Zea mays* L. *Journal of Plant Nutrition and Soil Science* 164: 445-450.

Grusak MA, Delrot S and Ntsika G (1990). Short-term effect of heat-girdles on source leaves of *Vicia faba*: Analysis of phloem loading and carbon partitioning parameters. *Journal of Experimental Botany* 41: 1371-1377.

Hammond JP, Bennett MJ, Bowen HC, Broadley MR, Eastwood DC, May ST, Rahn C, Swarup R, Woolaway KE and White PJ (2003) Changes in gene expression in Arabidopsis shoots during phosphate starvation and the potential for developing smart plants. *Plant Physiology* 132: 578-596.

Hermans C, Johnson GN, Strasser RJ and Verbruggen N (2004) Physiological characterisation of magnesium deficiency in sugar beet: acclimation to low magnesium differentially affects photosystems I and II. *Planta* 220: 344-355.

Hermans C, Bourgis F, Faucher M, Delrot S, Strasser RJ and Verbruggen N (2005) Magnesium deficiency in sugar beet alters sugar partitioning and phloem loading in young mature leaves. *Planta* 220: 441-449.

Hermans C and Verbruggen N (2005) Physiological characterization of magnesium deficiency in *Arabidopsis thaliana*. *Journal of Experimental Botany* 56: 2153-2161.

Hermans C, Hammond JP, White PJ and Verbruggen N (2006) How do deficiencies of essential mineral elements alter biomass allocation? *Trends in Plant Sciences* 11: 610-617.

Igamberdiev AU and Kleczkowski LA (2001) Implications of adenylate kinase-governed equilibrium of adenylates on contents of free magnesium in plant cells and compartments. *Biochemichal Journal* 360: 225-231.

Jiyun J, Lin B and Zhang W (1999) Improving nutrient management for sustainable development of agriculture in China, pp.157-174. *In*: Smaling EMA., Oenema O and Fresco LO (eds.) Nutrient disequilibria in agroecosystems. Concepts and case studies. CABI Publishing. University Press, Cambridge, UK.

Kaftan D, Brumfeld V, Nevo R, Scherz A and Reich Z (2002) From chloroplasts to photosystems: in situ scanning force microscopy on intact thylakoid membranes. *EMBO Journal* 21: 6246-6253.

Kim S, Zhao K, Jiang R, Molitor J, Borevitz JO, Nordborg M and Marjoram P (2006) Association mapping with single-feature polymorphisms. *Genetics* 173: 1125-1133.

Klevay LM and Milne DB (2002) Low dietary magnesium increases supraventricular ectopy. *The American Journal of Clinical Nutrition* 75: 550-4.

Lahner B, Gong J, Mahmoudian M, Smith EL, Abid B, Rogers EE, Guerinot ML, Harper JF, Ward JM, McIntyre L, Schroeder JI and Salt DE (2003) Genomic scale profiling of nutrient and trace elements in *Arabidopsis thaliana. Nature Biotechnology* 21: 1215-1221.

Laing W, Greer D, Sun O, Beets P, Lowe A and Payn T (2000) Pysiological impacts of Mg deficiency in *Pinus radiata*: growth and photosynthesis. *New Phytologist* 146: 47-57.

Li L, Tutone AF, Drummond RSM., Gardner RC and Luan S (2001) A novel family of magnesium transport genes in Arabidopsis. *The Plant Cell* 13: 2761-2775.

Liu C, Watanabe M and Wang Q (2008) Changes in nitrogen budgets and nitrogen use efficiency in the agroecosystems of the Changjiang River basin between 1980 and 2000. *Nutrient Cycling in Agroecosystems* 80: 19-37.

Mayer JE, Pfeiffer WH, Beyer P (2008) Biofortified crops to alleviate micronutrient malnutrition. *Current Opinion in Plant Biology* 11:166-70.

Marschner H (1995) *Mineral nutrition of higher plants*. Springer-Verlag, Berlin, Germany.

Mehne-Jakobs B (1995) The influence of magnesium-deficiency on carbohydrate concentrations in Norway spruce (*Picea abies*) needles. *Tree Physiology* 15: 577-584.

Meij IC, van den Heuvel LPWJ and Knoers NVAM (2002) Genetic disorders of magnesium homeostasis. *Biometals* 15: 297-307.

Misson J, Raghothama KG, Jain A, Jouhet J, Block MA, Bligny R, Ortet P, Creff A, Somerville S, Rolland N, Doumas P, Nacry P, Herrerra-Estrella L, Nussaume L and Thibaud MC (2005) A genome-wide transcriptional analysis using *Arabidopsis thaliana* Affymetrix gene chips determined plant responses to phosphate deprivation. *Proceedings of the National Academy of Science of the USA* 102: 11934-11939.

Mitchell AD, Loganathan P, Payn TW and Tillman RW (1999) Effect of calcined magnesite on soil and *Pinus radiata* foliage magnesium in pumice soils of New Zealand. *Australian Journal of Soil Research* 37: 545-560.

Morris J, Hawthorne M, Hotze T, Abrams SA, and Hirschi D (2008) Nutritional impact of elevated calcium transport activity in carrots. *Proceedings of the National Academy of Sciences of the USA* 105: 431-1435.

Muller R, Morant M, Jarmer H, Nilsson L and Nielsen TH (2007) Genome-wide analysis of the arabidopsis leaf transcriptome reveals interaction of phosphate and sugar metabolism. *Plant Physiology* 143: 156-171.

Nordborg M, Hu TT, IshinoY, Jhaveri J, Toomajian C, Zheng H, Bakker E, Calabrese P, Gladstone J, Goyal R, Jakobsson M, Kim S, Morozov Y, Padhukasahasram B, Plagnol V, Rosenberg NA, Shah C, Wall J, Wang J, Zhao K, Kalbfleisch T, Schultz V, Kreitman M, and Bergelson J (2005) The pattern of polymorphism in *Arabidopsis thaliana. PLoS Biology* 3:e196.

Pakrasi H, Ogawa T and Bhattacharrya-Pakrasi M (2001) Transport of metals: a key process in oxygenic photosynthesis. In Regulation of Photosynthesis, pp. 253-264. Aro EM and Anderson B (eds), Kluwer Academic Publishers.

Park SH, Kim CK, Pike LM, Smith RH and Hirschi KD (2004) Increased calcium in carrots by expression of an Arabidopsis H^+/Ca^{2+} transporter. *Molecular Breeding* 14: 275–282.

Pyle AM (2002) Metal ions in the structure and function of RNA. *Journal of Biological Inorganic Chemistry* 7: 679-690.

Quamme GA (2008) Recent developments in intestinal magnesium absorption. *Current Opinion in Gastroenterology* 24: 230-235.

Salt DE, Baxter I and Lahner B (2008) Ionomics and the study of the plant ionome. *Annual Review of Plant Biology* 59: 709-733.

Shaahan MM, El-Sayed AA and Abou El-Nour EAA (1999) Predicting nitrogen, magnesium and iron nutritional status in some perennial crops using a portable chlorophyll meter. *Scienta Horticulturæ* 82: 339-348.

Schlingmann KP, Waldegger S, Konrad M, Chubanov V and Gudermann T (2007) TRPM6 and TRPM7 - Gatekeepers of human magnesium metabolism. *Biochimica et Biophysica Acta* 1772: 813-21.

Schock I, Gregan J, Steinhauser S, Schweyen R, Brennicke A and Knoop V (2000) A member of a novel *Arabidopsis thaliana* gene family of candidate Mg^{2+} ion transporters complements a yeast mitochondrial group II intron-splicing mutant. *The Plant Journal* 24(4): 489-501.

Shaul O, Hilgemann DW, Aldmeida-Engler J, Van Montagu M, Inzé D, Galili G (1999) Cloning and characterization of a novel Mg^{2+}/H^{+} exchanger. *EMBO Journal* 18: 3973-3980.

Shaul O (2002) Magnesium transport and function in plants: the tip of the iceberg. *Biometals* 15: 309-323.

Sun OJ, Gielen GJHP, Tattersall Smith RSC and Thorn AJ (2001) Growth, Mg nutrition and photosynthetic activity of *Pinus radiata*: evidence that NaCl addition counteracts the impact of low Mg supply. *Trees* 15:335-340.

Troyanos YE, Hipps NA, Moorby J and Kingswell G (2000) The effects of external potassium and magnesium concentrations on the magnesium and potassium inflow rates and growth on micropropagated cherry rootstocks, 'F.12/1' (*Prunus avium* L.) and 'Colt' (*Prunus avium* L.) x (*Prunus pseudocerasus* L.). *Plant and Soil* 255: 73-82.

Wang R, Okamoto M, Xing X and Crawford NM (2003) Microarray analysis of the nitrate response in Arabidopsis roots and shoots reveals over 1,000 rapidly responding genes and new linkages to glucose, trehalose-6-phosphate, iron, and sulfate metabolism. *Plant Physiology* 132: 556-567.

Waters BM and Grusak MA (2008) Whole-plant mineral partitioning throughout the life cycle in *Arabidopsis thaliana* ecotypes Columbia, Landsberg *erecta*, Cape Verde Islands, and the mutant *ysl1ysl3*. *New Phytologist* 177: 389-405.

White PJ and Broadley MR (2005) Biofortifying crops with essential mineral elements. *Trends in Plant Science* 10: 586-593

Zhao K, Aranzana MJ, Kim S, Lister C, Shindo C, Tang C, Toomajian C, Zheng H, Dean C, Marjoram P and Nordborg M (2007) An Arabidopsis example of association mapping in structured samples. *PLoS Genetics* 3:e4.

Zhu C, Naqvi S, Gomez-Galera S, Pelacho AM, Capell T and Christou P (2007) Transgenic strategies for the nutritional enhancement of plants. *Trends in Plant Science* 12: 548-555.

Electronic References

http://walnut.usc.edu (Molecular and Computational Biology, University of Southern California, USA).

www.purdue.edu/dp/ionomics (Purdue Ionomics Information Management System, Purdue University, USA).

In: Dietary Magnezium: New Research
Editor: Andrew W. Yardley
ISBN 978-1-60692-109-8

Chapter VII

A Role for Magnesium in the Regulation of Ruminal Sodium Transport

Friederike Stumpff* and Holger Martens
Department of Veterinary Physiology, Free University of Berlin, Germany

Abstract

The ruminal epithelium is a stratified squamous epithelium that has evolved to display functions essential for the unique ability of cows and sheep to ferment dietary components like carbohydrates and protein, and to selectively absorb nutrients and minerals for the production of milk. A characteristic property of this tissue is its pronounced ability to transport magnesium against an electrochemical gradient. Absorption of magnesium is reduced by dietary elevation of ruminal potassium, leading to hypomagnesaemia that can reach clinical significance. Studies of the intact tissue and of isolated cells suggest that cellular magnesium uptake is decreased by apical depolarization of the ruminal membrane, resulting in both a lower cytosolic concentration and transepithelial transport of the element.

Another characteristic feature of this unusual epithelium is the expression of a sodium-conducting channel with functional properties that are clearly distinct from the epithelial sodium channel (ENaC) found in most mammalian epithelia. Thus, it has not been possible to demonstrate direct regulation of ruminal sodium transport by aldosterone, and the effects of amiloride are clearly limited to an inhibition of the sodium proton exchanger (NHE3) expressed by this tissue. Studies at the level of the animal and the tissue suggest that sodium conductance is enhanced by depolarization of the apical membrane. Recent *in vitro* studies have demonstrated that ruminal epithelial cells express non-selective cation channels in the apical membrane that are regulated by changes in cytosolic magnesium. We propose that the reduction in ruminal magnesium uptake observed after ingestion of high potassium fodder may be related to a role for magnesium

* Corresponding Author: Friederike Stumpff, M.D., Department of Veterinary Physiology, Free University of Berlin, Oertzenweg 19b, 14163 Berlin, Germany (0049 30 838 62595 (Office); 0049 30 838 62610 (Fax); E-Mail Address: stumpff@zedat.fu-berlin.de

in a signaling cascade that leads to an increase in the permeability of this non-selective cation channel for sodium, thus enhancing absorption of this ion from the rumen and restoring ruminal osmolarity, while contributing to the retention of potassium.

Introduction

Compared to the extensive research on various molecules involved in signal transduction, Mg^{2+} has not gotten much attention. One of the reasons for this may be that in man, hypomagnesaemia is a fairly rare condition and one that is easily treated by magnesium supplements when it does occur – as in pregnancy or lactation. Thus, the stimulus for research in the area has been limited. Conversely and due to the large amounts of magnesium lost in milk, hypomagnesaemia in cows and sheep continues to lead to deaths of afflicted animals or even part of entire herds [32, 47, 92, 104, 118]. As a result, there has been ongoing interest in the uptake of magnesium in this species.

In the following, the focus will be on the ruminant in general and on the very peculiar organ that gives this species its name. Thus, this topic may not appear to be of general interest. However, we feel that the story that is emerging from many decades of research on how the ruminant has adapted to a dramatically altered nutritional situation by utilizing the interactions of Mg^{2+} with uptake of other cations may have implications for other physiological situations.

The Ruminant Species: Adaptation to a Roughage Diet

The ruminant species and mankind evolved in parallel as survivors of a relatively short period of mass extinction during which the forests of the Oligocene perished and were replaced with vast grasslands [11]. During this era, the ancestral ruminant, a small and forest-dwelling species [60], perfected its ability to utilize poorly digestible fiber and adapted to uptake of grass and roughage for its nutritional requirements. This accomplishment has been essential for the survival of these animals, and probably also for that of the humanoid apes which left the dwindling forests and began to follow and hunt these herds of ruminants.

Central to the ability of ruminants to subsist on a diet of grass while excreting large amounts of milk is the development of an advanced digestive system with several specialized compartments (reticulum, rumen, and omasum) that precede the actual stomach (abomasum) and the lower digestive tract (Figure 1). The largest of these forestomaches, the rumen, fills almost half of the entire abdominal cavity of these animals with a volume reaching 60 to 100 l in cows [138]. Lined with squamous, stratified epithelium which is keratinized and non-glandular [48, 53], this pouch is probably of esophageal origin [98] and serves as both a water reservoir [138] and a fermentation chamber in which poorly digestible forage is broken down and reassembled into digestible nutrients by an abundant flora of microorganisms [8, 57, 58, 156]. Maintanance of a pH that should be slightly acidic (5.5 - 7.0) and an osmolarity that is marginally hypotonic before or slightly hypertonic after a meal (to blood) is central to this fermentation process. Ruminal homeostasis is ensured by a number of factors that include production of ample amounts of saliva, continuous mixing of saliva with ruminal content by ruminal contractions and rumination of roughage, and the ability of the rumen to serve as a barrier between blood and rumen content while absorbing certain minerals and organic compounds in a controlled manner.

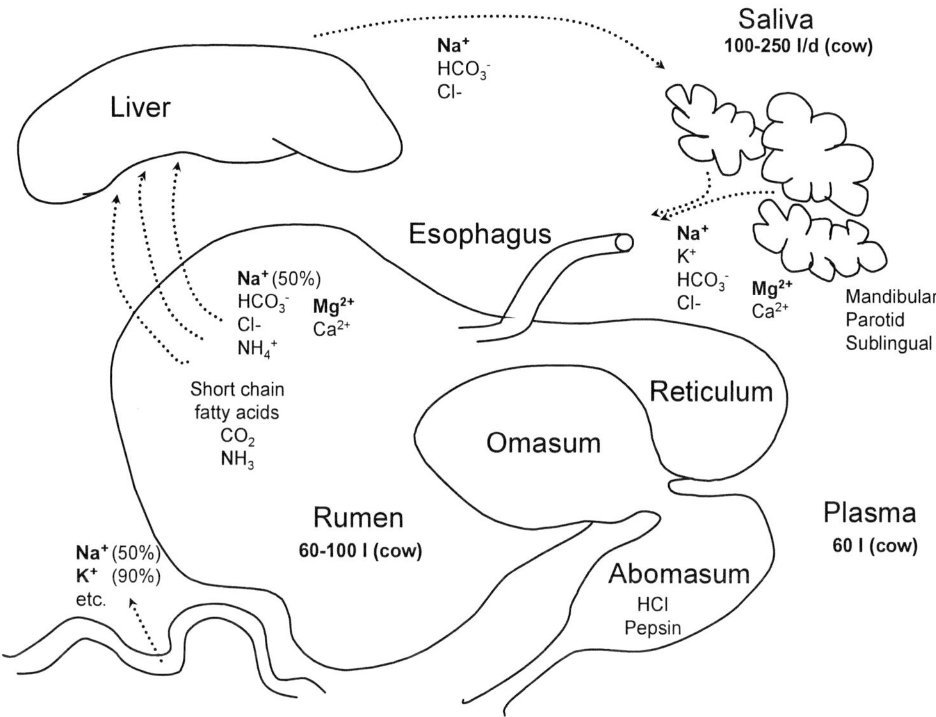

Fig 1: Schematic representation of the ruminant forestomach system: The glandular stomach (abomasum) is preceded by three compartments lined with stratified, squamous epithelium: the reticulum, the rumen, and the omasum. These forestomaches are involved in absorption of fermentation products and inorganic ions. Some 100 – 250 l/d of saliva are produced daily by the cow, representing 5 times the total plasma content of sodium, 50% of which is reabsorbed by the forestomaches. Over 30% of plasma Mg^{2+} content are excreted via saliva on a daily basis and are absorbed primarily in the rumen. Substantial amounts of both elements are secreted in milk (40 l/d).

Saliva

A striking difference between ruminants and most monogastric species is the ability to produce an extremely large stream of well buffered saliva that amounts to about 6 16 l/d in sheep [67] and 100 – 200 l/d in cattle [9, 15] with values of up to 250 l/d in lactating cows [23, 138] (Figure 1). This saliva is low in chloride (22 mmol/l) and contains large amounts of pH buffers such as HCO_3^- (120 mmol/l) and PO_4^- (30 mmol/l). After feeding, the flow rate but not the ionic composition of saliva increases, and can be so massive that the ADH and renin-angiotensin mechanism is activated [138]. Postprandial stimulation of salivary flow can be at least partially mimicked by the addition of volatile fatty acids to the rumen [15]. In contrast, in experiments in which ruminal pH was altered by addition of HCl, or ruminal osmolarity by addition of mannitol, no impact on the flow rate or composition of saliva could be observed in the sense of a feedback mechanism [15], although salivary secretion dropped when pH reached very low levels (<3.5) [15]. When strongly hypertonic solutions of sodium or potassium salts were infused into the rumen, or sodium salts or urea were infused into the blood, production of saliva decreased and the concentration of those substances increased in the saliva. Other treatments including physiological elevations of ruminal potassium content had little effect on salivary composition [157]. Thus, evidence for sensors in the gut or rumen are scarce and salivary flow appears to be regulated by the composition of the portal blood [21, 138], possibly via hepatic sensors [119, 151].

A major fact that emerged from these studies is that if experimentally obtained saliva is not returned to the rumen, flow rate decreases to 50% of the initial value within two hours [15]. This decrease can be prevented by administration of $NaHCO_3$ containing solution to the rumen [14] and points towards the importance of ruminal reabsorption of these elements.

With the saliva, the animal secretes an amount of Na^+ that is 1.2-1.5 mol/d in sheep and 15 – 30 mol/d in cows [82] and is thus five times higher than the sodium content of the body, and 15 times higher than the amount of sodium consumed with the fodder [139]. Salivary secretion of HCO_3^- reaches levels that can lead to acidaemia when salivary flow is high, as after a meal [111, 112, 129, 139], stressing the importance of a rapid reabsorption of HCO_3^-.

Sodium content of saliva is strongly regulated by aldosterone, which is of considerable importance given the fact that in the natural diet of the ruminant, sodium is a scarce element. In sodium depleted sheep, salivary content of this mineral can fall dramatically from concentrations of about 180 mmol/l to as low as 40 mmol/l. Potassium excretion rises concomitantly from a normal level of 4 to 6 mmol/l to values of over 130 mmol/l [14]. Conversely, ruminal reabsorption of Na^+ is not regulated by aldosterone [85].

Crisis situations can occur in spring, when animals are quickly transferred from a diet of hay, which is comparably low in potassium, to a diet of fresh spring grass which is rich in potassium. In these situations, potassium levels in the rumen can rapidly peak to over 100 mmol/l, while sodium levels drop to lows of 30 mmol/l. To restore the balance for sodium, animals thus have to be able to absorb sodium actively against this very high background of potassium, while any absorption of potassium has to be tightly coupled to its excretion in the kidney. Given the enormous surface area and volume of the rumen, and the huge quantities of potassium rich roughage, the demands on this organ are thus clear: it has to prevent potassium from entering the blood stream too quickly, and it has to be highly able to transport sodium, bicarbonate, magnesium and calcium from the rumen to the plasma against an electrochemical gradient.

The Rumen

Histology and Organogenesis

Interestingly, the esophagus of mammals including humans has been shown to posses transporting properties in that it forms a tight barrier against the efflux of K^+ [68] and has considerable potential for the active transport of Na^+ [109]. The physiological function of this pronounced transport of electrolytes across the esophagus is unclear and probably merely serves maintenance of cell equilibrium. However, it is tempting to speculate that these transporting properties may have facilitated the adaptation of the esophageal wall to the requirements of forming a chamber for fermentation in the evolutionary process.

Of course, dramatic differences between the two types of tissue predominate. From an electrophysiological point of view, one pronounced difference is the fact that while participation of the rumen in the total absorption of potassium is small [49, 113], the tissue is depolarized by high apical potassium [37, 38, 136]. This characteristic feature will be discussed in more detail further down.

The histology of ruminal epithelium has been studied in some detail [48] and shows a typical structure with stratum corneum, granulosum, spinosum and basale; tight junctions (claudin 1 and ZO1), gap junctions (connexin-43) and expression of increasing levels of the α subunit of the Na^+/K^+-ATPase towards the basal membrane of the multilayered epithelium. The surface area is enlarged by leaf-like papillae of 10 to 15 mm length in the cow. Conversely, the abomasum is lined with a glandular epithelium which secretes hydrochloric acid and pepsin and is comparable to the gastric mucosa of animal with simple stomachs.

Studies of organogenesis in ruminant embryos show that the forestomach system develops from an extension of the primordial esophagus to the dorsal side of the primordial stomach, and is subsequently separated from the proper esophagus by constriction [98].

Ruminal Osmoregulation

For short periods of time following the ingestion of a meal, an osmotic gradient between blood and rumen fluid may develop that can exceed 200 mosmol/kg [139], with prefeed values usually being reached within about 3 – 4 hours [129]. The survival both of the microorganisms that digest the roughage, and of the cells lining the rumen depends on a rapid restoration of ruminal osmolarity to the normal level and a number of mechanisms have been described that may facilitate this process. While saliva plays a major role in elevating ruminal osmolarity after drinking [139], hypertonicity cannot be restored by influx of saliva in a reasonable amount of time since saliva is isotonic with blood.

Hyperosmolarity after ingestion of a meal is based in part on an increase in fermentation products that can cross the membrane via lipid diffusion (Figure 1). These include short chain fatty acids (SCFA) [6, 75, 87, 108, 120, 132], ammonia, [1, 16, 17, 41, 54, 87, 93] and CO_2 [6, 87, 97]. Besides lowering ruminal osmolarity and preventing the influx of water and ruminal distention, absorption of SCFA is of essential importance for the energy metabolism of ruminants [12, 13].

Conversely, ruminal hyperosmolarity following ingestion of non-ionic, non-diffusible substances or fermentation of easily digestible carbohydrates such as glucose or starch can lead to problems such as loss of apetite or even ruminal damage in unadapted animals [22, 105]. *In vitro* and *in vivo* experiments have established that in these cases, osmolarity is restored by an increase in water influx into the rumen [31, 42, 78, 122, 129, 158, 160].

Of the electrolytes, potassium shows the biggest rise in concentration [129]. Surprisingly and in marked contrast to the problems that can occur when osmolarity rises after ingestion of easily digestible carbohydrates, the rumen is highly able to deal with the osmotic challenge of large amounts of fresh, potassium rich grass. As potassium in the rumen rises to values that can reach 100 mmol/l, sodium concentration falls so that osmolarity within the rumen remains constant (at about 130 mmol/l) (Figure 2). The inverse regulation of both ions seems to be a constant factor under many different feeding regimes [24, 50, 59, 61, 80, 96, 113, 130, 131, 136, 149, 159, 160]. However, we are only beginning to understand the mechanism by which this regulatory response occurs.

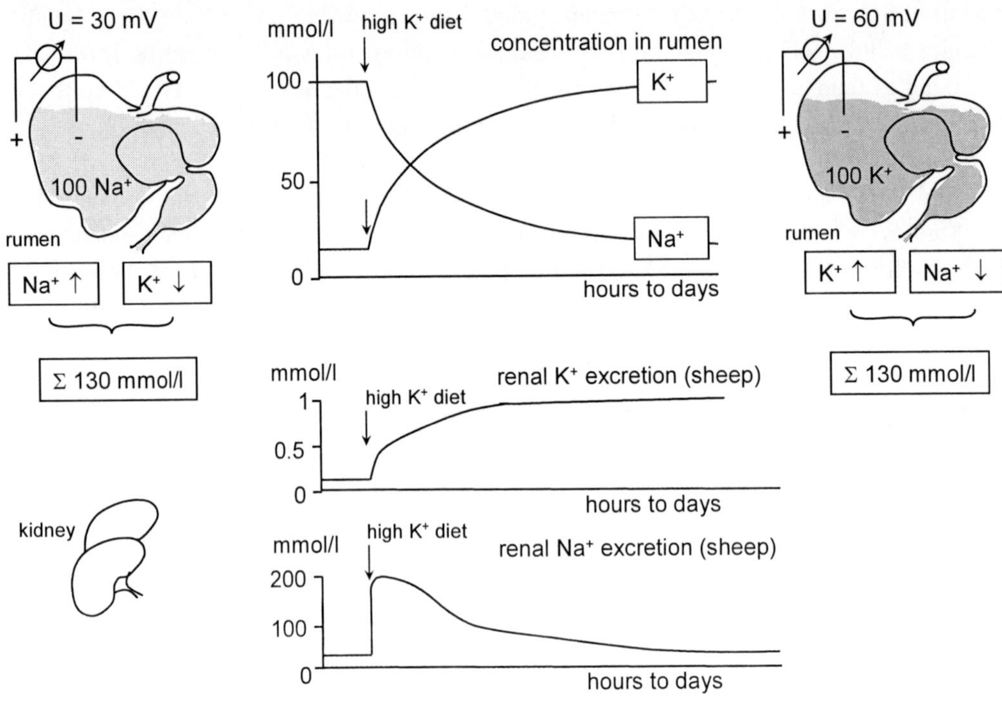

Fig 2: Ruminal osmoregulation: When sheep are transfered from a low potassium diet (i.e. hay) to a high potassium diet (i.e. grass), the concentration of potassium in the rumen continues to rise for a period of several hours to days. Concomittantly, ruminal concentration of sodium falls, so that the sum of both ions remains constant and ruminal osmolarity is restored. *In vivo* measurements show that the transepithelial potential increases with the concentration of potassium. Simultaneously, sodium excretion in urine peaks, while potassium excretion rises more slowly until maximum values are observed after about a week.

The Role of the Rumen in the Potassium Balance of Ruminants

Due to the large amounts of plant material that ruminants have to ingest to meet their energy requirements, daily intake of potassium can exceed 30 % of the total amount to be found in the body and is thus more than ten times higher than the dietary potassium intake of man (as related to body weight) [46, 69, 130]. As in man, about 90% of total potassium intake is absorbed [25, 46, 69, 112, 130, 149]. To prevent a rise to toxic concentrations in the plasma, potassium absorbed by the gut is rapidly redistributed to the cytosolic compartment of muscle, bone, liver and red blood cells, while the much slower renal corrections of disturbances in potassium balance require several hours [46, 70]. Thus, it should not come as a surprise that after a rapid transfer from a low potassium diet to one rich in potassium, the rumen is used as an additional storage space for this mineral [136] until urinary excretion of potassium has reached the level of intake. In the ruminant, this can take several hours or even days [149] (Figure 2).

Conversely, excretion of Na^+ sets in almost immediately after ingestion of a high potassium meal (1-3 hours) [25, 111, 112, 137, 149, 158, 160]. The sodium content of the diet does not appear to be related to this effect as natriuresis of sheep switched to a high potassium, low sodium diet is larger than that of sheep switched to a medium potassium, medium sodium diet [30]. The kidney of the sheep may retain sodium even when there are ample amounts in the diet, and lose sodium when intake is severely reduced [160], thus reflecting the replacement of Na^+ by K^+ due to ruminal osmoregulation.

From what is known about renal potassium excretion [46], an increase in the delivery of sodium to the distal nephron should stimulate uptake via ENaC, leading to a more lumen negative potential, and enhanced potassium excretion. Therefore, the sodium absorbed from the rumen should help to stimulate renal potassium excretion before ruminal K^+ reaches the gut and plasma potassium levels begin to rise. The ability of the rumen to absorb sodium thus appears central both for potassium balance and ruminal osmoregulation after ingestion of large amounts of potassium rich fodder.

Transport of Sodium and Chloride across the Rumen

Considering that the ability of ruminants to extract scarce sodium from grass and concentrate it in milk has been known for a long time, studies of Na^+ transport across the ruminal epithelium came relatively late. However, and perhaps for this reason, the ruminal epithelium was among the first tissues in which active transport of ions was investigated [143] following Hans Ussing's discovery of active sodium transport in frog skin [152]. The reasons for this interest are obvious: the ruminal epithelium is a moderately tight tissue [109] and thus, very suitable for determining active transport. An additional advantage of this organ is that due to its enormous size, experiments can easily be performed on animals *in vivo* by surgical fistulation of the rumen. Ruminal content can be removed by hand from such fistulas and exchanged for other solutions. It appears that animals adapt to this procedure reasonably well and will continue to ingest hay, if provided, during manipulations of the rumen. The solutions applied should not be dramatically out of the (considerable) physiological range and should contain appropriate amounts of Na^+, HCO_3^-, Ca^{2+} and Mg^{2+} if influx of saliva into the rumen is prevented in the technique of the isolated rumen.

The first study of ruminal transport was performed on goat rumen pouches in situ and left no doubt that chloride was being transported against a chemical gradient from rumen to blood [143]. In the same paper, and five years prior to the discovery of the Na^+/K^+-ATPase [142], the authors also noted absorption of Na^+ against an electrochemical gradient, and the secretion of a small amount of K^+ into the ruminal pouch. Subsequently, Dobson [27-29] published results from *in vivo* experiments in the sheep demonstrating that sodium is actively transported across the tissue. In these studies, electrodes were used to measure the potential difference, PD_t, generated across the ruminal epithelium. A mean PD_t of 30 mV with the blood side positive was observed, and many subsequent studies have confirmed the hypothesis that this potential is generated by active transport of sodium across the ruminal epithelium, with chloride following along the electrochemical gradient generated by this transport [36-39, 53, 81, 83, 85, 86, 128, 131, 136, 160]. Half of the sodium that is secreted by saliva is thus absorbed by the rumen [27], corresponding to a recirculation of total body sodium 2-3 times a day across this tissue [138]. Thus, water and electrolyte balance in the ruminant cannot be understood without taking the ruminal-portal-salivary exchanges into account (Figure 1).

It has since been demonstrated that the major part of ruminal Na^+ transport takes place by apical uptake of Na^+ via NHE3 exchange [42, 82, 83, 145], blockable by amiloride (1 mmol/l) (Figure 3). Conversely, bumetanide and furosemide have no effect on Na^+ transport across the intact ruminal epithelium, and there is no other indication of Na^+-K^+-Cl^- cotransport in the rumen [83, 87].

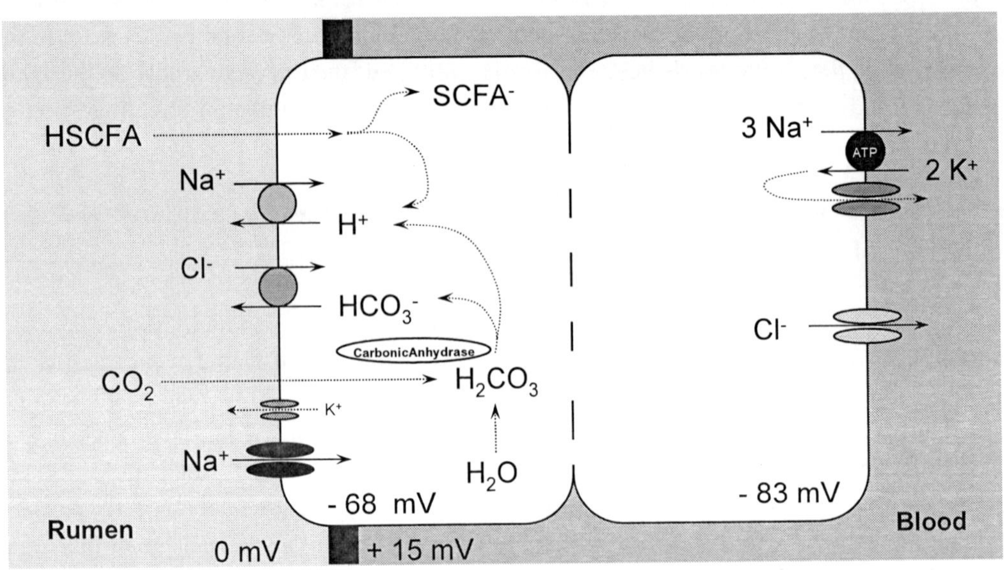

Fig 3: Current model of Na^+ transport across the ruminal epithelium: Na^+ transport from the rumen can occur both via sodium-proton exchange (NHE) coupled to chloride-bicarbonate exchange and via an electrogenic pathway. On the basolateral side, active transport of sodium occurs via the Na^+/K^+-ATPase which generates a potential (blood side positive) that drives basolateral efflux of chloride through a channel. This, in turn, stimulates apical uptake of Cl^- via Cl^-/HCO_3^- exchange and Na^+ via NHE. Carbondioxide and short chain fatty acids (HSCFA) are thought to diffuse freely through the lipid membrane and stimulate electroneutral sodium transport. (It should be noted that the ruminal epithelium consists of more than two layers. Potential levels are for orientation and can vary considerably from tissue to tissue.)

Basolateral extrusion of Na^+ takes place via the Na^+/K^+-ATPase mentioned above. Substantial evidence suggests that K^+ is mainly recycled via basolateral potassium channels, since apical potassium secretion is small [16, 39, 53, 73, 76]. The resulting negative cytosolic potential drives Cl^- out of the cell through a basolateral Cl^- channel [1, 74] and into the blood. This, in turn, may generate a chemical gradient for apical uptake of Cl^- via Cl^-/HCO_3^- exchange [27, 82], utilizing HCO_3^- that is continuously produced from CO_2 diffusing into the cell across the apical membrane. Accordingly, Cl^- transport is sensitive to acetazolamide in the manner known from many other transporting epithelia [36]. It should be noted that electroneutral coupling of chloride with bicarbonate exchange ensures that the potential gradient built up by the Na^+/K^+-ATPase does not break down. In line with this model, changes in chloride concentration do not lead to large changes of PD_t [52], although smaller effects of exchanging chloride for sulfate have been noted [37, 80]. However, any apical or paracellular conductance for chloride appears to be relatively small, or blocked by other ions under most circumstances.

Apical Na^+/H^+ exchange is stimulated both by CO_2 ($\Leftrightarrow$ H_2CO_3) and by the large amounts of short chain fatty acids (SCFA) found in the rumen. Both diffuse through the apical membrane in their lipophylic form, and donate a proton for exchange with Na^+ after dissociation [40, 43, 45, 75, 133-135].

In contrast, the response of ruminal epithelium to the third major fermentation product of the rumen, ammonia, depends on ruminal pH [1, 2]. At an (unphysiologically high) pH of 7.4, addition of ammonia to the ruminal epithelium *in vitro* inhibits the uptake of Na^+ via NHE due to the influx of NH_3 with subsequent reconstitution to NH_4^+ [1] and an increase of cellular pH [97]. At the more acidic values to be found physiologically (5.5-7.0), the amount of NH_3 is reduced greatly due to protonation, and the dominant observation is a stimulation of Na^+ uptake due to uptake of NH_4^+ with subsequent cytosolic release of protons for exchange in NHE [1]. Thus, in the healthy rumen with physiological pH values, the major products of fermentation, short chain fatty acids, bicarbonate and ammonium, all stimulate sodium reabsorption as a requirement for the postprandial stimulation of salivary flow.

Electrogenic Na^+ Conductance in the Rumen

The epithelial sodium channel (ENaC) is the channel that is responsible for the conductance of sodium across most mammalian transporting epithelia in the lung, gut and kidney [71, 115]. Characteristic features are block by low doses of amiloride in the micromolar range, stimulation by aldosterone and lack of voltage dependence (although a slightly higher open probability after *hyperpolarization* of the cell has been observed [114]).

In contrast, amiloride given in a dose as high as 1 mmol/l does not significantly affect the PD_t and the short circuit current across the ruminal epithelium, although Na^+ transport via NHE is significantly reduced. In addition and contrary to expectations, extensive *in vivo* [85] and *in vitro* experiments (unpublished results) by our laboratory failed to show any regulation of ruminal sodium transport by aldosterone. Likewise, adrenalectomy did not affect the PD_t of the ruminal epithelium *in vivo* [131]. In micropuncture experiments on the intact epithelium, it was found that *depolarization* of the apical membrane decreases the fractional apical resistance [72, 122] and increases the conductance of the ruminal epithelium for sodium. Thus, the electrogenic Na^+ conductance of ruminal epithelium has none of the properties associated with the expression of epithelial sodium channels (ENaC).

In an attempt to find further characteristics of the electrogenic sodium conductance of forestomach epithelia, it was observed in Ussing chamber experiments that removal of mucosal Ca^{2+}, Mg^{2+} or both increased the PD_t and the short circuit current across the omasal

[121] and ruminal epithelium [73]. At physiological concentrations of both divalent cations, the conductance saturates at a Na^+ concentration of about 30 mmo/l [116]. In light of the great physiological variability of ruminal Na^+ content (which varies from 25 mmol/l to above 100 mmol/l), this property is essential for maintaining sodium conductance at low levels of Na^+, while preventing a massive Na^+ influx at higher concentrations which might damage cell homeostasis.

It should be noted that these experiments were performed in absence of an electrochemical gradient for sodium and can thus not be explained by opening of a paracellular shunt pathway due to removal of divalent cations. Since both short circuit current and potential difference rose almost immediately after removal of divalent cations, it can also be concluded that the Na^+/K^+-ATPase is not the rate limiting step in sodium transport across the ruminal epithelium.

In microelectrode experiments on intact epithelia, removal of mucosal divalent cations led to a depolarization of the apical membrane [72], while paracellular conductance was not affected. Maneuvers that have been shown to reduce cytosolic Mg^{2+} concentration in isolated cells such as the elevation of cAMP [77, 126], magnesium deprivation [73, 124], or reduction of serosal Na^+ [121], can also increase Na^+ conductance through forestomach epithelia.

In patch clamp experiments on isolated cells of the ruminal epithelium, we have observed similar effects: conductance for both Na^+ and K^+ increases when external divalents cations are removed. Interestingly, a further opening could be achieved by hyperpolarization, and it was found that the voltage dependence of this conductance was altered by the cytosolic level of Mg^{2+} [77, 147]. A residual sodium conductance can also be observed in physiological solutions with normal concentrations of external divalent cations (Figure 4 A and B). However, when the Mg^{2+} concentration in the pipette is set to values at the upper end of the range reported for intact ruminal epithelial cells [123, 124, 126], no significant conductance for Na^+ can be seen (Figure 4 C). Under these high Mg^{2+} conditions, sodium conductance could be stimulated by elevation of cytosolic cAMP, either by direct application to the cytosol via the patch pipette, or via PGE2 [146]. The latter effect may rest both on a reduction of cytosolic magnesium [126], and/or upon direct effects on the channel protein. It is noteworthy that an endogenous production of prostaglandins has been observed in intact ruminal epithelium [40].

Although the precise nature of the Na^+ conducting channel in ruminal epithelium has yet to be identified, our experiments suggest that electrogenic uptake of Na^+ by the sheep rumen is regulated by voltage dependent binding of external and internal magnesium to sites in the pore of a non-selective cation channel.

Mg^{2+} Gating of Ion Channels

Regulation of channel conductance by intracellular or extracellular magnesium is known from a large number of ion channels, such as the inwardly rectifying potassium channel, the NMDA receptor, a number of non-selective cation channels from the TRP family [3, 100, 154] or the epithelial sodium channel, ENaC [26].

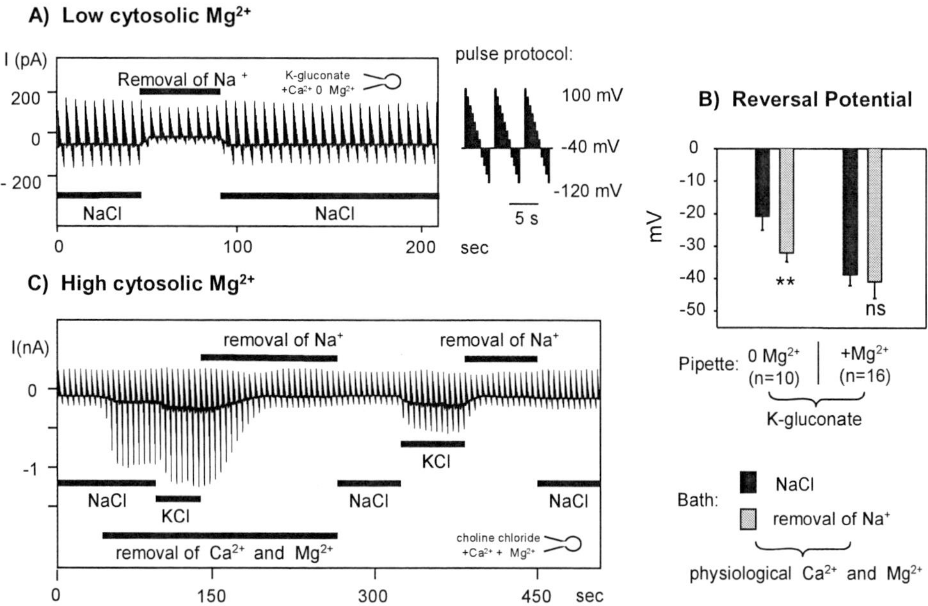

Fig 4: Sodium conductance of ruminal epithelial cells is blocked by external and internal Mg^{2+}: Original patch clamp recordings. Cells were filled with different pipette solutions, and currents in response to various voltages (pulse protocol) were measured. Removal of Na^+ from a bath solution with physiological concentrations of Ca^{2+} and Mg^{2+} resulted in a visable reduction of inward currents (A) and significant depolarization of the cells (B) when filled with a pipette solution that contained no Mg^{2+}. When Mg^{2+} was added to the cytosolic medium in a concentration of 0.9 mmol/l, effects of removing sodium from the bath solution were not significant. Removal of external Ca^{2+}, Mg^{2+}, or both increased both sodium and potassium conductance of the cells.

While voltage gated channels respond to a change in membrane voltage by changes in the conformation of the channel protein, in magnesium gated ion channels, removal of Mg^{2+} in the solution eliminates the voltage dependence. Inwardly rectifying potassium channels have been studied extensively for many decades [10, 56, 117], and it appears that voltage dependence is related to binding of Mg^{2+} to a binding site on the intracellular side (Figure 5 A). When the interior of the cell is hyperpolarized versus the outside, the resulting potential gradient will tend to push positively charged ions into the cell and away from the cell membrane. If the binding of Mg^{2+} to the internal mouth of the channel is weak, the probability that Mg^{2+} will dissociate and move into the cell lumen rises, and thus, the number of channels that are open at any given moment will increase. A characteristic and distinctive property of the inward rectifier is that the conductance change is a function not of the absolute potential E, but of the potential difference E – E(K^+) [56, 66] where E(K^+) is the reversal potential for potassium. The reason for this is that as the external potassium concentration rises, influx of potassium ions will push the blocking Mg^{2+} ion out of internal mouth of the channel pore [55] and the channel will open at voltages where it would otherwise have been closed. Thus, paradoxically, a channel that normally only opens when it is hyperpolarized to low levels will also open when the external side is exposed to a high concentration of potassium. The relatively simple mechanism of Mg^{2+} block allows depolarization of the cell when extracellular potassium concentration rises and allows influx of potassium when the membrane voltage is below the Nernst potential for this ion, but prevents efflux of potassium out of the cell at higher voltage levels.

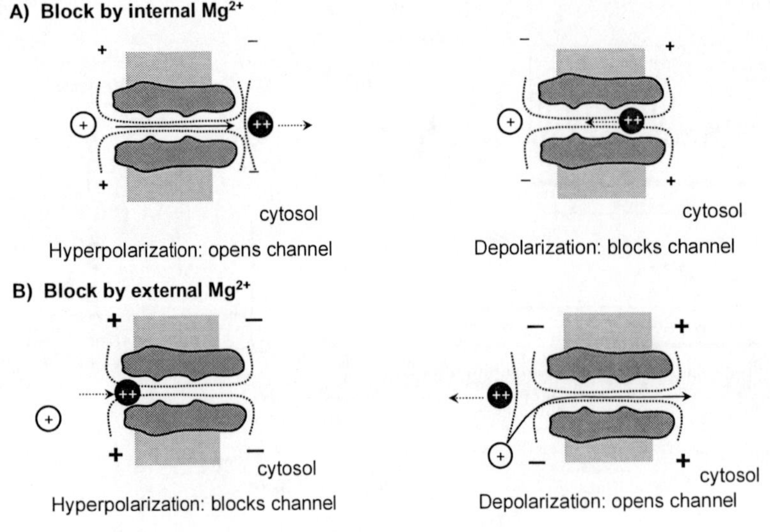

C) Hypothetical models for opening of bidirectional block

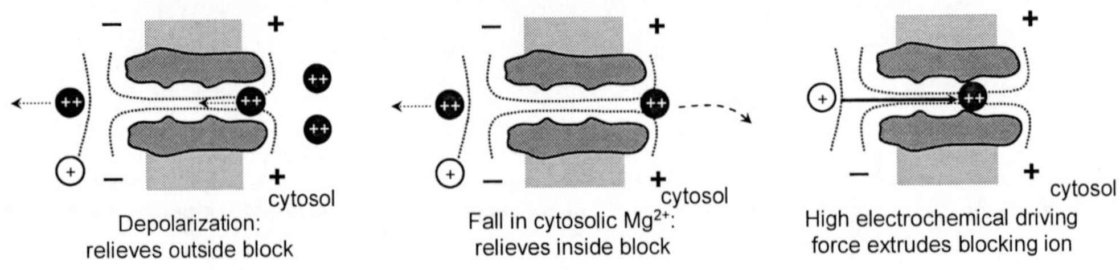

Fig 5: Voltage dependent block of ion channels by Mg^{2+}: some models (see text)

NMDA receptors of neurons are channels with a high permeability for calcium and have been studied extensively, facilitated undoubtedly in part by the low resting conductance of the neuron's cell membrane. These channels are opened by certain agonists, but conduct poorly in normal bathing medium with physiological concentrations of magnesium, even in the presence of an agonist [55]. However, when the cell is depolarized in the presence of an agonist, their conductance increases [4, 62]. In these channels, the binding sites for Mg^{2+} are thought to be inside the channel pore, within the region where transmembrane voltage drops from the external level to the level found on the internal side of the cell membrane. As above, it has been established that the affinity to Mg^{2+} changes as a function of membrane voltage (Figure 5 B). However, at depolarized membrane voltages, the probability of Mg^{2+} occupying these *external* sites is lower, the block is less pronounced, and the conductance of the NMDA receptor increases. Interestingly, this block appears to be modulated by binding of permeant monovalent cations to the external channel vestibule of NMDA receptors [110]. A further feature is an additional block with different binding affinity by *internal* Mg^{2+} [63]. It has been suggested that Mg^{2+} can permeate the channel at a low, voltage dependent rate and would thus impede the flow of other ions through the pore, with the number of channels blocked in this manner rising with the concentration of Mg^{2+}. The different blocking properties of external or internal Mg^{2+} can be explained by channel models in which several ions move in single file through a long narrow pore with asymmetrical energy barriers [63],

[56]. Note that the electrical field within the channel pore and thus, the forces that bind and repel the blocking Mg^{2+} ion, depend on the other ions within the pore. It has been proposed that the combination of block by internal and external Mg^{2+} make the NMDA-activated channel a bidirectional rectifier with an optimal voltage range for conductance [63] (Figure 5 C).

The epithelial calcium channels ECaC 1 (TRPV6) and ECaC 2 (TRPV5) are known for their extremely high Ca^{2+} selectivity (P_{Ca}/P_{Na} >100) *in vitro*, and appear to be involved in Ca^{2+} reabsorption in kidney and intestine [106, 154]. When divalent cations are removed, they become permeable to monovalent cations and open at negative potentials with strong inward rectification. As with the inward rectifier, this rectification depends at least in part on the presence of intracellular Mg^{2+}. Block by external divalent cations is decreased when intracellular Mg^{2+} levels drop. As with the NMDA receptor, interaction with permeant cations has been observed. At high potentials, Mg^{2+} block is relieved, indicating that Mg^{2+} may be able to permeate the selectivity filter of the channel if the driving force is high enough [154].

In terms of conductance for sodium and block by divalent cations, the ruminal conductance for sodium has striking similarity to channels belonging to the TRP family [106]. However, in isolated cells of the ruminal epithelium, the blocking effects of divalent cations are much larger than any currents that might be attributed to a conductance for Ca^{2+} and Mg^{2+}, even if the electrochemical driving force is set to very high levels in patch clamp experiments [148]. This is in line with the *in vitro* and *in vivo* observation that influx of Mg^{2+} into the cells and across the rumen saturates [85, 86, 123], although initial uptake rates are high and fast. Thus, while it cannot and should not be excluded that Mg^{2+} uptake by the rumen may involve channels from this group, these channels do not display the high rates of Mg^{2+} conductance reported for channels such as TRPM7 [95, 99].

Interestingly, low levels of messenger RNA of both TRPV5 and TRPV6 have been found in the rumen of sheep [162] where functionally, they may be involved in the transport of Ca^{2+} [120]. In the same study, a higher expression of both channels not just on the mRNA but also on the protein level was found in other parts of the gut of the sheep where absorption of Ca^{2+} is thought to play a minor role, and thus, the physiological role of these channels in the gastrointestinal tract needs to be clarified.

In the case of TRPV5, both high Ca^{2+} selectivity and sensitivity to extracellular divalent cations appear to depend on a single aspartate residue in the pore region between transmembrane domains 5 and 6 [101]. Point mutations can be expected to dramatically alter the conductance of ion channels, and the TRP family is no exception. Associated proteins may lead to further differences [153]. It should be noted that buffering of Ca^{2+} and Mg^{2+} in physiological solutions is by no means trivial [51, 79]. Since the cytosolic concentration of these ions has impacts on the selectivity of these channels, a prediction of their conductance *in vivo* from *in vitro* experiments has to be done with care. In most patch clamp studies [101] including our initial experiments with ruminal epithelial cells, [1, 101], the concentration of Mg^{2+} in the pipette solution is higher than the free concentration of the ion that is found in resting intact cells [123, 127], and the situation in the intact epithelium *in vivo* may be even more complex.

A recent study has shown that the esophageal epithelium of the rabbit possesses a sodium conductance with similar properties, and it has been suggested that in this tissue, ENaC subunits assemble to form a non-selective cation channel that is not blockable by amiloride [7]. Data from RT-PCR experiments in our laboratory suggest that alpha subunits of ENaC are expressed in ruminal epithelium (personal communication, Jatti Priesnitz). As mentioned, regulation of ENaC by intracellular Mg^{2+} has been demonstrated [26]. However, attempts to demonstrate other subunits have not been convincing so far, and while this is certainly an intriguing possibility, we do not feel that at this point that the involvement of other cation channels (i.e. TRP channels [100]) in ruminal sodium transport should be ruled out in light of the failure of aldosterone or amiloride to show any effects on electrogenic sodium conductance in the forestomach.

It may be argued that since the greater amount of sodium absorbed by the rumen is transported by the NHE as outlined above, any interest in a further mechanism is purely academic. However, the apical electrogenic entry of sodium determines the magnitude of the transepithelial potential (blood side positive), [27, 37-39, 82], and is thus an essential contributor to the total driving force for the basolateral efflux of choride and other anions such as bicarbonate [27]. Basolateral efflux of chloride drives apical uptake of chloride, which, in turn, should stimulate Na^+ uptake via coupling of NHE with Cl^-/HCO_3^- exchange. More importantly, perhaps, stimulation of electrogenic sodium transport should have a negative impact on the electrochemical driving force for potassium efflux from the rumen. The central importance of electrogenic sodium transport for transruminal potential thus makes it a gate-keeper for the transport of ions across the rumen, and since the electrogenic Na^+ conductance of ruminal epithelium is regulated by changes in cytosolic magnesium, the uptake of this ion by the ruminal epithelium should be of some interest.

Absorption of Magnesium

Interest in the uptake of magnesium by the ruminant is old and related to a surge of cases of an affliction known as "grass tetany" that led to widespread loss of cattle in the last century [90, 125]. After sudden transfer from normal winter rations to young spring grass, animals became afflicted with excitability, salivation, ataxia, recumbency, and tetanic muscle spasms [140, 141]. Despite normal magnesium content of the fodder, the animals were apparently unable to absorb this mineral and thus suffered from hypomagnesaemia. Sjollema's hypothesis that the surge in frequency was related to the introduction of fertilizers containing potash has since been confirmed by a solid body of evidence which has been reviewed elsewhere [34, 90]. It should be noted that a number of other factors are known to contribute to malabsorption of magnesium that include sodium deficiency [118] and high protein content of the diet with subsequent high levels of ruminal ammonia [41].

Absorption of magnesium from the rumen has been studied extensively at the level of the animal, the tissue, and the cell. It has been established that the main site for absorption of magnesium in the ruminant is the forestomach [107]. When the rumen is bypassed, decreased plasma Mg^{2+} concentrations, decreased urinary Mg^{2+} excretion and increased fecal Mg^{2+} excretion is observed. This negative magnesium balance cannot be compensated for by post-ruminal infusion of Mg^{2+} [150].

Given that the serosal side of the rumen is positive versus the mucosal side (30 mV), any paracellular transport will move Mg^{2+} from blood into the rumen [20]. Transport must thus be transcellular and active and was first demonstrated by Martens and Harmeyer in 1978 [86]. In the same study, it was shown that the transport is ouabain sensitive and saturable. The presence of basolateral Na^+/ Mg^{2+} exchange coupled to Na^+/K^+-ATPase has since been established [77, 126] as the mechanism underlying the active step of absorption (Figure 6 A).

A) Low ruminal potassium

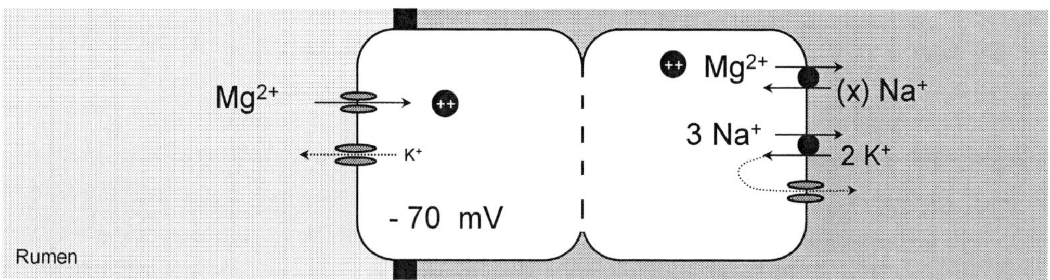

B) High ruminal potassium

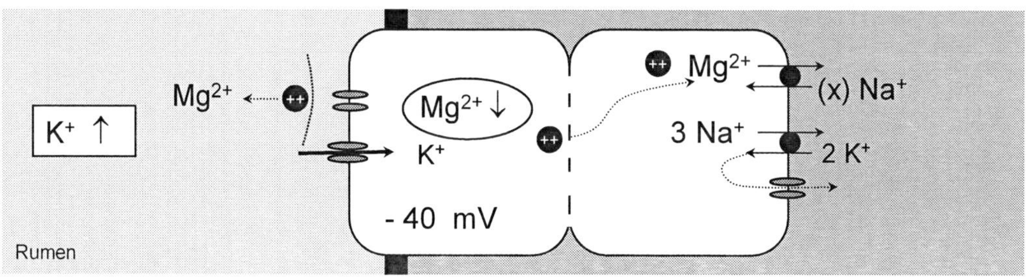

Fig 6: Reduction of Mg^{2+} uptake by elevation of ruminal potassium: Apical Mg^{2+} influx occurs down the electrochemical gradient, driven by the negative potential across the apical membrane (A). Basolateral efflux occurs in exchange for sodium. The stochiometry has not been identified.

After elevation of ruminal potassium (B), the apical membrane is depolarized and the gradient for uptake of Mg^{2+} decreases. Cytosolic Mg^{2+} concentration drops, and thus, also basolateral extrusion. Note that the relative contribution of the potassium conductance to total membrane permeability may rise as ruminal potassium levels increase.

In contrast, it has been shown that apical uptake depends on the electrochemical driving force for Mg^{2+} across the apical membrane (Figure 6 B). Depolarization of this membrane by potassium was found to reduce transport of Mg^{2+} across the rumen *in vivo* using various approaches that include the temporary isolation of the rumen from influx of saliva [19, 50, 80, 85, 87, 89, 94, 164]. Experiments across isolated ruminal epithelium in the Ussing chamber established that the potential difference, and not potassium concentration, were central to the reduction in the uptake of Mg^{2+} [76, 84]. Likewise, exposure of isolated cells of the ruminal epithelium in culture to high potassium solution resulted in a reduced uptake of Mg^{2+}[123, 124]. It has been shown that this maneuver depolarizes isolated cells of the ruminal epithelium via potassium channels [1]. In contrast, plasma magnesium concentration had no influence on the rate of Mg^{2+} absorption [91], and the effects of K^+ on Mg^{2+} absorption are not attributable to high levels of absorbed K^+, but rather to the concentration of K^+ present in the rumen [113]. From these experiments, a model has emerged that resembles that developed for the distal convoluted tubule, where absorption occurs via an apical Mg^{2+} channel in conjunction with a basolateral Na^+/ Mg^{2+} exchanger [65, 161]. In the context of this review, it is tempting to point out that in humans, a fall in plasma magnesium is known to lead to kaliuresis [161] [64] [105], and that reduction in plasma Mg^{2+} levels should thus help with excretion of potassium.

It should be noted that there is evidence for a second transporting process that is not potential dependent and which facilitates uptake of magnesium into depolarized cells at higher ruminal potassium concentrations of this mineral [61, 76, 124]. In addition, a number of factors are known to stimulate absorption of magnesium from the rumen, including a rise in bicarbonate, short chain fatty acids, and a low but physiological pH of around 6.4 [90].

Interestingly, reductions in the absorption of Mg^{2+} were also observed after acute exposure to ammonia [18, 41, 54, 87, 89]. For reasons that are not clear at present, compensatory mechanisms set in after a few days [41] in this case, so that hypomagnesaemia is transient. It is possible to speculate about the role that the electrogenic vacuolar H-ATPase might play in this regulatory response [124] or about up-regulation of enzymes which are involved in ammonia metabolism in the rumen epithelium [102, 103].

The practical implications of these physiological background facts are clear and have led to a reduction in the frequency of the affliction. Adjusting cattle to a high potassium and high protein diet with production of ammonia must be done slowly. Mg^{2+} concentration in the rumen must be elevated by feeding Mg^{2+} salts to activate the non-potential dependent magnesium uptake mechanism. Fertilization techniques which greatly raise potassium intake should be avoided. In addition, care has to be taken that animals are not sodium depleted, since this increases aldosterone levels, salivary excretion of potassium and thus, elevates ruminal levels of potassium [90] [118] with the detrimental effect on Mg^{2+} absorption from the forestomachs described above [88].

Ruminal transport of potassium

Given the high concentration of potassium in the ruminant diet and that the volume of the rumen can exceed that of the plasma, it is clear that any absorption of potassium from this organ has to be slow. When total potassium absorption is related to feed intake and recirculation of saliva is not considered, the contribution of the rumen to total potassium absorption is marginal, and most studies regard the small intestine as the major site for the absorption of dietary potassium [69, 164].

However, when the rate of absorption is related to the concentration found in the rumen, a certain permeability of the ruminal wall for potassium becomes apparent. Secretion of potassium under experimental conditions with very low ruminal potassium concentration was first noted by Sperber and Hyden [143], and this finding has been confirmed many times [35, 59, 80, 130, 160]. The simplest explanation for this observation is to assume a leak of potassium into the rumen paracellularly from the blood side (4-5 mmol/l K^+), driven by the positive PD_t of about 30 mV (blood side positive). In this case, an increase in ruminal potassium should lead to an increase in the potential across the ruminal wall, and such a potential was, indeed, measured in feeding experiments [136]. Subsequent parallel *in vivo* and *in vitro* investigations [37, 38] confirmed that the potential rose strongly with the luminal concentration of potassium both in the completely isolated rumen in anaesthetized sheep, and in isolated ruminal epithelium in the Ussing chamber. Conversely, raising Na^+ from a basal level of 20 mmol/l had little (*in vivo*) or no (*in vitro*) effect [37, 38]. Later *in vivo* studies (under more physiological conditions with HCO_3^- and acetate instead of Cl^- as the major anions [18, 80]) confirmed the finding that K^+ concentration contributes more to overall transepithelial potential than concentrations of Na^+ exceeding 20 mmol/l. However, it should be noted that the increasing transepithelial potential with falling ruminal sodium concentration in these experiments suggests that any paracellular leak of sodium into the rumen has to be small. Thus, the simple model of a hypothetic "leak" pathway postulated above cannot be quite so simple after all and must, at the very least, be highly selective for potassium over sodium.

At first glance, these results seem to suggest that the efflux of potassium has to be considerable since the transruminal potential has to be continuously maintained by a corresponding flux of ions under *in vivo* non-equilibrium conditions. This is very clearly not the case. The ability of the rumen to concentrate potassium has already been outlined above (Figure 2). When sheep are transferred from a low potassium diet of hay and meals to a diet of high potassium grass from a heavily fertilized meadow, ruminal potassium concentrations can rise from levels of about 30 mmol/l to peaks of 100 mmol/l [136]. Concomitantly, the concentration of sodium falls from levels as high as 100 mmol/l to values of 25 mmol/l. Thus, while there can be no doubt about the coupling of potassium and transruminal potential [37, 38, 61, 76, 80, 84, 131, 155], and while a small passive flux of potassium down its electrochemical gradient has been demonstrated [59,160], the major ion being absorped under these conditions is sodium [59, 130, 144, 158, 160]. In line with this, a complete removal of sodium (or application of ouabain) abolished the potential and the short circuit current across the ruminal epithelium [53], establishing Na^+ as the major ion responsible for the potential across the ruminal wall. An explanation for the failure to observe changes in transepithelial potential in response to the elevation of ruminal sodium above 20 mmol/l [37, 38] has since emerged: *in vitro*, electrogenic sodium conductance saturates at 30 mmol/l of Na^+ [116]. Thus, raising Na^+ concentration from 20 mmol/l to higher values should only have marginal effects.

These data do not support the originally proposed model of a major paracellular leak pathway for potassium and suggest a transcellular electrogenic uptake pathway highly selective for potassium over sodium, with potassium channels being ideal candidates. In line with this, a high concentration of potassium was found to depolarize the apical membrane of ruminal epithelium and decrease the fractional apical resistance [76]. *In vitro* studies showing that active, ouabain sensitive potassium secretion can take place under equilibrium conditions [39, 53, 76, 163], with evidence for the existence of additional basolateral potassium channels [76], support the model of channel mediated transcellular uptake.

A similar notion of apical potassium channels evolved independently from *in vivo* experiments on sheep, demonstrating that ruminal uptake of ammonia cannot be explained exclusively by assumption of lipophillic diffusion of NH_3 [17]. *In vitro* experiments in the Ussing chamber followed, that postulated electrogenic uptake of NH_4^+ via a quinidine sensitive potassium channel [16]. This suggestion is supported by a recent study demonstrating stimulating effects of NH_4^+ on sodium transport, thus establishing that transport of NH_4^+ has to be transcellular [1]. Using the patch clamp technique, it was possible to directly demonstrate corresponding quinidine sensitive potassium channels with a conductance for both potassium and NH_4^+ in isolated ruminal epithelial cells [1]. Interestingly and typically [5, 33, 55, 56, 165], the open probability of these channels [1] rose with the concentration of the permeant ion. This property of potassium channels may help to explain why the cell is depolarized with increasing levels of potassium and falling levels of sodium [39, 53, 76] despite the fact that in low potassium ringer, the conductance for sodium exceeds that for potassium.

The assumption of transcellular flux via potassium channels integrates certain observations in a satisfactory way, since uptake of NH_4^+ is favored by the electrochemical gradient across the apical membrane of the rumen, whereas passive influx of K^+ into the cytosol is not possible except at high ruminal potassium concentrations due to the high cytosolic concentration of potassium. This is very much in line with the *in vivo* observations of ammonia transport at low pH and low concentrations of ammonia [17], while very high concentrations of potassium are necessary in order to observe sizable transport rates for potassium [160]. However, the failure to observe a clear effect of quinidine on potassium transport across the rumen *in vivo* does leave some room for a debate that should include the very wide range of quinidine effects on cellular metabolism [35]. Despite this caveat, the *in vivo* and *in vitro* evidence for the existence of potassium channels with a substantial contribution to total conductance of the apical and basolateral membrane of the ruminal epithelium is solid, and a viable model is needed to explain why nevertheless, potassium movements across the ruminal wall remain small [69, 136, 160].

An attempt to integrate the various observations can be made by considering the interaction of the electrogenic sodium conductance with potassium transport (Figure 7). As stated before, this pathway is stimulated by the depolarization of the apical membrane [72] and part of the potential generated by an increase of potassium in the rumen should be due to stimulation of this sodium conductance. Now, the paradoxical observations fall into place: potassium depolarizes the apical membrane, opens the sodium conductance [72, 77], the transepithelial potential increases, the electrochemical driving force for the efflux of potassium from the rumen falls. Therefore, we see an increase in sodium transport, a rise in transepithelial potential, but potassium efflux from the rumen remains limited.

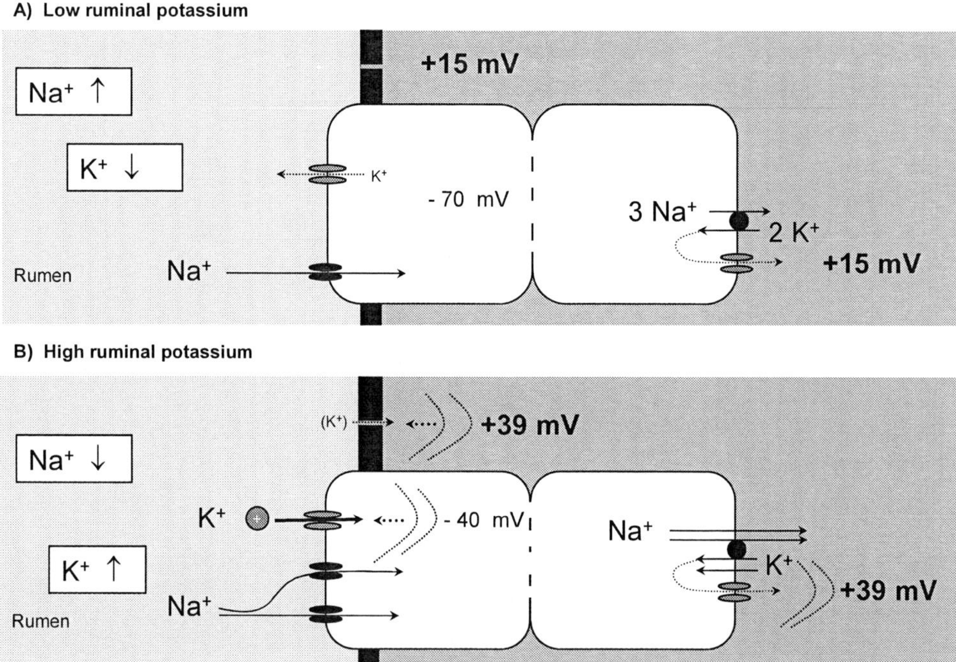

Fig 7: Uptake of K^+ by the ruminal epithelium: Flux of K^+ across the ruminal epithelium is passive and proportional to the transepithelial electrochemical driving force. With increasing concentration of ruminal K^+, the efflux of K^+ from the rumen into the plasma increases. However, stimulation of electrogenic Na^+ transport with depolarization of the apical membrane and generation of a strong, lumen positive transepithelial potential limits the amount of K^+ that leaks out of the rumen. In vivo, transepithelial potential can reach values of 60 – 70 mV.

A Role for Magnesium in Ruminal Osmoregulation

Numerous studies demonstrate that rising levels of potassium stimulate the absorption of sodium across the rumen *in vivo* [59, 130, 144, 158, 160]. Harrison notes that *in vitro* stimulation of Na^+ transport by elevation of K^+ only succeeded under open circuit conditions [52], and thus, a potential dependent mechanism appears to be involved. This effect cannot be attributed to a rise in osmotic pressure, since the effects of urea or mannitol on sodium absorption were discrete [160]. As has been outlined above, a high increase in osmotic pressure due to administration of non-ionic osmotic agents can even reduce Na^+ absorption, and induce water influx into the rumen [44, 78, 122]. Conversely, potassium stimulates absorption of sodium even in the absence of an osmotic gradient [85].

In light of the information we have at this point, it is possible to develop a fairly consistent model that may describe the events that occur when sheep or cows are transferred from a low potassium diet of hay to a diet higher in potassium, such as fresh spring grass (Figure 8). As the concentration of potassium in the rumen increases, the conductance of the apical membrane for potassium rises [1, 55] and the apical membrane is depolarized [76], the binding affinity of divalent cations at the external mouth of the non-selective cation channel is loosened, and simultaneously, uptake of magnesium decreases. Now, the non-selective cation channel begins to open [77, 147].

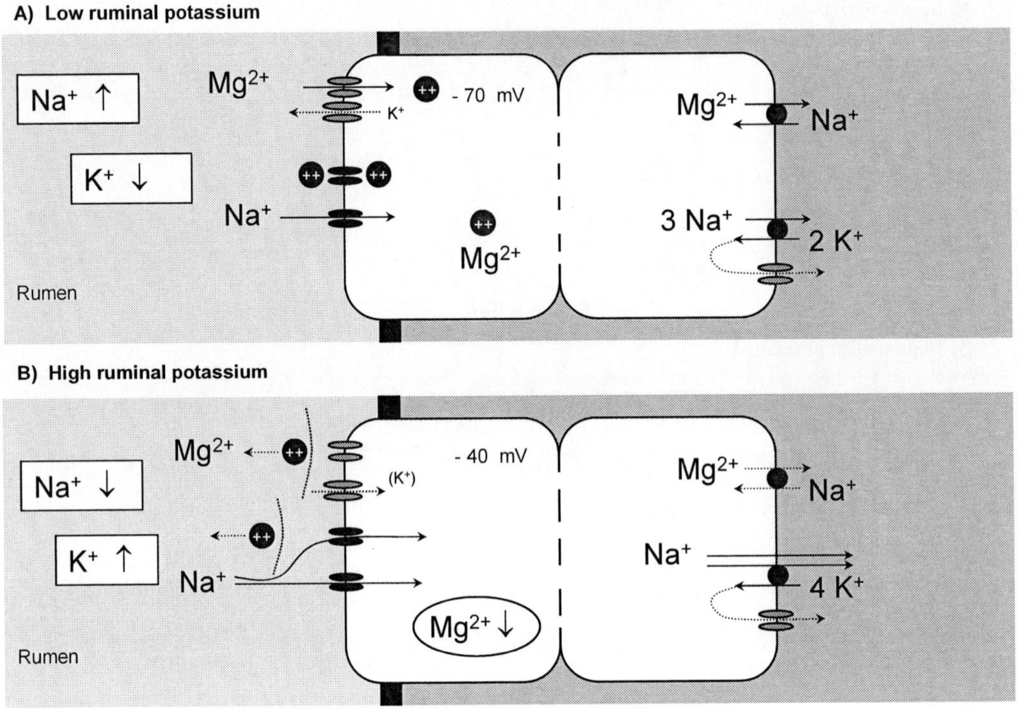

Fig 8: Stimulation of ruminal sodium transport by elevation of ruminal potassium: A) Divalent cations block many of the non-selective cation channels in the apical membrane, limiting electrogenic sodium influx. Despite a large concentration of apical Na^+, total sodium flux is low. After elevation of the ruminal K^+ concentration (B), the apical membrane is depolarized, uptake of Mg^{2+} decreases and cytosolic Mg^{2+} concentration drops. In addition, depolarization relieves the block of the non-selective cation from the external side. Electrogenic Na^+ transport rises creating an additional depolarizing stimulus and reducing the electrochemical gradient for the uptake of K^+.

As Na^+ rushes in, the apical membrane is depolarized even further and a catastrophic cascade of events would unfold but for the fact that at a certain potential level, residual internal Mg^{2+} begins to block the pore from the inside, thus limiting a further depolarization. It appears conceivable that at elevated cytosolic concentrations of sodium, basolateral Na^+/ Mg^{2+} exchange slows down so that internal Mg^{2+} levels begin to rise again despite reduced uptake. And thus, this model can predict that at medium levels of potassium, sodium transport is stimulated, while at very high levels of potassium, sodium transport is depressed [160].

An intriguing feature of this model is that as the transepithelial potential depolarizes due to the electrogenic efflux of sodium, the driving force for the flux of potassium through leaks from the rumen such as the paracellular pathway is decreased. Again, we can predict what happens when potassium levels rise: as sodium transport is depressed, potassium conductance begins to rise and this is, indeed, what is observed [160]. Thus, the introduction of potassium channels in the apical membrane of the rumen does make "sense" from an evolutionary point of view – or did, until potash fertilizers came up [140].

Conclusion

Ruminants can deal with abrupt and extremely large rises in potassium intake due to their ability to utilize the rumen as an additional reservoir for buffering K^+ until renal excretion of K^+ has set in. Ruminal concentrations of potassium can rise to values of 100 mmol/l in these situations, with sodium content decreasing in proportion so that osmolarity remains constant throughout. This is essential since rising osmolarity would interfere with ruminal fermentation processes and food uptake by the animal.

In contrast to the pronounced ability to maintain physiological ruminal osmolarity and plasma potassium levels, hypomagnesemia is a known complication with economic significance after transfer of ruminants to a high potassium diet. The pathogenesis of this condition has been shown to involve a decrease in Mg^{2+} absorption by the rumen after exposure to high ruminal potassium.

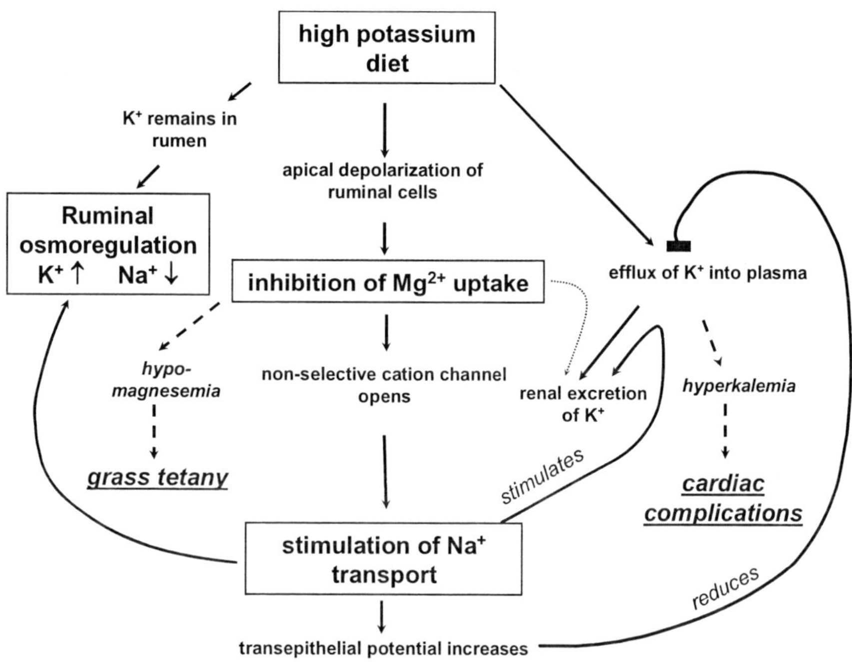

Fig 9: A role for magnesium in ruminal osmoregulation: The adverse effects of an inhibition of transcellular ruminal Mg^{2+} transport are balanced by the positive effects of a stimulation of Na^+ efflux from the rumen, namely, inhibition of K^+ efflux into the plasma, stimulation of renal K^+ excretion, and regulation of ruminal osmolarity.

We feel that the two phenomena may be causally linked via a signaling cascade that involves depolarization of the apical membrane by high potassium, reduced uptake of magnesium, and opening of a sodium conductance with subsequent rise in sodium transport out of the ruminal pouch (Figure 9). In evolutionary terms, the potassium-induced reduction in digestibility of Mg^{2+} may be balanced by the increased ability to quickly ingest very large amounts of fresh grass after a longer period of famine.

References

[1] Abdoun K, Stumpff F, Wolf K, and Martens H. Modulation of electroneutral Na transport in sheep rumen epithelium by luminal ammonia. *Am J Physiol Gastrointest Liver Physiol* 289: G508-520, 2005.

[2] Abdoun K, Wolf K, Arndt G, and Martens H. Effect of ammonia on Na^+ transport across isolated rumen epithelium of sheep is diet dependent. *Br J Nutr* 90: 751-758, 2003.

[3] Albitz R, Magyar J, and Nilius B. Block of single cardiac sodium channels by intracellular magnesium. *Eur Biophys J* 19: 19-23, 1990.

[4] Antonov SM and Johnson JW. Permeant ion regulation of N-methyl-D-aspartate receptor channel block by Mg(2+). *Proc Natl Acad Sci U S A* 96: 14571-14576, 1999.

[5] Aqvist J and Luzhkov V. Ion permeation mechanism of the potassium channel. *Nature* 404: 881-884, 2000.

[6] Ash RW and Dobson A. The Effect of Absorption on the Acidity of Rumen Contents. *J Physiol* 169: 39-61, 1963.

[7] Awayda MS, Bengrine A, Tobey NA, Stockand JD, and Orlando RC. Nonselective cation transport in native esophageal epithelia. *Am J Physiol Cell Physiol* 287: C395-402, 2004.

[8] Bach A, Calsamiglia S, and Stern MD. Nitrogen metabolism in the rumen. *J Dairy Sci* 88 Suppl 1: E9-21, 2005.

[9] Bailey CB. Saliva secretion and its relation to feeding in cattle. 4. The relationship between the concentrations of sodium, potassium, chloride and inorganic phosphate in mixed saliva and rumen fluid. *Br J Nutr* 15: 489-498, 1961.

[10] Balser JR, Roden DM, and Bennett PB. Single inward rectifier potassium channels in guinea pig ventricular myocytes. Effects of quinidine. *Biophys J* 59: 150-161, 1991.

[11] Beja-Pereira A, Luikart G, England PR, Bradley DG, Jann OC, Bertorelle G, Chamberlain AT, Nunes TP, Metodiev S, Ferrand N, and Erhardt G. Gene-culture coevolution between cattle milk protein genes and human lactase genes. *Nat Genet* 35: 311-313, 2003.

[12] Bergman EN. Energy contributions of volatile fatty acids from the gastrointestinal tract in various species. *Physiol Rev* 70: 567-590, 1990.

[13] Bergman EN, Reid RS, Murray MG, Brockway JM, and Whitelaw FG. Interconversions and production of volatile fatty acids in the sheep rumen. *Biochem J* 97: 53-58, 1965.

[14] Blair-West JR, Coghlan JP, Denton DA, Goding JR, and Wright RD. The effect of aldosterone, cortisol, and corticosterone upon the sodium and potassium content of sheep's parotid saliva. *J Clin Invest* 42: 484-496, 1963.

[15] Boda JM, McDonald PG, and Walker JJ. Effects of the Addition of Fluids to the Empty Rumen on the Flow Rate and Chemical Composition of Bovine Mixed Saliva. *J Physiol* 177: 323-336, 1965.

[16] Bödeker D and Kemkowski J. Participation of NH_4^+ in total ammonia absorption across the rumen epithelium of sheep (Ovis aries). *Comp Biochem Physiol A Physiol* 114: 305-310, 1996.

[17] Bödeker D, Winkler A, and Holler H. Ammonia absorption from the isolated reticulo-rumen of sheep. *Exp Physiol* 75: 587-595, 1990.

[18] Care AD, Brown RC, Farrar AR, and Pickard DW. Magnesium absorption from the digestive tract of sheep. *Q J Exp Physiol* 69: 577-587, 1984.

[19] Care AD, Farrar AR, and Pickard DW. Factors affecting the absorption of magnesium from the rumen in sheep. *Journal of Physiology* 325, 1982.

[20] Care AD and van't Klooster AT. In Vivo Transport of Magnesium and Other Cations across the Wall of the Gastro-Intestinal Tract of Sheep. *J Physiol* 177: 174-191, 1965.

[21] Carr DH and Titchen DA. Post prandial changes in parotid salivary secretion and plasma osmolality and the effects of intravenous of saline solutions. *Q J Exp Physiol Cogn Med Sci* 63: 1-21, 1978.

[22] Carter RR, Allen OB, and Grovum WL. The effect of feeding frequency and meal size on amounts of total and parotid saliva secreted by sheep. *Br J Nutr* 63: 305-318, 1990.

[23] Cassida KA and Stokes MR. Eating and resting salivation in early lactation dairy cows. *J Dairy Sci* 69: 1282-1292, 1986.

[24] Denton DA. The effect of variation in the concentration of individual extracellular electrolytes on the response of the sheep's parotid gland to Na^+ depletion. *J Physiol* 140: 129-147, 1958.

[25] Dewhurst JK, Harrison FA, and Keynes RD. Renal excretion of potassium in the sheep. *J Physiol* 195: 609-621, 1968.

[26] Diakov A and Korbmacher C. A novel pathway of epithelial sodium channel activation involves a serum- and glucocorticoid-inducible kinase consensus motif in the C terminus of the channel's alpha-subunit. *J Biol Chem* 279: 38134-38142, 2004.

[27] Dobson A. Active transport through the epithelium of the reticulo-rumen sac. *J Physiol* 146: 235-251, 1959.

[28] Dobson A. The forces moving sodium ions through rumen epithelium. *J Physiol* 128: 39-40P, 1955.

[29] Dobson A and Phillipson AT. The forces moving chloride ions through rumen epithelium. *J Physiol* 125: 26-27P, 1954.

[30] Dobson A, Scott D, and Bruce JB. Changes in sodium requirement of the sheep associated with changes of diet. *Q J Exp Physiol Cogn Med Sci* 51: 311-323, 1966.

[31] Dobson A, Sellers AF, and Gatewood VH. Dependence of Cr-EDTA absorption from the rumen on luminal osmotic pressure. *Am J Physiol* 231: 1595-1600, 1976.

[32] Donovan GA, Steenholdt C, McGehee K, and Lundquist R. Hypomagnesemia among cows in a confinement-housed dairy herd. *J Am Vet Med Assoc* 224: 96-99, 54, 2004.

[33] Doyle DA. Structural themes in ion channels. *Eur Biophys J* 33: 175-179, 2004.

[34] Dua K and Care AD. Impaired absorption of magnesium in the aetiology of grass tetany. *Br Vet J* 151: 413-426, 1995.

[35] Dua K and Care AD. Lack of effect of quinidine on divalent mineral absorption from the reticulorumen of sheep. *Res Vet Sci* 56: 114-115, 1994.

[36] Emanovic D, Harrison FA, Keynes RD, and Rankin JC. The effect of acetazolamide on ion transport across isolated sheep rumen epithelium. *Journal of Physiology* 254: 803-812, 1976.

[37] Ferreira HG, Harrison FA, and Keynes RD. The potential and short-circuit current across isolated rumen epithelium of the sheep. *J Physiol* 187: 631-644, 1966.

[38] Ferreira HG, Harrison FA, Keynes RD, and Nauss AH. Observations on the potential across the rumen of sheep. *J Physiol* 187: 615-630, 1966.

[39] Ferreira HG, Harrison FA, Keynes RD, and Zurich L. Ion transport across an isolated preparation of sheep rumen epithelium. *J Physiol* 222: 77-93, 1972.

[40] Gäbel G, Butter H, and Martens H. Regulatory role of cAMP in transport of Na^+, Cl^- and short-chain fatty acids across sheep ruminal epithelium. *Exp Physiol* 84: 333-345, 1999.

[41] Gäbel G and Martens H. The effect of ammonia on magnesium metabolism in sheep. *J Anim Physiol Anim Nutr* 55: 278-287, 1986.

[42] Gäbel G, Martens H, Suendermann M, and Galfi P. The effect of diet, intraruminal pH and osmolarity on sodium, chloride and magnesium absorption from the temporarily isolated and washed reticulo-rumen of sheep. *Q J Exp Physiol* 72: 501-511, 1987.

[43] Gäbel G and Sehested J. SCFA transport in the forestomach of ruminants. *Comp Biochem Physiol A Physiol* 118: 367-374, 1997.

[44] Gäbel G, Suendermann M, and Martens H. The influence of osmotic pressure, lactic acid and pH on ion and fluid absorption from the washed and temporarily isolated reticulo-rumen of sheep. *J Vet Med A* 34: 220-226, 1987.

[45] Gäbel G, Vogler S, and Martens H. Short-chain fatty acids and CO_2 as regulators of Na^+ and Cl^- absorption in isolated sheep rumen mucosa. *J Comp Physiol [B]* 161: 419-426, 1991.

[46] Giebisch G. Renal potassium transport: mechanisms and regulation. *Am J Physiol* 274: F817-833, 1998.

[47] Goff JP. Macromineral disorders of the transition cow. *Vet Clin North Am Food Anim Pract* 20: 471-494, v, 2004.

[48] Graham C and Simmons NL. Functional organization of the bovine rumen epithelium. *Am J Physiol Regul Integr Comp Physiol* 288: R173-181, 2005.

[49] Greene LW, Webb KE, Jr., and Fontenot JP. Effect of potassium level on site of absorption of magnesium and other macroelements in sheep. *J Anim Sci* 56: 1214-1221, 1983.

[50] Grings EE and Males JR. Effects of potassium on macromineral absorption in sheep fed wheat straw-based diets. *J Anim Sci* 64: 872-879, 1987.

[51] Günzel D, McGuigan JA, and Schlue WR. Use of Mg^{2+} and Ca^{2+} macroelectrodes to measure binding in extracellular-like physiological solutions. *Front Biosci* 10: 905-918, 2005.

[52] Harrison FA. Ion transport across rumen and omasum epithelium. *Philos Trans Royal Soc Lond B Biol Sci* 262: 301-305, 1971.

[53] Harrison FA, Keynes RD, Rankin JC, and Zurich L. The effect of ouabain on ion transport across isolated sheep rumen epithelium. *J Physiol* 249: 669-677, 1975.

[54] Head MJ and Rook JA. Hypomagnesaemia in dairy cattle and its possible relationship to ruminal ammonia production. *Nature* 176: 262-263, 1955.

[55] Hille B. Ion Channels of Excitable Membranes. *Sinauer Associates, Inc*: Chapter 15, pg. 482, 2001.

[56] Hille B and Schwarz W. Potassium channels as multi-ion single-file pores. *J Gen Physiol* 72: 409-442, 1978.

[57] Hoover WH and Miller TK. Rumen digestive physiology and microbial ecology. *Vet Clin North Am Food Anim Pract* 7: 311-325, 1991.

[58] Hungate RE, Bryant MP, and Mah RA. The rumen bacteria and protozoa. *Annu Rev Microbiol* 18: 131-166, 1964.

[59] Hyden S. Observations on the absorption of inorganic ions from the reticulo-rumen of the sheep. *Kugl Lantbrukshögkolans Annaler* 27: 273-285, 1961.

[60] Janis CM, Damuth J, and Theodor JM. Miocene ungulates and terrestrial primary productivity: Where have all the browsers gone? *Proc Natl Acad Sci U S A* 97: 7899-7904, 2000.

[61] Jittakhot S, Schonewille JT, Wouterse HS, Yuangklang C, and Beynen AC. The relationships between potassium intakes, transmural potential difference of the rumen epithelium and magnesium absorption in whethers. *Br J Nutr* 91: 183-189, 2004.

[62] Johnson JW and Ascher P. Glycine potentiates the NMDA response in cultured mouse brain neurons. *Nature* 325: 529-531, 1987.

[63] Johnson JW and Ascher P. Voltage-dependent block by intracellular Mg^{2+} of N-methyl-D-aspartate-activated channels. *Biophys J* 57: 1085-1090, 1990.

[64] Kamel KS, Harvey E, Douek K, Parmar MS, and Halperin ML. Studies on the pathogenesis of hypokalemia in Gitelman's syndrome: role of bicarbonaturia and hypomagnesemia. *Am J Nephrol* 18: 42-49, 1998.

[65] Kamel KS, Oh MS, and Halperin ML. Bartter's, Gitelman's, and Gordon's syndromes. From physiology to molecular biology and back, yet still some unanswered questions. *Nephron* 92 Suppl 1: 18-27, 2002.

[66] Katz B. Les constantes électriques de la membrane du muscle. *Arch Sci Physiol* 2: 285-299, 1949.

[67] Kay RN. The rate of flow and composition of various salivary secretions in sheep and calves. *J Physiol* 150: 515-537, 1960.

[68] Khalbuss WE, Alkiek R, Marousis CG, and Orlando RC. Potassium conductance in rabbit esophageal epithelium. *Am J Physiol* 265: G28-34, 1993.

[69] Khorasani GR, Janzen RA, McGill WB, and Kennelly JJ. Site and extent of mineral absorption in lactating cows fed whole-crop cereal grain silage of alfalfa silage. *J Anim Sci* 75: 239-248, 1997.

[70] Koeppen BM and Stanton BA. Renal Physiology. (Third edition, Mosby Inc, St. Louis, Missouri, ISBN 0-323-01242-01246). 2001.

[71] Kunzelmann K and Mall M. Electrolyte transport in the mammalian colon: mechanisms and implications for disease. *Physiol Rev* 82: 245-289, 2002.

[72] Lang I and Martens H. Na^+ transport in sheep rumen is modulated by voltage-dependent cation conductance in apical membrane. *Am J Physiol* 277: G609-618, 1999.

[73] Leonhard-Marek S. Divalent cations reduce the electrogenic transport of monovalent cations across rumen epithelium. *J Comp Physiol [B]* 172: 635-641, 2002.

[74] Leonhard-Marek S, Breves G, and Busche R. Effect of chloride on pH microclimate and electrogenic Na^+ absorption across the rumen epithelium of goat and sheep. *Am J Physiol Gastrointest Liver Physiol*, 2006.

[75] Leonhard-Marek S, Gäbel G, and Martens H. Effects of short chain fatty acids and carbon dioxide on magnesium transport across sheep rumen epithelium. *Exp Physiol* 83: 155-164, 1998.

[76] Leonhard-Marek S and Martens H. Effects of potassium on magnesium transport across rumen epithelium. *Am J Physiol* 271: G1034-1038, 1996.

[77] Leonhard-Marek S, Stumpff F, Brinkmann I, Breves G, and Martens H. Basolateral Mg^{2+}/Na^+ exchange regulates apical nonselective cation channel in sheep rumen epithelium via cytosolic Mg^{2+}. *Am J Physiol Gastrointest Liver Physiol* 288: G630-645, 2005.

[78] Lodemann U and Martens H. Effects of diet and osmotic pressure on Na^+ transport and tissue conductance of sheep isolated rumen epithelium. *Exp Physiol* 91: 539-550, 2006.

[79] Luthi D, Günzel D, and McGuigan JA. Mg-ATP binding: its modification by spermine, the relevance to cytosolic Mg^{2+} buffering, changes in the intracellular ionized Mg^{2+} concentration and the estimation of Mg^{2+} by 31P-NMR. *Exp Physiol* 84: 231-252, 1999.

[80] Martens H and Blume I. Effect of intraruminal sodium and potassium concentrations and of the transmural potential difference on magnesium absorption from the temporarily isolated rumen of sheep. *Q J Exp Physiol* 71: 409-415, 1986.

[81] Martens H and Blume I. Studies on the absorption of sodium and chloride from the rumen of sheep. *Comp Biochem Physiol A* 86: 653-656, 1987.

[82] Martens H and Gäbel G. Transport of Na and Cl across the epithelium of ruminant forestomachs: rumen and omasum. A review. *Comp Biochem Physiol A* 90: 569-575, 1988.

[83] Martens H, Gäbel G, and Strozyk B. Mechanism of electrically silent Na and Cl transport across the rumen epithelium of sheep. *Exp Physiol* 76, 1991.

[84] Martens H, Gäbel G, and Strozyk H. The effect of potassium and the transmural potential difference on magnesium transport across an isolated preparation of sheep rumen epithelium. *Q J Exp Physiol* 72: 181-188, 1987.

[85] Martens H and Hammer U. [Magnesium and sodium absorption from the isolated sheep rumen during intravenous aldosterone infusion (author's transl]. *Dtsch Tierarztl Wochenschr* 88: 404-407, 1981.

[86] Martens H and Harmeyer J. Magnesium transport by isolated rumen epithelium of sheep. *Res Vet Sci* 24: 161-168, 1978.

[87] Martens H, Heggemann G, and Regier K. Studies on the effect of K, Na, NH_4^+, VFA and CO_2 on the net absorption of magnesium from the temporarily isolated rumen of heifers. *Zentralbl Veterinarmed A* 35: 73-80, 1988.

[88] Martens H, Kubel OW, Gäbel G, and Honig H. Effects of low sodium intake on magnesium metabolism in sheep. *J agric Sci*: 237-243, 1987.

[89] Martens H and Rayssiguier Y. Magnesium metabolism and hypomagnesaemia. In: Proceedings of the 5th International Symposium on Ruminant Physiology (ed. Ruckebush, Y and Thivend, P.). 447-466, 1980.

[90] Martens H and Schweigel M. Pathophysiology of grass tetany and other hypomagnesemias. Implications for clinical management. *Vet Clin North Am Food Anim Pract* 16: 339-368, 2000.

[91] Martens H and Stossel EM. Magnesium absorption from the temporarily isolated rumen of sheep: no effect of hyper- or hypomagnesaemia. *Q J Exp Physiol* 73: 217-223, 1988.

[92] McCoy MA. Hypomagnesaemia and new data on vitreous humour magnesium concentration as a post-mortem marker in ruminants. *Magnes Res* 17: 137-145, 2004.

[93] McDonald IW. The absorption of ammonia from the rumen of the sheep. *Biochem J* 42: 584-587, 1948.

[94] McLean AF, Buchan W, and Scott D. Magnesium absorption in mature ewes infused intrarumenally with magnesium chloride. *Br J Nutr* 52: 523-527, 1984.

[95] Monteilh-Zoller MK, Hermosura MC, Nadler MJ, Scharenberg AM, Penner R, and Fleig A. TRPM7 provides an ion channel mechanism for cellular entry of trace metal ions. *J Gen Physiol* 121: 49-60, 2003.

[96] Morris JG and Gartner RW. The effect of potassium on the sodium requirements of growing steers with and without alpha-tocopherol supplementation. *Br J Nutr* 34: 1-14, 1975.

[97] Muller F, Aschenbach JR, and Gäbel G. Role of Na^+/H^+ exchange and HCO_3^- transport in pH_i recovery from intracellular acid load in cultured epithelial cells of sheep rumen. *J Comp Physiol [B]* 170: 337-343, 2000.

[98] Mutoh K and Wakuri H. Early organogenesis of the caprine stomach. *Nippon Juigaku Zasshi* 51: 474-484, 1989.

[99] Nadler MJ, Hermosura MC, Inabe K, Perraud AL, Zhu Q, Stokes AJ, Kurosaki T, Kinet JP, Penner R, Scharenberg AM, and Fleig A. LTRPC7 is a Mg.ATP-regulated divalent cation channel required for cell viability. *Nature* 411: 590-595, 2001.

[100] Nilius B, Vennekens R, Prenen J, Hoenderop JG, Bindels RJ, and Droogmans G. Whole-cell and single channel monovalent cation currents through the novel rabbit epithelial Ca^{2+} channel ECaC. *J Physiol* 527 Pt 2: 239-248, 2000.

[101] Nilius B, Vennekens R, Prenen J, Hoenderop JG, Droogmans G, and Bindels RJ. The single pore residue Asp542 determines Ca^{2+} permeation and Mg^{2+} block of the epithelial Ca^{2+} channel. *J Biol Chem* 276: 1020-1025, 2001.

[102] Nocek JE and Polan CE. Influence of ration form and nitrogen availability on ruminal fermentation patterns and plasma of growing bull calves. *J Dairy Sci* 67: 1038-1042, 1984.

[103] Oba M, Baldwin RLt, Owens SL, and Bequette BJ. Metabolic fates of ammonia-N in ruminal epithelial and duodenal mucosal cells isolated from growing sheep. *J Dairy Sci* 88: 3963-3970, 2005.

[104] Odette O. Grass tetany in a herd of beef cows. *Can Vet J* 46: 732-734, 2005.

[105] Owens FN, Secrist DS, Hill WJ, and Gill DR. Acidosis in cattle: a review. *J Anim Sci* 76: 275-286, 1998.

[106] Owsianik G, Talavera K, Voets T, and Nilius B. Permeation and selectivity of TRP channels. *Annu Rev Physiol* 68: 685-717, 2006.

[107] Pfeffer E, Thompson A, and Armstrong DG. Studies on intestinal digestion in the sheep. 3. Net movement of certain inorganic elements in the digestive tract on rations containing different proportions of hay and rolled barley. *Br J Nutr* 24: 197-204, 1970.

[108] Phillipson AT. Absorption of acetate from the rumen of sheep. *J Physiol* 109: Proc, 31, 1949.

[109] Powell DW, Morris SM, and Boyd DD. Water and electrolyte transport by rabbit esophagus. *Am J Physiol* 229: 438-443, 1975.

[110] Qian A, Antonov SM, and Johnson JW. Modulation by permeant ions of Mg(2+) inhibition of NMDA-activated whole-cell currents in rat cortical neurons. *J Physiol* 538: 65-77, 2002.

[111] Rabinowitz L. Aldosterone and potassium homeostasis. *Kidney Int* 49: 1738-1742, 1996.

[112] Rabinowitz L, Green DM, Sarason RL, and Yamauchi H. Homeostatic potassium excretion in fed and fasted sheep. *Am J Physiol* 254: R357-380, 1988.

[113] Rahnema SH and Fontenot JP. Effects of intravenous infusion of high levels of potassium and sodium on mineral metabolism in sheep. *J Anim Sci* 68: 2833-2838, 1990.

[114] Rossier BC. The epithelial sodium channel: activation by membrane-bound serine proteases. *Proc Am Thorac Soc* 1: 4-9, 2004.

[115] Rossier BC, Pradervand S, Schild L, and Hummler E. Epithelial sodium channel and the control of sodium balance: interaction between genetic and environmental factors. *Annu Rev Physiol* 64: 877-897, 2002.

[116] Rübbelke MK. In vitro Untersuchungen des Pansenepithels von Schafen zur Characterisierung eines elektrogenen, calcium-sensitiven Natriumtransportes (Inaugural-Dissertation, Institut für Veterinär-Physiologie, Freie Universität Berlin). Berlin, 1998 (Journal-Nr: 2169), 1998.

[117] Sakmann B and Trube G. Conductance properties of single inwardly rectifying potassium channels in ventricular cells from guinea-pig heart. *J Physiol* 347: 641-657, 1984.

[118] Sargison ND, Macrae AI, and Scott PR. Hypomagnesaemic tetany in lactating Cheviot gimmers associated with pasture sodium deficiency. *Vet Rec* 155: 674-676, 2004.

[119] Sawchenko PE and Friedman MI. Sensory functions of the liver--a review. *Am J Physiol* 236: R5-20, 1979.

[120] Schröder B, Vossing S, and Breves G. In vitro studies on active calcium absorption from ovine rumen. *J Comp Physiol [B]* 169: 487-494, 1999.

[121] Schultheiss G and Martens H. Ca-sensitive Na transport in sheep omasum. *Am J Physiol* 276: G1331-1344, 1999.

[122] Schweigel M, Freyer M, Leclercq S, Etschmann B, Lodemann U, Bottcher A, and Martens H. Luminal hyperosmolarity decreases Na transport and impairs barrier function of sheep rumen epithelium. *J Comp Physiol [B]* 175: 575-591, 2005.

[123] Schweigel M, Lang I, and Martens H. Mg(2+) transport in sheep rumen epithelium: evidence for an electrodiffusive uptake mechanism. *Am J Physiol* 277: G976-982, 1999.

[124] Schweigel M and Martens H. Anion-dependent Mg^{2+} influx and a role for a vacuolar H^{+}-ATPase in sheep ruminal epithelial cells. *Am J Physiol Gastrointest Liver Physiol* 285: G45-53, 2003.

[125] Schweigel M and Martens H. [Electrophysiologic changes in rumen epithelium in their effect on magnesium transport--a review]. *Berl Munch Tierarztl Wochenschr* 113: 97-102, 2000.

[126] Schweigel M, Park HS, Etschmann B, and Martens H. Characterization of the Na^{+}-dependent Mg^{2+} transport in sheep ruminal epithelial cells. *Am J Physiol Gastrointest Liver Physiol* 290: G56-65, 2006.

[127] Schweigel M, Vormann J, and Martens H. Mechanisms of Mg(2+) transport in cultured ruminal epithelial cells. *Am J Physiol Gastrointest Liver Physiol* 278: G400-408, 2000.

[128] Scott D. Absorption of chloride from the rumen of the sheep. *Res Vet Sci* 11: 291-293, 1970.

[129] Scott D. Changes in mineral, water and acid base balance associated with feeding and diet. Digestion and metabolism in the ruminant: Proceedings of the IV International Symposium on Ruminant Physiology (1974). ed: I.W. McDonald and A.C.I. Warner. The University of New England Publishing Unit (1975), 1975.

[130] Scott D. The effects of potassium supplements upon the absorption of potassium and sodium from the sheep rumen. *Q J Exp Physiol Cogn Med Sci* 52: 382-391, 1967.

[131] Scott D. The effects of sodium depletion and potassium supplements upon electrical potentials in the rumen of the sheep. *Q J Exp Physiol Cogn Med Sci* 51: 60-69, 1966.

[132] Sehested J, Diernaes L, Moller PD, and Skadhauge E. Interaction between absorption of sodium and acetate across the rumen epithelium of cattle. *Acta Vet Scand Suppl* 89: 107-108, 1993.

[133] Sehested J, Diernaes L, Moller PD, and Skadhauge E. Ruminal transport and metabolism of short-chain fatty acids (SCFA) in vitro: effect of SCFA chain length and pH. *Comp Biochem Physiol A Mol Integr Physiol* 123: 359-368, 1999.

[134] Sehested J, Diernaes L, Moller PD, and Skadhauge E. Transport of butyrate across the isolated bovine rumen epithelium--interaction with sodium, chloride and bicarbonate. *Comp Biochem Physiol A Mol Integr Physiol* 123: 399-408, 1999.

[135] Sehested J, Diernaes L, Moller PD, and Skadhauge E. Transport of sodium across the isolated bovine rumen epithelium: interaction with short-chain fatty acids, chloride and bicarbonate. *Exp Physiol* 81: 79-94, 1996.

[136] Sellers AF and Dobson A. Studies on reticulo-rumen sodium and potassium concentration and electrical potentials in sheep. *Res Vet Sci* 1: 95, 1960.

[137] Sellers AF, Gitis TL, and Roepke MH. Studies of electrolytes in body fluids of dairy cattle. III. Effects of potassium on electrolyte levels in body fluids in midlactation. *Am J Vet Res* 12: 296-301, 1951.

[138] Silanikove N. The struggle to maintain hydration and osmoregulation in animals experiencing severe dehydration and rapid rehydration: the story of ruminants. *Exp Physiol* 79: 281-300, 1994.

[139] Silanikove N and Tadmor A. Rumen volume, saliva flow rate, and systemic fluid homeostasis in dehydrated cattle. *Am J Physiol* 256: R809-815, 1989.

[140] Sjollema B. On the nature and therapy of grass staggers. *Vet Rec* 10: 425, 1930.

[141] Sjollema B. Untersuchungen über die Ursache der Grastetanie und der großen Frequenzzunahme dieser Krankheit. *Deutsche Tierärztliche Wochenzeitschrift* 15, 1932.

[142] Skou JC. The influence of some cations on an adenosine triphosphatase from peripheral nerves. *Biochim Biophys Acta* 23: 394-401, 1957.

[143] Sperber I and Hyden S. Transport of chloride through the ruminal mucosa. *Nature* 169: 587, 1952.

[144] Stacy BD and Warner AC. Balances of water and sodium in the rumen during feeding: osmotic stimulation of sodium absorption in the sheep. *Q J Exp Physiol Cogn Med Sci* 51: 79-93, 1966.

[145] Stevens CE. Transport of sodium and chloride by the isolated rumen epithelium. *Am J Physiol* 206: 1099-1105, 1964.

[146] Stumpff F, Brinkmann I, and Martens H. Regulation of a non-selective cation channel in cells of the ovine rumen epithelium by PGE2 and Forskolin. *Pflügers Arch* 449 (Suppl.): S116, 2005.

[147] Stumpff F, Brinkmann I, Schweigel M, and Martens H. High potassium diet, sodium and magnesium in ruminants: the story is not over. *Production diseases in farm animals*: 284-285, 2004.

[148] Stumpff F, Martens H, and Schweigel M. A patch-clamp and furaptra study of electrodiffusive Mg uptake into cells of the ruminal epithelium. *Acta Physiol* 186 (Suppl): 232 (PW203A-217), 2006.

[149] Suttle NF and Field AC. Studies on magnesium in ruminant nutrition. 8. Effect of increased intakes of potassium and water on the metabolism of magnesium, phosphorus, sodium, potassium and calcium in sheep. *Br J Nutr* 21: 819-831, 1967.

[150] Tomas FM and Potter BJ. The site of magnesium absorption from the ruminant stomach. *Br J Nutr* 36: 37-45, 1976.

[151] Tsuchiya Y, Nakashima S, Banno Y, Suzuki Y, and Morita H. Effect of high-NaCl or high-KCl diet on hepatic Na^+- and K^+-receptor sensitivity and NKCC1 expression in rats. *Am J Physiol Regul Integr Comp Physiol* 286: R591-596, 2004.

[152] Ussing HH and Zerahn K. Active transport of sodium as the source of electric current in the short-circuited isolated frog skin. *Acta Physiol Scand* 23: 110-127, 1951.

[153] van de Graaf SF, Hoenderop JG, and Bindels RJ. Regulation of TRPV5 and TRPV6 by associated proteins. *Am J Physiol Renal Physiol* 290: F1295-1302, 2006.

[154] Voets T, Janssens A, Prenen J, Droogmans G, and Nilius B. Mg^{2+}-dependent gating and strong inward rectification of the cation channel TRPV6. *J Gen Physiol* 121: 245-260, 2003.

[155] Wadhwa DR and Care AD. The absorption of calcium ions from the ovine reticulo-rumen. *J Comp Physiol [B]* 170: 581-588, 2000.

[156] Wallace RJ. Ruminal microbial metabolism of peptides and amino acids. *J Nutr* 126: 1326S-1334S, 1996.

[157] Warner AC and Stacy BD. Influence of ruminal and plasma osmotic pressure on salivary secretion in sheep. *Q J Exp Physiol Cogn Med Sci* 62: 133-142, 1977.

[158] Warner AC and Stacy BD. Intraruminal and systemic responses to variations in intake of sodium and potassium by sheep. *Q J Exp Physiol Cogn Med Sci* 57: 89-102, 1972.

[159] Warner AC and Stacy BD. Solutes in the Rumen of the Sheep. *Q J Exp Physiol Cogn Med Sci* 50: 169-184, 1965.

[160] Warner AC and Stacy BD. Water, sodium and potassium movements across the rumen wall of sheep. *Q J Exp Physiol Cogn Med Sci* 57: 103-119, 1972.

[161] Warnock DG. Renal genetic disorders related to K^+ and Mg^{2+}. *Annu Rev Physiol* 64: 845-876, 2002.

[162] Wilkens M, Kunert-Keil C, and Schröder B. Expression of the epithelial Ca^{2+} channels TRPV5 and TRPV6 in ovine Ca^{2+} transporting tissues. *Acta Physiol* 186(Suppl): 232 (PW203A-215), 2006.

[163] Wolffram S, Frischknecht R, and Scharrer E. Influence of theophylline on the electrical potential difference and ion fluxes (Na, Cl, K) across the isolated rumen epithelium of sheep. *Zentralbl Veterinarmed A* 36: 755-762, 1989.

[164] Wylie MJ, Fontenot JP, and Greene LW. Absorption of magnesium and other macrominerals in sheep infused with potassium in different parts of the digestive tract. *J Anim Sci* 61: 1219-1229, 1985.

[165] Yellen G. The voltage-gated potassium channels and their relatives. *Nature* 419: 35-42, 2002.

In: Dietary Magnezium: New Research
Editor: Andrew W. Yardley
ISBN 978-1-60692-109-8

Chapter VIII

Zinc, Copper, Manganese and Magnesium in Liver Cirrhosis

***Dario Rahelic*[1], *Milan Kujundzic*[2] *and Velimir Bozikov*[1]**
[1]Division of Endocrinology, Diabetology and Metabolic Disorders,
[2]Division of Gastoenterology,
Dubrava University Hospital, Zagreb, Croatia.

Abstract

The role of trace elements in the pathogenesis of liver cirrhosis and its complications is still not clearly understood.

Zinc, copper, manganese and magnesium are essential trace elements whose role in liver cirrhosis and its complications is still a matter of research.

Zinc is associated with more than 300 enzymatic systems. Zinc is structured part of Cu-Zn superoxide dismutase, important antioxidative enzyme. Zinc acts as an antioxidant, a membrane and cytosceletal stabilizator, an anti-apoptotic agent, an important co-factor in DNA synthesis, an anti-inflammatory agent, etc. Copper is an essential trace element which participates in many enzymatic reactions. Its most important role is in redox processes. Reactive copper can participate in liver damage directly or indirectly, through Kupffer cell's stimulation. Scientists agree that copper's toxic effects are related to oxidative stress. Manganese is a structural part of arginase, which is an important enzyme in the urea metabolism. Manganese acts as an activator of numerous enzymes in Krebs cycle, particularly in the decarboxilation process.

Magnesium is important for the protein synthesis, enzyme activation, oxidative phosphorilation, renal potassium and hydrogen exchange etc.

Since zinc, copper, manganese and magnesium have a possible role in the pathogenesis of liver cirrhosis and cirrhotic complications, the aim of our study was to investigate the serum concentrations of mentioned trace elements in patients with liver cirrhosis and compare them with concentrations in controls.

Serum concentrations of zinc, copper, manganese and magnesium were determined in 105 patients with alcoholic liver cirrhosis and 50 healthy subjects by means of plasma sequential spectrophotometer. Serum concentrations of zinc were significantly lower (median 0.82 vs. 11.22 µmol/L, p<0.001) in patients with liver cirrhosis in comparison to controls. Serum concentrations of copper were significantly higher in patients with liver cirrhosis (median 21.56 vs. 13.09 µmol/L, p<0.001) as well as manganese (2.50 vs. 0.02 µmol/L, p<0.001). The concentration of magnesium was not significantly different between patients with liver cirrhosis and controls (0.94 vs. 0.88 mmol/L, p=0.132). There were no differences in the concentrations of zinc, copper, manganese and magnesium between male and female patients with liver cirrhosis. Only manganese concentration was significantly different between Child-Pugh groups (p=0.036). Zinc concentration was significantly lower in patients with hepatic encephalopathy in comparison to cirrhotic patients without encephalopathy (0.54 vs. 0.96 µmol/L, p=0.002). The correction of trace elements concentrations might have a beneficial effect on complications and maybe progression of liver cirrhosis. It would be recommendable to provide analysis of trace elements in patients with liver cirrhosis as a routine.

Keywords: zinc, copper, manganese, magnesium, liver cirrhosis, trace elements.

1. Liver Cirrhosis

1.1. Epidemiology

According to data from the World Health Organization (WHO) chronic liver disease causes more than 1.4 million death outcomes per year. Liver cirrhosis mortality rates vary across the countries. A cirrhosis mortality rate in Great Britain is now among the highest in Europe (28.9 per 100.000 in man and 12.8 in women). Between 1987-1991 and 1997-2001, cirrhosis mortality in man in Scotland doubled more than once (112% increase) and in women increase almost by two-thirds (67%) (Leon et al., 2006 a,b). On the contrary, in Sweden decrease in liver cirrhosis mortality has been observed. In the last fifteen years an age standardized mortality rate of liver cirrhosis was about 4 per 100.000 deaths per year (Stokkeland et al., 2006).

The regional differences in cirrhosis mortality rates follow a north-south gradient, with the lowest rates in Northern and the highest in Southern Europe. In 1995 cirrhosis mortality rates in Northern Europe for men were about 12.2 per 100.000 and for women 4.8. On the contrary, in Southern Europe cirrhosis mortality rates were about 33.7 for men and 12.1 for women. Some exceptions were noticed in order to obtain general pattern. France has substantially higher death rates than other southern European countries like Greece, Spain and Italy (Ramstedt, 2002).

Taking into account that liver cirrhosis has important impact on overall mortality, even small progress in explaining the liver cirrhosis pathogenesis could have positive influence on disease progression.

1.2. Definition

Liver cirrhosis is, according to the WHO, a diffuse process characterized by fibrosis and conversion of normal liver architecture to structural abnormal nodules without normal lobular organization.

1.3. Etiology

There are numerous causes of liver cirrhosis. Alcohol is the most common cause in the Western countries but viral infection is the most common cause world-wide. Other causes, like hereditary hemochromatosis, Wilson's disease, α1-antitrypsin deficiency, galactosemia, autoimune disease, Budd-Chiari syndrome, secondary biliary cirrhosis, hepatic venous congestion, thrombosis of portal vein, infection, sarcoidosis, drugs, etc. are less common.

1.4. Alcoholic Liver Disease

Ethanol is metabolized in the liver through three pathways, by alcohol dehydrogenase / aldehyde dehydrogenase (ADH), microsomal ethanol oxidative system (MEOS) and by catalase.

More than 80% of ethanol is metabolized through first pathway. Consequently, an increase in the NADH/NAD ratio occurs, what inhibits many NAD+ dependent enzymes.

Liver changes caused by alcohol consumption include fatty liver, alcoholic hepatitis and alcoholic (Laenec's) liver cirrhosis. Fatty liver is initial, reversible phase of alcoholic liver disease characterized by the development of fatty vacuole in hepatocytes due to the impaired fatty acid metabolism.

Alcoholic hepatitis is characterized by hepatocyte necrosis, infiltration of polymorphonuclear leucocytes mainly in zone 3, then by dense cytoplasmic inclusions called Mallory bodies and by hiatal sclerosis (Jensen et al, 1994 a,b). Mallory bodies are not specific for alcoholic liver disease, because they can be found also in Wilson's disease and primary biliary cirrhosis.

Liver cirrhosis is pathohystological term characterized by necrosis of liver parenchyma, fibrosis and development of regeneratory lobules. According to the lobular size, liver cirrhosis can be divided on micronodular, macronodular and mixed cirrhosis. Micrinodular cirrhosis is characterized by lobules smaller than 3 mm in diameter and macronodular by lobules above 3 mm in diameter.

Alcoholic liver cirrhosis is usually micronodular, but during the time can transform to macronodular cirrhosis.

1.5. Pathogenesis of Alcoholic Liver Disease

Alcoholic liver cirrhosis is caused by toxic effects of alcohol on the liver, lipid peroxidation and immunologic alterations. After absorption, alcohol is transformed to acetaldehyde. Accumulation of acetaldehyde alters hepatocyte function. Also, the product of alcohol metabolism is reduced nicotinamide-adenine dinucleotide (NADH) which accumulates in the cytosol and mitochondria of hepatocytes. That results in inhibition of many NAD+ dependent enzymes like the enzymes of β-oxidation. All that cause decreased oxidation of fatty acids with increased export of very low density lipoprotein (VLDL) and hypertriglyceridemia which are commonly associated with alcohol use (Crabb & Estonius, 1998). Consequently, fat deposition occurs within the liver what cause so called *fatty liver*. Acetaldechide can also modify liver proteins and DNA forming neoantigens which can be recognized by the immune system and cause immunological reaction. Acetaldechyde stimulates collagen synthesis by stellate cells. Acetaldechyde reduces mitochondrial glutathione concentration. Alcohol by itself causes increased oxygen consumption with consequent centrilobular hypoxia.

In the condition of low blood and tissue alcohol concentration, ADH has a key role in the metabolism of alcohol. When tissue concentration increases above 10 mmol/L MEOS starts to metabolize alcohol. MEOS is situated in microsomes of smooth endoplasmic reticulum. Chronic alcohol consumption causes an increase in MEOS activity 5 to 10 times. Main role in MEOS has isoenzyme CYP2E1 from cytochrom P450 family. CYP2E1 metabolizes ethanol but also acetaldechyde and many other drugs what explains the increased toxicity of therapeutic doses of some drugs in alcoholics (Vucelic et al., 2002).

Chronic alcohol consumption leads to the induction of CYP2E1 with generation of oxygen radicals and lipid peroxidation. Also, alcohol sensitizes Kupffer cells and stellate cells and probably inhibits regeneration of injured hepatocytes (Crabb & Estonius, 1998). Reactive oxygen species cause hepatocyte injury by lipid peroxidation.

In pathogenesis of liver cirrhosis important occurrences are necrosis of hepatocytes, hepatocellular regeneration, fibrosis and destruction of lobular structure with forming pseudolobules.

In fibrogenesis, necrosis of hepatocytes occurs first. In the early phase, as mentioned above, products of cell inflammation, like proteinases and free oxygen radicals, cause necrosis of hepatocytes with consequent release of numerous cytokines. Changes of extracellular matrix occur in further phase. Those changes include non-proportional increase in a concentration of some extracelular matrix molecules, changes on molecules and their transposition within the matrix.

There is a multiple increase in concentration of extracellular matrix molecules like collagen, glycoproteins and proteoglycans. Chronic alcohol intake also stimulates production and releasing of numerous cytokines by stimulated Kupffer cells. One of the most important cytokine in fibrogenesis is certainly transforming growth factor β (TGF-β). Released cytokines stimulate stellate cells on proliferation and collagen synthesis.

On the other hand, degradation of protein matrix has also important role in fibrogenesis (Sherlock et al., 2002). Matrix degradation is regulated by metalloproteinase (Arthur & Iredale, 1994; Arthur, 2000). The most important metalloproteinases are collagenases (MMP-

1 and MMP-13, which disolve type I, II and III collagen), gelatinase (MMP-2 and MMP-9, which disolve type IV collagen) and stromelisins (MMP-3 and MMP-10, which disolve proteoglycans, laminin, fibronectin, etc.) (Takahara et al., 1995). All these enzymes are synthesized by Kupffer cells and activated stellate cells. Metalloproteinases are inhibited by tissue metalloproteinase inhibitors (TIMP). Activated stellate cells synthesize TIMP-1. Therefore, stellate cells have important role in degradation and synthesis of connective tissue (Iredale et al., 1992).

Fibrosis alters the liver structure and obstructs biliary and vascular pathways with clinical consequences.

1.6. Clinical Manifestations of Liver Cirrhosis

Fatty infiltration causes nonspecific symptoms or abnormal laboratory results of liver function. The liver is usually enlarged. In advanced alcoholic liver disease common symptoms are loss of appetite, weight loss, nausea, jaundice, abdominal pain and edema. Liver cirrhosis is characterized by an enlarged liver in the beginning and small, fibrous liver in advanced stages, enlarged spleen, portal hypertension with esophageal varices, hepatic encephalopathy, anemia, etc.

1.7. Treatment of Patients with Liver Cirrhosis

Treatment of liver cirrhosis is mostly symptomatically. Usually, the main problem in patients with liver cirrhosis is the treatment of complications like hepatic encephalopathy, hepatorenal syndrome and bleeding from esophageal varices.

Numerous studies have tried to focus on prevention of alcoholic liver cirrhosis and progression of alcoholic liver disease to liver cirrhosis. There were also numerous studies which have tried to slow down progression of liver disease and prevent complications. As the oxidative stress has important role in pathogenesis of liver cirrhosis, trace elements have become important substrate for investigations of pathogenesis of liver cirrhosis and its complications.

Trace elements certainly have important role in pathogenesis of liver cirrhosis and its complications.

2. Trace Elements

2.1. Definition

Trace elements are present in human body in very small concentration *(ppm - pars per million)*.

Development of new laboratory methods has allowed better quality and quantity determination of trace elements, as well as better understanding of their role in numerous metabolic processes.

There are essential and nonessential trace elements. Essential trace elements are those necessary for life and normal body function. According to Cotzias (Cotzias, 1967), essential trace elements are iron (Fe), zinc (Zn), copper (Cu), manganese (Mn), cobalt (Co), iodine (J), molybdenum (Mo), selenium (Se) and chromium (Cr). There is an additional division of trace elements on incontestable essential trace elements and »probably essential trace elements for humans«. Incontestably essential trace elements are iron (Fe), zinc (Zn), copper (Cu), chromium (Cr), iodine (I), cobalt (Co), molybdenum (Mo) and selenium (Se). Probably essential trace elements are manganese (Mn), tin (Sn), nickel (Ni), fluor (F), silicon (Si), vanadium (Va), calcium (Ca) and magnesium (Mg).

Trace elements entry includes ingestion by food and water. Normal nutrition satisfies requirements of human body for trace elements.

Concentration of trace elements is different in different drinking waters. Food processing, especially industrial, influences (mostly decrease) concentration of trace elements. There is also a question of trace element supplementation in patients with long-term parenteral nutrition.

All above mentioned suggests that an intake of trace elements in human body by food or by drink water varies.

Trace elements form moderately stable complexes with enzymes, nucleic acids and other ligands, changing and controlling their function, while other form compact static complexes and become integral functional components of enzymes (Speech et al., 2001). Therefore, it is obvious that some trace elements participate in numerous biochemical reactions which are necessary for life, like oxygen transport and release, redox processes, etc.

Optimal concentration of trace elements is within narrow range between their deficiency and toxicity.

Deficiency of trace elements is usually caused by the inadequate intake or other factors, like an increased loss caused by diarrhea, malabsorption after surgical resection of small intestine, by forming metal complexes with food ingredients which do not allow absorption, increase urinary losses, increase losses caused by pancreatic juices or other exocrine secretions, etc. The deficiency can as well be caused by the antagonistic actions of some trace elements on absorption or transportation of other trace elements, for example, in the case of intake of zinc and copper or copper and molibden. The intake of one trace element can also cause the deficiency of the other trace elements.

Toxic effects of trace elements depend on chemical shape, way of entry in the body, biological ligands, tissue distribution, concentration and velocity of elimination.

Toxicity mechanisms include enzyme inhibition by binding to essential amino-acid residuum, changing both function and structure of nucleic acids, inhibition of synthesis, influence on membrane permeability, inhibition of phosphorilation, etc (Kasper et al., 2005).

As it would be difficult to present role of all trace elements in liver cirrhosis we choose to present only zinc, copper, manganese and magnesium according to data from our research.

2.2. Zinc, Copper, Manganese and Magnesium in Liver Cirrhosis

The role of trace elements in pathogenesis of liver cirrhosis and its complications is still not clearly understood. In fibrogenesis the initial occurrence is hepato-cellular necrosis. In the early phase, inflammation cell products, proteinases and reactive oxygen radicals, may initiate hepato-cellular necrosis with consecutive releasing of numerous cytokines. Following hepatic injury, there is an increase in extracellular matrix, the activation of stellate cells, the increase in rough endoplasmatic reticulum and expression of smooth muscle specific α-actin (Friedman, 1993).

Activated stellate cells are influenced by numerous cytokines. Some of them have proliferative effect on stellate cells while others stimulate fibrogenesis (Pinzani, 1995).

Zinc, copper, manganese and magnesium are essential trace elements whose role in liver cirrhosis and its complications is still a matter of research. There are contrary reports about their serum concentrations in patients with liver cirrhosis.

2.2.1. Zinc

Zinc is incontestably essential trace element in humans. In nature zinc is especially present in sea food, cereals, vegetable, milk, walnuts etc. Average daily intake is approximately 12-15 mg. From oral intake, only 20-30% will be absorbed. In the enteric cell zinc induces synthesis of metalothionein, low molecular weight protein and when this process ends further absorption of zinc decreases. About two thirds of absorbed zinc is bounded on albumin and other is bounded on ß-2 microglobulin. Normal plasma concentration of zinc is 0.85-1.10 µg/mL.

In adult people renal excretion is approximately 300-600 µg per day. Renal tubular absorption decreases with tiazid diuretics administration (Prasad et al., 1996). Increased urinary losses are common in nephrotic syndrome, liver cirrhosis and other hypoalbuminic states, during penicillamine administration, catabolic states after burning, trauma, surgery, hemolytic anemia, etc. Decreased serum concentration of zinc is common in patient with acute myocardial infarction, infection, hepatitis, etc. (Kasper et al., 2005).

Lower serum concentration of zinc is common in patients with liver cirrhosis due to decreased intake, decreased absorption, decreased bioavailability and increased losses due to malabsorption, diarrhea or increased urinary losses.

There is a reduced liver protein synthesis in patients with liver cirrhosis with consequently decreased zinc bioavailability.

Zinc participates in more than 300 enzymatic systems (Christianson, 1991). Zinc is involved in synthesis of nucleic acid, protein synthesis, testosterone secretion, cerebral function etc. Zinc presents natural defense from reactive oxygen radicals through antioxidative enzyme, Cu-Zn superokside dysmutase (Speich et al., 2001). Its role in storage and release of hormones, neurotransmision, visual processes and cognitive processes were also described (Truong-Tran et al., 2000; Vallee et al., 1993).

Zinc acts as an antioxidant, membrane and cytoskeletal stabilizator, anti-apoptotic agent, important cofactor in DNA synthesis, anti-inflamatory agent etc. (Truong-Tran et al., 2001).

In the last decade role of zinc in apoptosis was considered intensively (Truong-Tran et al., 2000; Zalewski et al., 1993; Sunderman, 1995; Wyllie, 1997). Apoptosis is important in early embryonic development, what has been found in investigations with zinc deficient rats (Record et al., 1985).

Ethanol consumption induces apoptosis in liver and lymphoid tissue as well as many other. According to the published data it seems that zinc has influence on apoptosis of blood mononuclear cells by inhibiting the mitochondrial pathway of cell death. It was suggested that mitochondrial pathway of ethanol-related immune cell death may be inhibited by zinc supplementation (Szuster-Ciesielska et al., 2005).

On the other hand, it seems that zinc at pharmacologic concentrations stimulates cytokine expression and induces apoptosis of peripheral blood mononuclear cells (Chang et al., 2006).

The role of zinc in Alzheimer disease has also been investigated (Anderson et al., 1996).

Zinc has also role in glucose metabolism. Decreased secretion of insulin and impaired glucose tolerance were found in zinc deficient patients (Marchesini et al., 1998). Zinc is also integral part of insulin molecule and crucial for the synthesis, storage and secretion of insulin in pancreatic islet cells (Grungreiff et al., 2005; Chausmer, 1998; Blostein-Fuji et al., 1997). There has been hypothesed that zinc deficiency could be a link between liver cirrhosis and "liver" diabetes mellitus (Grungreiff et al., 2005). Zinc supplementation increases glucose disposal due to the increased non-insulin-mediated glucose uptake, without any systematic effect on insulin secretion and sensitivity (Marchesini et al., 1998).

Zinc has an important role in fibrogenesis. Some of zinc metalloenzymes, like DNA and RNA polymerases, have a great impact on regeneration of liver parenchyma. In fibrogenesis, zinc acts antagonistically to copper (Arakawa et al., 2003).

Zinc inhibits the cross-linking of covalent bonds in collagen through lysyl oxidase (Sato et al., 2005).

Zinc is a structure part of collagenasis. On the other hand, zinc is the inhibitor of prolyl hydroxilase, which is important enzyme in collagen synthesis (Camps et al., 1992).

In some studies, in the early phase a positive correlation between liver regeneration and zinc tissue concentration was found (Milin et al., 2005). In regenerated liver translocation of metallothionein to the nuclei is noticed where zinc participate in cell cycle processes (Tsujikawa et al., 1994).

Zinc is an activator of ornithin transcarbomoilase which participates in ammonia metabolism.

Zinc also participates in amino-acid metabolism, therefore its role in portal encephalopathy was investigated. Studies have showed that long-term oral zinc supplementation in patients with liver cirrhosis improve urea synthesis from ammonia and amino-acids with consequently decrease in concentration of ammonia and improvement clinical features of liver cirrhosis (Marchesini et al., 1996).

According to the results from clinical trials, zinc has a positive effect on the oxydative stress. Zinc supplementation in protein deficient rats resulted in increased activity of catalase, glutathion peroxidase, glutathion reductase and glutathion-S-transferase (Sidhu et al., 2005).

Zinc supplementation in those patients leads to significant increase in reduced glutathion concentration (GSH) and increased superoxide dismutase (SOD) activity in comparison to control group. By zinc supplementation in mentioned research serum concentration of copper, iron and selenium were normalized.

The results suggested possible influence of zinc on antioxidative enzymes activity and its possible effect on concentration of other trace elements.

The research on animal models showed that zinc supplementation has a protective effect on ethanol induced liver damage.

Zinc supplementation decreases ethanol induced zinc depletion and decrease in cytochrom P450 2E1 (CYP2E1) activity. Also, zinc supplementation increases activity of alcohol dehydrogenase in liver. That partially can explain zinc influence on the oxidative stress.

Zinc has also the important role in preserving of intestinal integrity as well as in prevention of endotoxemia with consequent inhibition of TNF-α synthesis induced by endotoxine (Kang et al., 2005).

Mentioned effects of zinc are independent from metallothioneine. Zinc supplementation has protective effect on ethanol induced decreasing of glutathione concentration, decreasing glutathione peroxidase activity and increasing glutathione reductase activity in liver (Zhou et al., 2005).

Zinc inhibits free oxygen radicals generation and increases antioxidative pathways activity.

According to Camps (Camps et al., 1992) zinc supplementation leads to decreased lipid peroxidation, collagen deposition, inhibition of prolyl-hydroxilase and increased collagenase activity.

Zinc induces synthesis of metallothionein. Metallothionein is effective cytoprotective agent against ethanol induced liver damage. Its protective effect can be explained by its influence on oxidative stress (Zhou et al., 2002).

Also, ZNF 267 (*zinc finger protein* 267) mRNA expression is increased in stellate cells of patients with liver cirrhosis. ZNF 267 is binding for MMP-10 and presents negative regulator of transcription MMP-10 and indirectly enhances fibrogenesis in the liver (Schnabl et al., 2005). The role of MMP-10 was mentioned above. All mentioned suggests the important role of zinc in fibrogenesis and pathogenesis of liver cirrhosis and its complications.

2.2.2. Copper

Copper is an essential trace element which participates in many enzymatic reactions. Copper has the most important role in redox processes, where presents donator of electron on mitochondrial level.

Copper absorbed in duodenum, binds for ceruloplasmin, albumin and transcuprein. More than 90% of copper in plasma binds for ceruloplasmin, and the rest binds for albumin and transcuprein (Luza et al., 1996).

In hepatocite copper is incorporated into ceruloplasmin and metallothionein, cistein rich protein, which binds also other heavy metals, like cadmium and mercury. Metallothionein acts as a factor of detoxicaton in gastrointestinal mucosa, but also prevents copper induced cytotoxicity (Luza et al., 1996; Sato et al., 2005). Copper enters into the cell by two copper transporting enzymes, ATP-ase ATP7A i ATP7B, products of genes for Menkel and Wilson's disease. Copper elimination is mainly through hepatobiliary tract, and around 4% by urinary tract.

Copper participates in gene expression. Copper is a cofactor of many enzymes, like superoxide dismutase, important antioxidative enzime, furthermore enzyme tirosinase, which is necessary for melanin synthesis in human body, as well as many other enzymes. Copper influences on metabolism of iron, its absorption, incorporation in hemoglobin, etc.

Toxic effect of copper was focus of interest of many scientists. One of proposed model was that metallothionein saturated with copper entry to lysosomes, where is incompletely demolished and polymerized, forming insoluble material containing reactive copper which, together with iron, run lisosomal lipid peroxidation. That consequently causes hepatocyte necrosis.

Reactive copper participates in liver damage directly or indirectly, through stimulation of Kupffer and other cells (Klein et al., 1998). Toxic effect of copper is explained through its role in production of oxygen radicals (Bremner, 1998). Oxygen radicals can cause destruction of cell lipids, nucleic acids, proteins and carbohydrates, what results in the impairment of cell function and cell integrity.

Copper is also very important in fibrogenesis. Copper is the cofactor of lysil oxidase, which is involved in the formation of molecular bridges in collagen. An excessive accumulation of copper in the liver and an increase in the copper concentration promote hepatic fibrosis (Arakawa and Suzuki, 1993; Sato et al., 2005).

2.2.3. Manganese

Manganese is an essential trace element discovered in 1774. Manganese entries the human body by ingestion. Only 3-4% of ingested manganese is absorbed. Proportion of absorbed manganese can increase in specific states, like hypochromic anemia. In plasma manganese is transported by transmanganin (Kasper et al., 2005). In the body manganese is accumulated in mitochondria. The highest concentration of manganese is in enteric system, liver, pancreas, kidney, lungs and muscles. It passes hemato-encephalic barrier and can be accumulated in the brain in the state of prolonged exposition. Mainly, manganese is excreted through hepatobiliary system. Partly is reabsorbed in small intestine and the rest is excreted by feces.

Ingestion of manganese substances can cause destruction of gastrointestinal mucosa with bleeding. Chronic intoxication with manganese leads to degenerative changes in basal ganglia, especially in globus pallidus and corpus striatum (Spahr et al., 1996; Rose et al., 1999). Decreased synthesis of dopamine and decreased conversion causes decreased concentration of dopamine in corpus striatum. Possible explanation could be decreased activity of tyrosine kinase and other oxidative enzymes situated in mitochondria, where manganese is especially accumulated. Gradually, in three phases, symptoms like those in Parkinson disease develop in patients intoxicated with manganese.

Manganese is a structural part of arginase, which is an important enzyme in the urea metabolism. Manganese acts as an activator of numerous enzymes in Krebs cycle, particularly in the decarboxilation process.

Glutamine synthesis is also manganese metalloenzyme what confirms the role of manganese in antioxidative system. Manganese influences on skeletal growth, synthesis of nucleic acids, proteins, hemoglobin, lipid and carbohydrates metabolism, etc.

According to the results of the studies, there is a common increased serum concentration of manganese in patients with hepatic encephalopathy. There are opinions that toxicity of manganese contributes to occurrence of hepatic encephalopathy. Prevention of manganese accumulation and decrease in serum manganese concentration could have beneficial effect on mental status of patients with liver cirrhosis (Hauser et al., 1996).

Several studies have showed accumulation of manganese in basal ganglia in patients with liver cirrhosis. Extrapyramidal symptoms could be explained as a result of copper toxicity on dopaminergic function of basal ganglia (Spahr et al., 1996; Rose et al., 1999).

2.2.4. Magnesium

Magnesium is the fourth frequent cation in human body. It occurs in soft tissues and bones. Only 1-5% of magnesium is situated extracellularly. The main part of magnesium originates from ingested food. About 1/3 of ingested magnesium will be absorbed. Mostly, magnesium will be excreted through urinary system. Around 30% is bounded to serum proteins, 15% is in complexes and around 50% is available in ionized form. Magnesium bounded to serum proteins is mainly (75%) bounded to albumins, α-1 and α-2 globulins. Parathyroid hormone is important regulator of magnesium concentration acting through regulation of renal tubular reabsorption.

Magnesium is important in protein synthesis, activation of enzymes, oxidative phosphorilation, etc.

Magnesium also has an important role on the level of neuromuscular connection where slows down neuromuscular impulse inhibiting acetylcholine. That is the main reason why disturbance in magnesium equilibrium causes neuromuscular symptoms.

Magnesium deficiency is usually caused by kidney disease, chronic alcoholism, excessive diuresis, malabsorption, sever diarrhea, etc. Magnesium deficiency causes increased muscular excitability due to the increased acetylcholine activity, with consequent muscular tremor. Mental disorders include confusion and hallucinations. Magnesium influences on heart conductive system and magnesium deficiency can cause arrhythmia. Magnesium intoxication usually caused by acute or chronic renal insufficiency, cause hyporeflexity, cardiac arrhythmia, respiratory depression and coma.

According to the results of published studies, there is a decreased serum concentration of magnesium in patients with liver cirrhosis (Rocchi et al., 1994). Study of Stergiou has showed that spironolactone decreases magnesium excretion by decreasing furosemide-induced renal excretion of potassium and magnesium (Stergiou et al., 1993).

Since zinc, copper, manganese and magnesium have the possible role in the pathogenesis of liver cirrhosis and cirrhotic complications, the aim of our study was to investigate the serum concentrations of mentioned trace elements in patients with liver cirrhosis and compared them with concentrations in controls.

3. Material and Methods

3.1. Subjects

The study included 105 patients with diagnosed liver cirrhosis of ethylic etiology who were hospitalized from 2000 to 2005 in the Division of Gastroenterology at Dubrava University Hospital, with median age 55 years. Seventy eight (74%) of them were male and twenty seven (26%) were female. According to the Child-Pugh classification patients with liver cirrhosis were divided in Child-Pugh A, B and C group. There were 35 subjects in every Child-Pugh group.

Inclusion criteria were alcoholic liver cirrhosis (diagnosed by anamnestic data of alcohol consumption, laboratory and pathohistological findings, negative markers of viral hepatitis and normal values of ceruloplasmine), ability to sign the Informed consent and age 18 to 70.

Exclusion criteria were vegetarianism, Wilson's disease, malign disease, acute liver failure, impaired renal function (creatinine clearance <60 ml/min), multiorganic failure and inability to sign the Informed consent.

The control group consisted of 50 healthy subjects (median age 52 years) who were performed laboratory analysis as part of systematic medical examinations. There were 35 (70%) males and 15 (30%) females.

The Informed consent was obtained from all study subjects. The study protocol was approved by the Ethics Committee of Dubrava University Hospital. The protocol was carried out in accordance with the ethics guidelines of the Helsinki Declaration.

3.2. Methods

Blood samples were collected without anticoagulans and serum was stored in a freezer on -20°C until processing. In processing 1 ml of serum was taken, 1.5 ml of concentrated nitric acid and 0.5 ml 30% H_2O_2 were added on account of the digestion. After the digestion the sample was cooling for 20 minutes. The solution was transferred into a 10 ml container and was supplemented with ultra clean water. The concentrations of trace elements were determined by means of plasma sequential spectrophotometer TraceScan (Thermo Jarrell Ash, USA). Data were presented with median and 5-95 percentile range and compared using Wilcoxon and Kruskal-Wallis non-parametric tests. Statistics was done using MedCalc software (MedCalc Software, Mariakerke, Belgium). Only $p<0.05$ was considered significant.

4. Results

The serum concentrations of zinc, copper, manganese and magnesium in patients with liver cirrhosis and controls are presented in Table 1. The serum concentration of zinc was significantly lower in patients with liver cirrhosis in comparison to the controls (0.82 μmol/L vs. 11.22 μmol/L, $p<0.001$). The serum concentration of copper was significantly higher in patients with liver cirrhosis in comparison to the controls (21.56 μmol/L vs. 13.09 μmol/L, p<0.001) as well as manganese concentration (2.50 μmol/L vs. 0.02 μmol/L, p<0.001). The concentration of magnesium was not significantly different between patients with liver cirrhosis and controls (Table 1, p=0.132). There were no differences in the concentrations of zinc, copper, manganese and magnesium between male and female patients with liver cirrhosis (Table 2).

Table 1. Serum concentrations of zinc, copper, manganese and magnesium in patients with liver cirrhosis and controls

Trace elements	Subjects (N=105) median and 5 - 95 percentiles	Controls (N=50) median and 5 - 95 percentiles	Statistics	
			z	p
Zinc (μmol/L)	0.82 (0.24–1.74)	11.22 (9.23–15.10)	10.05	<0.001
Copper (μmol/L)	21.56 (11.17–30.60)	13.09 (11.17–19.95)	-7,66	<0.001
Manganese (μmol/L)	2.50 (0.01–29.65)	0.02 (0.01–0.40)	-8,21	.001
Magnesium (mmol/L)	0.94 (0.63–1.36)	0.88 (0.56–1.12)	-1.51	132

Table 2. Serum concentrations of zinc, copper, manganese and magnesium in male and female patients with liver cirrhosis

Trace elements	Male (N=78) median and 5 - 95 percentiles	Female (N=27) median and 5 - 95 percentiles	Statistics	
			z	p
Zinc (μmol/L)	0.84 (0.25–1.70)	0.74 (0.20–1.99)	-0.32	0.750
Copper (μmol/L)	21.18 (9.86–30.07)	23.56 (15.49–32.12)	1.58	0.113
Manganese (μmol/L)	2.10 (0.01–31.20)	3.70 (0.08–29.55)	1.45	0.146
Magnesium (mmol/L)	0.96 (0.58–1.40)	0.88 (0.71–1.36)	-1.05	0.293

Table 3. Serum concentrations of trace elements in Child-Pugh groups

Trace elements	Child-Pugh A (N=35) median and 5 - 95 percentiles	Child-Pugh B (N=35) median and 5 - 95 percentiles	Child-Pugh C (N=35) median and 5 - 95 percentiles	Statistics	
				H	p
Zinc(μmol/L)	1.06 (0.38–1.49)	0.78 (0.26–1.94)	0.54 (0.14–1.45)	19.24	0.053
Copper (μmol/L)	19.98 (13.75–29.84)	22.30 (10.51–31.65)	23.20 (9.75–29.76)	1.00	0.608
Manganese (μmol/L)	2.00 (0.12–9.42)	2.10 (0.01–27.62)	6.30 (0.01–35.75)	9.21	0.036
Magnesium (mmol/L)	0.93 (0.65–1.18)	0.96 (0.65–1.38)	0.88 (0.40–1.53)	5.34	0.084

The data in Table 3 show that the serum levels of manganese were significantly different between Child-Pugh groups (H=9.21, p=0.036). An additional analysis showed that the serum levels of manganese were significantly higher in patients with Child-Pugh C liver cirrhosis (6.30 μmol/L) in comparison to patients with Child-Pugh A (2.00 μmol/L , z=-3.09, p=0.002) and B liver cirrhosis (2.10 µmol/L, z=-2.06, p=0.039). The concentrations of zinc, copper, and magnesium did not differ significantly between Child-Pugh groups (Table 3).

The serum concentrations of zinc, copper, manganese and magnesium in cirrhotic patients with and without hepatic encephalopathy are represented in Table 4. The concentration of zinc was significantly lower in patients with hepatic encephalopathy in comparison to cirrhotic patients without encephalopathy (0.54 µmol/L vs. 0.96 µmol/L, p=0.002). There were no differences in serum concentrations of other trace elements between patients with or without encephalopathy. The serum concentrations of zinc, copper, manganese and magnesium in cirrhotic patients with and without ascites are represented in Table 5. Only manganese concentration was significantly different between patients with and without ascites. Namely, serum manganese concentration was higher in cirrhotic patients with ascites in comparison to the cirrhotic patients without ascites (4.10 µmol/L vs. 1.80 µmol/L, p<0.001).

Table 4. Serum concentrations of trace elements in cirrhotic patients with and without hepatic encephalopathy

Trace elements	Without encephalopathy (N=83) median and 5 - 95 percentiles	With encephalopathy (N=22) median and 5 - 95 percentiles	Statistics z	p
Zinc (µmol/L)	0.96 (0.25–1.77)	0.54 (0.19–1.11)	-3.07	0.002
Copper (µmol/L)	21.56 (13.07–31.43)	21.31 (9.85–29.31)	-1.21	0.227
Manganese (µmol/L)	2.20 (0.01–31.38)	4.90 (0.01–26.94)	0.66	0.506
Magnesium (mmol/L)	0.95 (0.63–1.36)	0.90 (0.53–1.37)	-1.72	0.086

Table 5. Serum concentrations of trace elements in cirrhotic patients with and without ascites

Trace elements	Without ascites (N=45) median and 5 - 95 percentiles	With ascites (N=60) median and 5 - 95 percentiles	Statistics z	p
Zinc (µmol/L)	0.97 (0.36–1.57)	0.69 (0.18–1.78)	1.77	0.077
Copper (µmol/L)	20.25 (11.84–30.47)	22.42 (10.74–30.82)	-0.28	0.778
Manganese (µmol/L)	1.80 (0.01–11.20)	4.10 (0.01–31.80)	-3.43	< 0.001
Magnesium (mmol/L)	0.92 (0.64–1.13)	0.94 (0.54–1.46)	-0.58	0.564

5. Discussion

Mechanisms linked on ethanol metabolism, especially oxidative stress, redox potentials and acetaldehyde, participate in the emergence of liver damage. Trace elements play an important role in oxidative stress and redox potentials. A possible role of zinc, copper, manganese and magnesium in pathogenesis of liver cirrhosis and its complications is still subject of researches.

In our research the serum levels of zinc were significantly lower in patients with liver cirrhosis in comparison to controls (Table 1, median 0.82 μmol/L in patient with liver cirrhosis and 11.22 μmol/L in controls, $p<0.001$). The results confirm Kugelmans' research (Kugelmas et al., 2000), which explained low zinc levels with low ingestion due to protein reluctance, increased loss in gastroenterological system due to diarrhea or intestinal malabsorption and increased urinary losses. The assumption is also based on the research of McClain (McClain et al., 1991) and Extremera (Extremera et al., 1990). Protein deficiency occurs frequently due to the poor dietary intake. Our results confirm findings of decreased serum concentrations of zinc in patients with liver cirrhosis. Possible explanations for the decreased zinc levels in cirrhotic patients are mentioned above.

In Celik's research (Celik et al., 2002) the decrease in both serum and ascites zinc content was found in patients with liver cirrhosis. The interaction between zinc and copper in their intestinal absorption and their competition for binding sites on the carrier proteins and cellular uptake may be regulators of their homeostasis. Maybe this can explain inverse concentrations of zinc and copper. Zinc binds on albumin, transferrin and metalloproteins in the cell, so relative concentrations of these proteins might regulate the serum concentration of zinc (Celik et al., 2002; Mertz, 1981).

The serum copper content was found significantly increased in patients with liver cirrhosis in comparison to the control group (Table 1, median 21.56 μmol/L in patient with liver cirrhosis and 13.09 μmol/L in controls, $p<0.001$). It could be explained with copper's role in the redox process. Redox cycling between Cu^{2+} and Cu^{1+} can catalyze the production of toxic hydroxyl radicals (Askwith et al., 1998; Harrison et al., 2000). It is a well known fact that redox processes and oxidative stress play an important role in the pathogenesis of liver cirrhosis.

Serum concentrations of manganese were significantly higher in cirrhotic patients in comparison to the controls (Table 1, median 2.50 μmol/L in cirrhotic patients and 0.02 μmol/L in controls, $p<0.001$). Higher serum levels of manganese in Krieger's research (Krieger et al., 1995) as well as in research of Layrargues and co. (Layrargues et al., 1998) were also found in cirrhotic patients.

Moscarella did not find any significant difference in the concentrations of manganese between the cirrhotic patients and the controls (Moscarella et al., 1994). After all, it seems that serum levels of manganese are higher in patients with liver cirrhosis than in healthy people. Manganese is secreted in bile so the concentration of manganese increases in cholestatic liver disease, which could be one of the possible explanations why manganese accumulation is common in liver cirrhosis (Krieger et al., 1995).

It has been suggested that a possible mechanism responsible for manganese accumulation in the pallidum of patients include a decrease in biliary excretion and increased systemic availability due to the portosystemic shunting.

Intrahepatic shunting or portosystemic shunting also have an additional effect on manganese accumulation. In the study of Rose and co. (Rose et al., 1999) pallidal manganese concentrations were the highest in shunted rats, which confirms that shunting is a major determinant of manganese accumulation in the brain. Manganese accumulation in the brain was confirmed by several clinical studies (Krieger et al., 1995; Rose et al., 1999; Hauser et al., 1996, Spahr et al., 1996).

The difference between serum concentrations of magnesium in cirrhotic patients and controls was not significant (Table 1, median 0.94 mmol/L in cirrhotic patients and 0.88 mmol/L in controls, p= 0.132). Results are opposite to Kosch's research (Kosch et al., 2000). In that research serum levels of magnesium were lower in patients with liver cirrhosis in comparison to patients with liver steatosis and controls. In addition, the research of Rocchi (Rocchi et al., 1994) and Suzuki (Suzuki et al., 1996) confirmed the same. Our research did not confirm lower concentrations of magnesium in patients with liver cirrhosis. That partially could be explained with influence of spironolactone on magnesium levels. Namely, in Stergiou's research (Stergiou et al., 1993) spironolactone in health subjects decreased urine excretion of magnesium and in cirrhotic patients antagonized magnesiuric effect of furosemide. Our patients with liver cirrhosis mostly have spironolactone in their standard therapy. However, there were no differences in serum concentration of magnesium between patients who were taking spironolactone and those who were not taking spironolactone.

There was a slight decrease in serum zinc concentrations in patients with more severe clinical state of liver cirrhosis according to Child-Pugh classification but these differences in our research were not significant.

As zinc is bound to albumin in the serum, it has been thought that the serum zinc concentration would decrease with advancing grades of hepatic fibrosis (Hatano et al., 2000). Yoshida found that patients with decompensated liver cirrhosis have lower levels of zinc than patients with compensated cirrhosis (Yoshida et al., 2001). However, in Hatano's research (Hatano et al., 2000) serum zinc levels did not differ significantly between grades of hepatic fibrosis.

Copper levels in our research were similar in all three Child-Pugh groups (Table 3), as well as in Hatano's research.

Serum levels of manganese were higher in patients with Child-Pugh C liver cirrhosis in comparison to those in Child-Pugh A and B cirrhosis. Our results are contrary to Spahr's research (Spahr et al., 1996) who found similar concentrations of manganese in all three Child-Pugh groups. It seems that manganese concentrations are higher in patients with severe liver cirrhosis possible due to the advanced intrahepatic and portosystemic shunting.

In our study magnesium levels were similar in all Child-Pugh groups. Moscarella's research (Moscarella et al., 1994) also confirms similar levels in compensated and decompensated liver cirrhosis. However, Wang found that magnesium deficiency occurs more frequently in severe liver disease (Wang et al., 2004). Significantly lower zinc levels were found in cirrhotic patients with hepatic encephalopathy

(Table 4, median 0.54 μmol/L in patients with encephalopathy and 0.96 μmol/L without encephalopathy, p= 0.002), which was confirmed in other studies (Grungreiff et al., 2000; Riggio et al. 1992). There are some findings that zinc supplementation can cause increased releasing of glutamine from skeletal muscle and also activate glutamine synthetasis, which can decrease the level of ammonia and improve hepatic encephalopathy (Grungreiff et al., 2000). That can be explained with the fact that zinc supplementation increases the hepatic activity of ornithine transcarbamoylase, key enzyme of the urea cycle, which consecutively increases urea formation and decreases ammonia levels (Riggio et al., 1992). The rationale for use of zinc is also its ability to induce intestinal and hepatic metallothionein synthesis. Zinc decreases copper absorption by increasing the formation of Cu-metallothionein in intestinal epithelial cells (Friedman, 2004). However, Riggio found that short-term zinc supplementation has no influence on hepatic encephalopathy (Riggio et al., 1991).

Considering all, zinc supplementation could have a positive influence on hepatic encephalopathy but before the implementation of this result in the treatment, further researches are necessary.

The levels of manganese were not significantly different between patients with liver cirrhosis and hepatic encephalopathy and patients without encephalopathy (Table 4, $p=0.506$), which is opposite to the researches of Hauser (Hauser et al., 1996) and Krieger (Krieger et al., 1995). They found increased concentrations of manganese and suggested a beneficial effect of prevention of accumulation or decreasing manganese concentration in patients with liver cirrhosis. Rose and Layrargues found increased concentrations of manganese in basal ganglia of cirrhotic patients in comparison to the controls (Rose et al., 1999; Layrargues et al., 1998).

Manganese concentrations were significantly higher in cirrhotic patients with ascites in comparison to those without ascites (Table 5, median 4.10 μmol/L in patients with ascites and 1.80 μmol/L in patients without ascites, $p<0.001$). The levels of zinc, copper and magnesium were within reference range. Our results are contrary to the research of Pasqualetti and co. who found significantly lower magnesium concentrations in patients with ascites (Pasqualetti et al., 1987). Therefore, it is necessary to research the possible role of manganese in emergence of ascites in patients with liver cirrhosis.

Finally, decreased serum concentrations of zinc and increased levels of manganese in patients with liver cirrhosis could have an important role in the pathogenesis of liver cirrhosis and its complications, especially in hepatic encephalopathy. The supplementation of zinc could improve hepatic encephalopathy. The decrease in manganese levels could also have a beneficial effect on the neurological status in patients with liver cirrhosis and hepatic encephalopathy. Increased concentrations of manganese in cirrhotic patients with ascites inspire further researches about a possible role of manganese in the pathogenesis of ascites in patients with liver cirrhosis. Maybe, decreasing of manganese levels might also have beneficial effect on prevention or volume of ascites.

6. Conclusion

Considering all that, the correction of serum trace elements concentrations would have a beneficial effect on some complications of liver cirrhosis and maybe on progression of the disease, so it would be recommendable to provide laboratory analysis of trace elements in patients with liver cirrhosis as a routine.

References

Anderson, AJ; Su, JH; Cotman, CW. DNA damage and apoptosis in Alzheimer's disease: colocalization with c-Jun immunoreactivity, relationship to brain area, and effect of postmortem delay. *J. Neurosci*, 1996, 16, 1710-16.

Arakawa, Y; Suzuki, I. Hepatic disease and trace elements. *The Journal of Therapy*, 1993, 75, 894-905.

Arthur, MJP; Iredale, JP. Hepatic lipocytes, TIMP-1 and liver fibrosis. *J.Roy.Coll.Phys*., 1994, 28, 200.

Arthur, MJP. Fibrogenesis II. Metalloproteinases and their inhibitors in liver fibrosis. *Am J Physiol Gastrointest Liver Physiol*, 2000, 279 (2), 245-9.

Askwith, CC; Kaplan, J. Iron and copper transport in yeast and its relevance to human disease. TIBS, 1998, 23, 135-8.

Blostein-Fuji, A; DiSilvestro, RA; Frid, D; Katz, C; Malarkey, W. Short-term zinc supplementation in women with non-insulin-dependent diabetes mellitus effects on plasma 5' nucleotididase activity, insulin-like growth factor-1 concentrations and lipoprotein oxidation rates in vitro. *Am J Clin Nutr*, 1997, 66, 639-42.

Bremner, I. Manifestation of copper excess. *Am J Clin Nutr*, 1998, 67 (5), 1069s-1073s.

Camps, J; Bargallo, T; Gimenez, A; Alie, S; Caballeria, J; Pares, A; Joven, J; Masana, L; Rodes, J. Relationship between hepatic lipid peroxidation and fibrogenesis in carbon tetrachloride-treated rats: effect of zinc administration. *Clin Sci*., 1992, 83(6), 695-700.

Celik, HA; Aydin, HH; Ozsaran, A; Kilincsoy, N; Batur, Y; Ersoz, B. Trace elements analysis of ascitic fluid in benign and malignant disease. *Clin Biochem*, 2002, 35(6), 477-81.

Chang, KL; Hung, TC; Hsieh, BS; Chen, YH; Chen, TF; Cheng, HL. Zinc at pharmacologic concentrations affects cytokine expression and induces apoptosis of human peripheral blood mononuclear cells. *Nutrition,* 2006, 22(5), 465-74.

Chausmer, AB. Zinc, insulin and diabetes. *J Am Coll Nutr*, 1998, 17, 109-15.

Christianson, DW. The structure biology of zinc. *Adv. Prot. Chem*., 1991, 42, 281-335.

Cotzias, GC. Trace Substances. Eviron Health-Proc, *Univ. Mo. Annu Conf*, 1967, 5.

Crabb, DW; Estonius M. Alcoholic Liver Disease and Nonalcoholic Steatohepatitis. In: Stein JH. *Internal Medicine*. St. Louis: Mosby; 1998; 2194-99.

Extremera, B; Maldonado, MA; Martinez, MR; Hinojosa, JC; Ruiz, AD; Moreno, R. Zinc and liver cirrhosis. *Acta Gastroenterologica Belgica*, 1990, 53 (3), 292-8.

Friedman, SL. The cellular basis of hepatic fibrosis: mechanisms and treatment strategies. *N Engl J Med*, 1993, 328, 1828-35.

Friedman, SL; Keeffe EB. *Handbook of liver disease*. Second edition. Philadelphia: Churchill Livingstone, Sabre Zagreb; 2004.

Grungreiff, K; Grungreiff, S; Reinhold, D; Zinc deficiency and hepatic encephalopathy: Results of long-term follow-up on zinc supplementation. *Journal of Trace Elements in Experimental Medicine*, 2000, 13 (1), 21-31.

Grungreiff, K; Reinhold, D. Liver cirrhosis and "liver" diabetes mellitus are linked by zinc deficiency. *Medical hypothesis*, 2005, 64, 316-7.

Harrison, MD; Jones, CE; Solioz, M; Dameron, CT. Intracellular copper routing: the role of copper chaperones. *TIBS*, 2000, 25, 29-32.

Hatano, R; Ebara, M; Fukuda, H; Yoshikawa, M; Sugiura, N; Kondo, F; Yukawa, M; Saisho, H. Accumulation of copper in the liver and hepatic injury in chronic hepatitis C. *Journal of Gastroenterology & Hepatology*, 2000, 15 (7), 786-91.

Hauser, RA; Zesiewich, TA; Martinez, C; Rosemurgy, AS; Olanow, CW. Blood manganese correlates with brain magnetic resonance imaging changes in patients with liver disease. *Can J Neur Sci*., 1996, 23 (2), 95-8.

Iredale, JP; Murphy, G; Hembry, RM et al. Human hepatic hepatocytes synthesise tissue inhibitor of metalloproteinases-1 (TIMP-1): implications for regulation of matrix degradation in liver. *J.Clin.Invest*. 1992, 90, 282.

Jensen, K (a); Gluud, C. Mallory body: morphological, clinical and experimental studies (part 1 of a literature survey). *Hepatology*, 1994, 20, 1061.

Jensen, K (b); Gluud, C. Mallory body: theories on development and pathological significance (part 2 of a literature survey). *Hepatology*, 1994, 20, 1330.

Kang, YJ; Zhou, Z. Zinc prevention and treatment of alcoholic liver disease. *Mol Aspects Med*. 2005, 26(4-5), 391-404.

Kasper, DL; Braumwald, E; Fauci, A; Hauser, S; Longo, D; Janeson, JL. *Harrison's Principles of Internal Medicine*. 16th edition. New York: McGraw-Hill; 2005.

Klein, D; Lichtmannegger, J; Heinzmann, U; Muller-Hocker, J; Michaelsen, S; Summer, KH. Association of copper to metallothionein in hepatic lysosomes of Long-Evans cinnamon (LEC) rats during the development of hepatitis. *Eur J Clin Invest*, 1998, 28 (4), 302-10.

Kosch, MA; Nguyen, SQ; Tokmak, F; Schodjaian, K; Hausberg, M; Rahn, KH; Kisters, K. Zinc and magnesium status in patients with liver disease due to chronic alcoholism. *Journal of Trace & Microprobe Techniques*, 2000, 18 (4), 529-33.

Krieger, D; Krieger, S; Jansen, O; Gass, P; Theilmann, L; Lichtnecker, H. Manganese and chronic hepatic encephalopathy. *Lancet*, 1995, 346, 270-4.

Kugelmas, M. Preliminary Observation: Oral Zinc Sulfate Replacement is effective in Treating Muscle Cramps in Cirrhotic Patients. *J Am Coll Nutr*, 2000, 19 (1), 13-15.

Layrargues, GP; Rose, C; Spahr, L; Zayed, J; Normandin, L; Butterworth, RF. Role of manganese in pathogenesis of portal-systemic encephalopathy. *Metabolic Brain Disease*, 1998, 13 (4), 311-7.

Leon, DA (a); McCambridge. J. Liver cirrhosis mortality rates in Britain from 1950 to 2002: an analysis of routine data. *Lancet*, 2006, 367, 52-6.

Leon, DA (b); McCambridge. J. Liver cirrhosis mortality rates in Britain, 1950 to 2002. *Lancet*, 2006, 367, 645.

Luza, SC; Speisky, HC. Liver copper storage and transport during development: implication for cytotoxicity. *Am J Clin Nutr*, 1996, 63 (5), 812s-20s.

Marchesini, G; Fabri, A; Bianchi, G; Brizi, M; Zoli, M. Zinc Supplementation and Amino Acid-Nitrogen Metabolism in Patients With Advanced Cirrhosis. *Hepatology*, 1996, 23, 1084-92.

Marchesini, G; Bugianesi, E; Ronchi, M; Flamia, R; Thomaseth, K; Pacini, G. Zinc Supplementation Improves Glucose Disposal in Patients With Cirrhosis. *Metabolism*, 1998, 47 (7), 792-8.

McClain, CJ; Marsano, L; Burk, RF; Bacon, B. Trace elements in liver disease. *Semin Liver Dis.*, 1991, 11, 321-39.

Mertz, W. Essential trace elements. *Science*, 1981, 213 (4514), 1332-8.

Milin, C; Tota, M; Domitrovic, R; Giacometti, J; Pantovic, R; Cuk, M; Mrakovcic-Sutic, I: Jakovac, H; Radosevic-Stasic, B. Metal Tissue Kinetics in Regenerating Liver, Thymus, Spleen and Submandibular Gland After Partial Hepatectomy in Mice. *Biol Trace Elem Res*, 2005, 108, 225-43.

Moscarella, S; Duchini, A; Buzzelli, G. Eur. J. Gastroenterol. *Hepatol.*, 1994, 6 (7), 633.

Pasqualetti, P; Casale, R; Colantonio, D; Di Lauro, G; Festuccia, V; Natali, L; Natali, G. Serum levels of magnesium in hepatic cirrhosis. *Quad Sclavo Diag*, 1987, 23 (1), 12-7.

Pinzani, M. Hepatic stellate (Ito) cells: expanding roles for a liver-specific pericyte. *J Hepatol.*, 1995, 22, 700.

Prasad, R; Kaur, G; Nath, R; Walia, BN. Molecular basis of pathophysiology of Indian childhood cirrhosis: role of nuclear copper accumulation in liver. *Molecular & Cellular Biochemistry*, 1996, 156 (1), 25-30.

Ramstedt, M. Alcohol-Related Mortality in 15 European Countries in the Postwar Period. *Eur J Popul*, 2002, 18, 307-23.

Record, IR; Tulsi, RS; Dreosti, IE; Fraser, FJ. Cellular necrosis in zinc-deficient rat embryos. *Teratology*, 1985, 32, 397-405.

Riggio, O; Ariosto, F; Merli, M; Caschera, M; Zullo, A; Balducci, G; Ziparo, V. et al. Short-term oral zinc supplementation does not improve chronic hepatic encephalopaty. Results of a double-blind crossover trial. *Dig Dis Sci*, 1991, 36, 1204-8.

Riggio, O; Merli, M; Capocaccia, L; Caschera, M; Zullo, A; Pinto, G; Gaudio, E. et al. Zinc supplementation reduces blood ammonia and increase liver ornithine trancarbamylase activity in experimental cirrhosis. *Hepatology*, 1992, 16, 785-9.

Rocchi, E; Borella, P; Borghi, A; Paolillo, F; Pradelli, M; Farina, F; Casalgrandi, G. Zinc and magnesium in liver cirrhosis. *Eur J Clin Invest*, 1994, 24 (3), 149-55.

Rose, C; Butterworth, RF; Zayed, J; Normandin, L; Todd, K; Michalak, A; Spahr, L; Huet, PM; Pomier-Layrargues, G. Manganese Deposition in Basal Ganglia Structures Results From Both Portal-Systemic Shunting and Liver Dysfunction. *Gastroenterology*, 1999, 117, 640-4.

Sato, C; Koyama, H; Satoh, H; Hayashi, Y; Chiba, T; Ohi, R. Concentrations of Copper and Zinc in Liver and Serum Samples in Biliary Atresia Patients at Different Stages of Traditional Surgeries. *Tohoku J. Exp. Med.*, 2005, 207, 271-7.

Schnabl, B; Hu, K; Muhlbauer, M; Hellerbrand, C; Stefanovic, B; Brenner, DA; Scholmerich, J. Zinc finger protein 267 is up-regulated during the activation process of human hepatic stellate cells and functions as a negative transcriptional regulator of MMP-10. *Biochem Biophys Res Commun*, 2005, 335(1), 87-96.

Sherlock, S; Dooley, J. *Disease of the liver and biliary system.* 11th edition. Oxford: Blackwell Science Ltd.; 2002.

Sidhu, P; Garg, ML; Dhawan, DK. Protective effects of zinc on oxidative stress enzymes in liver of protein-deficient rats. *Drug Chem Toxicol*, 2005, 28(2), 211-30.

Spahr, L; Butterworth, RF; Fontaine, S; Bui, L; Therrien, G; Milette, PC; Lebrun, LH; Zayed, J; Leblanc, A; Pomier-Layrargues, G. Increased Blood manganese in Cirrhotic Patients: Relationship to Pallidal Magnetic Resonance Signal Hyperintensity and Neurological Symptoms. *Hepatology*, 1996, 24, 1116-20.

Speich, M; Pineau, A; Ballereau, F. Minerals, trace elements and related biological variables in athlets and during physical activity.*Clin Chim Acta*, 2001, 321(1-2), 1-11.

Stergiou, GS; Mayopoulousymvoulidou, D; Mountokalakis, TD. Attenuation by spironolactone of the magnesiuric effect of acute fursemid administration in patients with liver cirrhosis and ascites. *Mineral & Electrolyte Metabolism*, 1993, 19 (2), 86-90.

Stokkeland, K; Brandt, L; Ekbom, A; Ösby, U; Hultcrantz, R. Morbidity and mortality in liver cirrhosis in Sweden 1969-2001 in relation to alcohol consumption. *Scand J Gastroenterol*, 2006, 41, 463-8.

Sunderman, FW. The influence of zinc on apoptosis. *Ann. Clin. Lab. Sci.*, 1995, 25, 134-42.

Suzuki, K; Oyama, R; Hayashi, E; Arakawa, Y. Liver disease and essential trace elements. Nippon Rinsho. *Japanese Journal of clinical medicine*, 1996, 54 (1), 85-92.

Szuster-Ciesielska, A; Daniluk, J; Bojarska-Junak, A. Apoptosis of blood mononuclear cells in alcoholic liver cirrhosis. The influence of in vitro ethanol treatment and zinc supplementation. *Toxicology*, 2005, 212, 124-34.

Takahara, T; Furui, K; Funaki, J; Nakayama, Y; Itoh, H; Miyabayashi, C. Increased expression of matrix metalloproteinase-II in experimental liver fibrosis in rats. *Hepatology*, 1995, 21, 787-95.

Truong-Tran, AQ; Ho, LH; Chai, F; Zalewski, PD. Celular zinc fluxes and the regulation of apoptosis / gene-directed cell death. *J.Nutr.*, 2000, 130 (Suppl.), 1459 S - 66 S.

Troung-Tran, AQ; Carter, J; Ruffin, R; Zalewski PD. New insights into the role of zinc in the respiratory epithelium. *Immunol Cell Biol*, 2001, 79, 170-7.

Tsujikawa, K; Suzuki, N; Sagawa, K. Induction and subcellular localization of metallothionein in regenerating rat liver. *Eur J Cell Biol*, 1994, 63, 240-6.

Vallee, BL; Falchuk; KH. The biochemical basis of zinc physiology. *Physiol. Rev.*, 1993, 73, 79-118.

Vucelic, B; Hrstic, I. Ciroza jetre. In: Vucelic B. et al. *Gastroenterologija i hepatologija*. Zagreb: Medicinska naknada; 2002; 1269-80.

Wang, F; Cao, J; Ma, L; Jin, Z. Study on cellular and serum concentration of calcium and magnesium in periferal blood cells of cirrhosis. *Chin J Hepatol*, 2004, 12 (3), 144-7.

Wyllie, AH. Apoptosis: an overview. *Br. Med. Bull.*, 1997, 53, 451-65.

Yoshida, Y; Higashi, T; Nouso, K; Nakatsukasa, H; Nakamura, S; Watanabe, A; Tsuji, T. Effects of zinc deficiency/zinc supplementation on ammonia metabolism in patients with decompensated liver cirrhosis. *Acta Medica Okayama*, 2001, 55 (6), 349-55.

Zalewski, PD; Forbes, IJ; Betts, WH. Correlation of apoptosis with change in intracellular labile Zn using Zinquin a new specific fluoroscent probe for zinc. *Biochem. J.*, 1993, 296, 403-8.

Zhou, Z; Sun, X; Kang, J. Metallothionein Protection against Alcoholic Liver Injury through Inhibition of Oxidative stress. *Experiment. Biol. Med.*, 2002, 227, 214-22.

Zhou, Z; Wang, L; Song, Z; Saari, JT; McClain, CJ; Kang, YJ. Zinc supplementation prevents alcoholic liver injury in mice through attenuation of oxidative stress. *Am J Pathol*, 2005, 166(6), 1681-90.

Index

B

C

D

E

F

G

H

I

J

K

L

M

N

O

P

Q

R

S

T

U

V

W

X

Z